# POWER,
# POLITICS,
## — AND —
# UNIVERSAL
# HEALTH
# CARE

# POWER, POLITICS, AND UNIVERSAL HEALTH CARE

## THE INSIDE STORY OF A CENTURY-LONG BATTLE

STUART ALTMAN AND DAVID SHACTMAN

FOREWORD BY
SENATOR JOHN KERRY

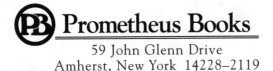 Prometheus Books

59 John Glenn Drive
Amherst, New York 14228–2119

Published 2011 by Prometheus Books

Cover image © 2011 Media Bakery
Cover design by Grace M. Conti-Zilsberger

Inquiries should be addressed to
Prometheus Books
59 John Glenn Drive
Amherst, New York 14228–2119
VOICE: 716–691–0133
FAX: 716–691–0137
WWW.PROMETHEUSBOOKS.COM

15  14  13  12  11    5  4  3  2  1

Library of Congress Cataloging-in-Publication Data

Altman, Stuart H.
    Power, politics, and universal health care : the inside story of a century-long battle / by Stuart H. Altman and David Shactman.
        p.  cm.
    Includes bibliographical references and index.
    ISBN 978–1–61614–456–2 (cloth : alk. paper)
    ISBN 978–1–61614–457–9 (ebook)
    1. Medical policy—United States. 2. Health care reform—United States. I. Shactman, David. II. Title.
    [DNLM: 1. Health Care Reform—history—United States. 2. Health Policy—United States. 3. History, 20th Century—United States. 4. History, 21st Century—United States. 5. Politics—United States. 6. Universal Coverage—United States. WA 11 AA1]

RA395.A3.A485  2011
362.10973—dc23

2011019051

Printed in the United States of America on acid-free paper

# CONTENTS

Foreword
*by Senator John Kerry*     7

Introduction
*by Stuart Altman*     11

Prologue: Barack Obama and the Challenge of Health Care Reform     17

Acknowledgments     23


**Part 1:  The Hard Road to Success:
             One Hundred Years of Past Failures**

    1. Nixon Comes Close: Our Plan Looks Like a Slam Dunk,     27
       but Ends with Just a Dunk
    2. Clinton Chooses Wrong: The Colossal Defeat     62
       of Managed Competition
    3. The Past Foreshadows the Present:     97
       Early Attempts with Little Success


**Part 2:  Expanding Health Coverage Piece by Piece**

    4. The Hill–Burton Program: How America's Uninsured Poor     111
       Got a Right to Free Hospital Care
    5. The Three-Layer Cake: Lyndon Johnson, Wilbur Mills,     122
       and the Epic Battle to Enact Medicare

6. Ooops! The Brief Life and Death of Medicare Catastrophic    149
7. Ted Kennedy and the Republican Congress:    162
   HIPAA and SCHIP Add Two More Pieces to the Puzzle
8. The Unlikely Saga of the Medicare Prescription Drug Benefit  177


**Part 3: Why Can't Americans Afford Their Health Care?
The Battle to Control Health Care Costs**

9. Controlling Health Costs: Many Attempts but Few Successes   203
10. The Last Twenty Years:
    Health Care Spending Keeps Growing    230


**Part 4: Success at Last!**

11. Obama Develops His Plan    245
12. Early Players and Done Deals    254
13. Baucus, Grassley, and the Gang of Six    274
14. The Summer of Death Panels    278
15. The Speaker Carries the Day    285
16. The Senate and the Christmas Eve Health Bill    292
17. Success at Last    314
18. How He Did It: A Political Strategy Learned from History    330
19. The Future Is Cost Control    338

Epilogue    343

Endnotes    347

Glossary    381

Bibliography    395

Index    407

# FOREWORD

## By Senator John Kerry

"What's past is prologue," William Shakespeare wrote—and it seems that's especially true when it comes to health care. The history of health reform in America spans a century of false starts, near misses, and historic advances that culminated when President Obama signed the Patient Protection and Affordable Care Act into law on March 23, 2010. It was a day that a lot of people thought would never come and a moment that almost didn't happen—and the story of how we got there is one of the most important stories in modern politics and public–policy making.

Stuart Altman is the man to tell that story. He's an expert who made a career of overseeing federal health programs and designing proposals to boost health care coverage. He's advised five presidents from both parties. He was there by my side when I ran for president in 2004, helping design a program that became a cornerstone of my health care plan. And in 2009, he was there again, lending his unbiased expertise to a health care debate that too often devolved into partisan antics and baseless claims.

This book navigates it all, from Teddy Roosevelt's 1912 pledge to guarantee government protection against "the hazards of sickness" to the historic debate that finally reformed our health care system nearly a century later. In between, generations of Americans worked for the day when health care would be viewed as a fundamental right instead of a privilege for those fortunate enough to afford it.

It wasn't an easy journey, but bit by bit our country was remade. Congress passed the Social Security Act in 1935, the G.I. Bill in 1944, the Civil Rights Act in 1964, and Medicare and Medicaid in 1965. Now, the Affordable Care Act will join this list of landmark laws that made America a stronger, fairer, and more prosperous country.

There were tough lessons along the way. Health care reform's greatest champion, Ted Kennedy, often said his biggest political mistake was turning down a health care deal with Richard Nixon in 1971 that, for the first time, would have required all companies to provide a health plan for their employees, with federal subsidies for low-income workers. He backed away from it under heavy pressure from fellow Democrats who made the perfect the enemy of the very good—and who believed we could achieve a bolder reform once our Party recaptured the White House in the wake of the Watergate scandal. The lesson Teddy learned was that when it comes to historic breakthroughs in America, you make the best deal you can and immediately start pushing for ways to improve the deal.

I was in the Senate in 1993 when President Clinton tried again for universal health coverage. Again, we learned lessons the hard way—lessons that we carried with us in 2009.

This time around, we were determined to have Congress craft the plan, with the relevant committees working in unison. This time around we were going to bring industries to the table rather than facing them as opponents. And this time around we were going to work our hardest to find a bipartisan solution.

I became deeply involved in 2008 when the Senate Finance Committee began holding hearings on comprehensive health reform and convened a summit with experts to discuss our policy options. We spent nearly two years attempting to forge a bipartisan solution. We held the longest Finance Committee markup in twenty-two years. But even then, only one Republican voted for the America's Healthy Future Act out of committee. By the time the bill reached the Senate floor, health reform had become even more politicized as we moved closer to the 2010 election.

The Senate spent twenty-five consecutive days in session—the second longest consecutive session in history—debating the Patient Protection and Affordable Care Act. It all came down to a rare Christmas Eve vote in 2009. That early morning vote to pass comprehensive health reform was one of the proudest votes of my Senate career. The one thing that made that day bittersweet was knowing that Ted Kennedy wasn't there to share it with us, but I knew he was looking down from above, confident that we had learned enough not to let a very good opportunity slip through our fingers.

Champions of universal coverage had a decision to make. Were we going to let another historic opportunity pass us by, or would we take meaningful steps toward a new tomorrow?

The choice was simple. We'd come too far to stop; we wouldn't let the perfect be the enemy of the good. So, in a rare display of bicameral trust, we found the way forward. The House passed the Senate bill and then we used a reconciliation bill to make some more important changes.

By the end of March 2010, President Obama had done what no other president in American history had been able to do. He signed comprehensive health legislation that makes insurance more affordable for families and small businesses, ends egregious and discriminatory practices from insurance companies, and extends coverage to thirty-four million uninsured Americans. Today the Affordable Care Act is already delivering much-needed health care stability and security to Americans and making our country more competitive across the globe.

The work isn't over, of course. As we've learned from our ever-winding journey with Medicare and Medicaid, these programs will always evolve and improve over time. Now, much of our future debate will focus on the need to control health care costs through additional health care delivery and payment reforms.

It took nearly a century to pass universal health coverage, and I know we won't figure out all the solutions to long-term cost containment overnight. But as we move forward, it's critically important to understand where we've been—and there's no better expert to navigate the history of health policy than Stuart Altman. The Altman/Shactman book is an important chronicle of America's history with health reform. It contains lessons we should all keep in mind as we continue our ongoing journey to build a stronger, fairer, and more efficient health care system for all of our citizens.

# INTRODUCTION

## By Stuart Altman

"**S**tuart, you make sure Medicare covers prescription drugs. Your father and I paid enough when we were working. They promised to pay for all my medical care, so don't tell me there isn't enough money." My mother was eighty-two years old, a four-foot-eleven-inch, feisty, red-headed Jewish mother from the Bronx. I had just been appointed by President Clinton to the National Bipartisan Commission on the Future of Medicare when she gave me those instructions, and she was dead serious. At that time, there was no Medicare drug benefit, and while my mother wanted more benefits, the commission was established to keep it from going broke. There was a clear disconnect between what my mother and most other seniors wanted and what taxpayers were willing to support. Although I tried to get my mother what she wanted, the majority of the commission had other thoughts. They wanted to reduce the cost of the Medicare program and shift the responsibility of taking care of my mother to the private sector.

Americans have always been conflicted about the role that government should assume in providing something as personal as health care. Every national poll shows that a substantial majority of Americans favor universal health care. After all, we are the only industrialized country in the world without it. Unfortunately, every poll also shows that most Americans think government is wasteful and bureaucratic, and that we pay too much in taxes. As a result, it has been very difficult to convince the 85 percent of people who have health insurance to pay more in taxes for the 15 percent who don't.

Many Americans assume that people without health insurance can get adequate care at hospitals and community health clinics. However, research clearly disproves that notion. The Institute of Medicine reports that "safety-net services are not enough to prevent avoidable illness, worse health outcomes, and premature death."[1] "The uninsured receive less preventive care, are diagnosed at more advanced disease stages, and, once diagnosed, tend to receive less therapeutic care (drugs and surgical interventions). Having health insurance would reduce mortality rates for the uninsured by 10 to 15 percent."[2]

Although they are ambivalent about government, polls also reveal that Americans are very happy to have Medicare, a government program that provides health insurance to citizens sixty-five years and older. In fact, older Americans would like Medicare to cover even more of their health expenses, including all of their prescription drugs, nursing home care, bone marrow transplants—you name it. However, those Americans who finance Medicare don't want higher taxes, and they think the program should just cut out waste and unnecessary services—unless, of course, those services happen to be for members of their families.

When my mother was ninety-two, the doctors told us she needed triple bypass surgery and a new heart valve. Like most families in similar circumstances, we were conflicted. We didn't know what to do. What were the chances that a ninety-two-year-old could survive a triple bypass, and even if she did, would she have a reasonable quality of life? My mother had had a good life. Should we make her go through this major procedure and risk causing her pain and suffering when there might be little or no benefit?

We consulted with all the specialists, considered the available options, and finally decided to go ahead with the surgery. The one thing we never considered was the cost. We didn't have to. Medicare paid the bill, and it was large. It included a month in the ICU, two months in a rehab facility, and home nurses around the clock. Initially, my mother appeared to come through the operation remarkably well, but complications developed including lung problems, pneumonia, and loss of reasoning. In the end, she never regained her strength and died seven months later.

Ten years later I found myself testifying before the Senate Finance Committee about the Obama health plan. The country was divided over national health reform because of the projected cost: about a trillion dollars over ten years. Conservative members of Congress, both Democrats and Republicans, insisted that we had to "bend the cost curve" (i.e., reduce the rate of increase in health care spending) before they would support a major expansion of health coverage. US citizens, reeling from the 2008–2009 recession, were seeing health costs eat up larger and larger parts of their family budgets and were reluctant to support universal coverage without meaningful cost control. In my testimony, I suggested we had to be more critical about the way we spent our health dollars. I cited the amount we spent in the last year of life for heroic procedures that often have no benefit.

You would have thought I euthanized my mother! Despite the fact I never advocated reducing any care that could be beneficial, the volume of hate mail and threatening e-mail astonished me. Bloggers depicted me as some sort of Doctor Death. The dichotomy in peoples' responses was evident. Americans do not want the government to spend too much on health care, but they also do not trust the government to set limits. Neither do they trust private insurance companies.

In the '90s, Americans rejected national health reform, preferring private market competition to government regulation. Then, when private Health Maintenance Organizations (HMOs) competed and began to regulate costs, an enormous backlash occurred and people called for the government to regulate private HMOs. I remember the furor over one-day hospital stays for mothers who were giving birth.

A poll taken on August 10, 2009, during the Obama administration's push for health care reform, revealed that 51 percent of Americans feared the federal government more than private insurance.[3] Forty-one percent felt the opposite. Not surprisingly, 67 percent of Democrats feared private insurance more while 82 percent of Republicans expressed more fear of the government.

In reality, we simply cannot have a reasonable health care system without the government. We want to know our doctors are licensed and our medicines are safe. Furthermore, a substantial minority of the population (some estimate about one-third) will not be able to afford health insurance or health care without government assistance because of factors such as poverty, unemployment, sickness, disability, and old age.

Yet, as a society we have mixed feelings. Nearly everyone—Republicans, Democrats, conservatives, and liberals—wants to help the poor and less fortunate, but we have always been reluctant to give too much power to the federal government. We prefer private enterprise or, if necessary, administering public programs through the states. Hence, while many countries enacted national health care systems, Americans opted for private insurance.

Private insurance works fine for most of us, but not all. Insuring old people is prohibitively expensive because they get sick far more often than the young. Hence we developed Medicare, a separate government insurance program to serve the elderly. Private insurance cannot provide charity to everyone who cannot afford health insurance, so we developed Medicaid, a separate, state-run, federally subsidized program to serve the poor. We also have the Veterans Administration, a separate government program that specializes in care for those injured in war. We have special programs for poor children, for kidney disease, and for people with AIDS.

As a result, we developed a piecemeal system that is often hard to coordinate, difficult to change, and nearly impossible to comprehend. Not many people understand the Obama health plan, and fewer can predict its eventual impact. People ask me all the time, "How did we get here? Why is it so complicated? Why are we so bitterly divided and wildly emotional about something as mundane as health care reform?" I tell them there is no simple answer. To understand the Obama health care saga, you have to understand the history of how we got here. Our health care system is a result of blending our best intentions with a wide spectrum of political ideals. It encompasses our oldest fears about powerful, centralized government, private versus public enterprise, competition versus regulation, and personal responsibility versus paternalism. It is Ayn Rand versus Franklin Roosevelt. It impacts the way we choose and interact with our doctors, our hospitals, and our nursing homes. It conjures up pictures of Marcus Welby and of Jack Kevorkian.

I hope that the stories we tell and the history we recount in this book will answer the many questions that people have. We wrote this book for a general audience, so readers who are not familiar with the intricacies of health policy can enjoy reading the history and easily understand the issues. But we also delve into the myriad of political, policy, and economic issues that make health reform so complex and so difficult to enact. In that sense, the book is intended to be a resource for students and practitioners of health care policy.

I have been fortunate to be a part of many of the efforts to reform our health care system. In the '70s, I helped formulate Richard Nixon's proposals for national health care—proposals that closely resemble the program enacted by Barack Obama. In the '80s and '90s, I chaired the commission that recommended Medicare payment policies to Congress. I served on Bill Clinton's transition team and on his National Bipartisan Commission on the Future of Medicare. And, as mentioned earlier, I testified before Congress on the Obama health plan and served on the group that advised Obama during the presidential campaign.

Over that period of time I have watched our health care system evolve into one of the best in the world. Advances in technology and in the capabilities of modern medicine have grown beyond our dreams. Who would have imagined the computer-assisted microsurgery techniques that are now commonplace or the magic of pharmaceuticals to alleviate sickness, depression, and pain? Despite our piecemeal systems of coverage, most Americans have comprehensive health insurance and, aside from the cost, they are generally pleased with what they have. But the system also has many holes. Too many of us fall through the cracks and remain uninsured. The cost of health care is too high, and it continues to rise. Piecemeal systems fail to interact, and care can be inefficient and uncoordinated. Whatever results from Obama's health care bill, we will still have a long journey to travel before we have the system we want.

That journey for me has been very personal, not only within my family but as the central focus of my life's work. As fortunate as I have been to play a role in the national arena, the long and complicated history of US health policy precedes even the few of us who reluctantly admit dating back to the Nixon administration. And, of course, between Nixon and Obama, there were many issues in which I was simply not involved. Hence, the story we tell in this book is not just my story but a story the country has struggled with for nearly a hundred years. It also is not just my writing, but a collaboration with David Shactman, my colleague and coauthor, who wrote some of the stories about me. We decided to relate these stories in the third person even though, in a few places, I had to write about myself.

At the time I write this, the Obama health plan has recently become law. Assuming it survives political opposition, it will be gradually phased in, and much of it will not take effect for several years. It will still leave approximately fifteen million American citizens uninsured. If it is to succeed in the long run, it will require much more significant cost control. Whether it is a significant step in solving the problems of our health care system remains to be seen.

There is an old joke that is frequently told in health care conferences. An aging health economist, who has spent his entire life trying to get the United States to enact universal health care, dies and goes to heaven. One day, he meets God and beseeches him to answer one question. "God," he asks, "will Americans ever have affordable, universal health care?" And God answers, "Yes, my son, but not in my lifetime."

Perhaps, someday, some reader of this book will render that joke obsolete.

# PROLOGUE

# Barack Obama
# and the Challenge of
# Health Care Reform

"**I** am not that leader and will not be a distraction," said Tom Daschle, withdrawing his nomination as President Obama's Secretary of the Department of Health and Human Services (DHHS)—the man chosen to shepherd universal health care through the 111th Congress. The assembled media had not expected the sudden turn of fortune for the former Senate majority leader, who had somehow neglected to pay some $140,000 of federal income tax. Stunned by the sudden announcement, they rushed to transmit the story over their laptops and Blackberries®.

But to Stuart Altman, it was déjà vu all over again. The seventy-one-year-old professor and Washington insider had seen it all before. He had been one of the architects of Richard Nixon's universal health plan. Nixon had relied on Wilbur Mills, the all-powerful chairman of the Senate Ways and Means Committee, to push his health plan through the Ninety-Third Congress. Mills planned to report the bill out of committee immediately after the 1973 summer recess, but Nixon became involved in that "third-rate burglary" called Watergate. Then, in October, Mills was found at the Washington Tidal Basin with a stripper named Fannie Fox, and health care reform drowned along with Nixon's presidency and Wilbur Mills's political career.

It was eighteen years since Altman sat in the governor's mansion in Little Rock with President-elect Bill Clinton. He had worked day and night with the Clinton transition team to craft a proposal for universal health care. Then he watched painfully as Clinton made the fateful decision to develop a complex plan to restructure the entire health care system, practically disdaining input from Congress. After the 1,300-page proposal failed to garner support, Clinton sought a compromise bill from the divided Congress. By that time, however, Clinton was weakened from the Whitewater scandal and the

Lewinsky affair. He sought support from another powerful chairman of the House Ways and Means Committee, Dan Rostenkowski, the consummate dealmaker. However, on May 31, 1994, "Rosty" was indicted by a federal grand jury on seventeen counts of conspiring to defraud the government. Altman's and most Americans' dream of universal health care disappeared and would not receive serious reconsideration for another fifteen years.

"Could this all be happening again?" he asked himself, watching Daschle on the evening news. Obama had made universal health care a prominent issue in his campaign. Altman had been a member of the group that helped Obama create his plan. At the time, he felt there was a real chance to pass a comprehensive health plan that combined the right balance of government involvement and private sector reform. Outside events could also help. The ensuing economic crisis, peaking at the time of his inauguration, offered the rare opportunity for large-scale, Roosevelt-type reforms. It was in this kind of atmosphere that FDR was able to enact social security (although he withdrew his plan for universal health care, afraid it would drag his social security proposal down to defeat).

Altman had worked on health care reform in and out of Washington since 1971, often conferring with Ted Kennedy, the "Lion of the Senate," and the one individual in the country who was most associated with the effort to enact universal care. Kennedy had already been working with Daschle to achieve his lifetime goal. But Daschle was now out of the picture, and Kennedy, who was diagnosed with a malignant brain tumor in 2008 and who collapsed with a seizure during the Obama inauguration, might not be healthy enough to lead the fight.

Altman's optimism was beginning to wane. He wondered whether the new Obama administration could avoid the pitfalls that had frustrated the repeated attempts of its predecessors. Had the young president learned the right lessons from past failures to ensure that this final piece of America's social contract could become a reality? The current system was in serious need of repair. The health care industry was one-seventh of the entire US economy and the largest employer in many localities. Costs were rising at an unsustainable rate, such that many individuals and businesses could not afford health insurance. Government health programs were devouring a huge part of federal and state budgets and driving up the deficit. And, despite the fact that the United States was spending twice as much on health as other industrial countries, forty-six million Americans were uninsured and health outcomes were ranked thirty-seventh in the world (behind Saudi Arabia, Morocco, and Costa Rica, and just one place ahead of Slovenia).[1]

Given the situation, one might assume that nearly everyone would favor reform. However, Altman knew better because he had been there before and understood the history. He picked up the telephone and called his colleague David Shactman to discuss his thoughts. Altman and Shactman had worked together for more than a decade to help design programs to make the US health care system more efficient. They talked about all the obstacles that Obama would have to overcome.

## Economic Constraints

First, there was the economy. As Obama assumed the presidency, a full-blown financial crisis was exploding across the globe. The United States was about to experience its worst recession and highest unemployment since the Great Depression. The president knew he would have to incur enormous budget deficits to rescue the financial system and to stimulate the economy. Health care reform would no longer resonate with the public as it had in the presidential campaign. The economy would become the overriding issue, and hardly anyone would want to consider a program that would add to the deficit or raise taxes. Obama's health plan was going to cost about a trillion dollars over ten years. Where was he going to get the money?

## Interest Group Opposition

Second, there were the interest groups. Opposition from various interest groups had been sinking health reform proposals for nearly a hundred years. The health insurance industry was instrumental in killing the Clinton plan, and Obama wanted to win their support. However, he wanted the government to offer a public plan to compete with private companies; a policy that liberal supporters were demanding but that private insurance companies strongly opposed. Furthermore, he wanted insurance companies to stop restricting, refusing, or terminating coverage for people with preexisting conditions. In order to do so, however, he would have to find a way to get more healthy people to buy insurance.[2] Obama had opposed the plan advanced by his challenger, Hillary Clinton, to require every American to have some form of coverage, but his advisors knew he needed to modify his position. This would not be easy, however, because business groups and political conservatives opposed such a government mandate. It could also create opposition among liberal supporters unless he could provide substantial subsidies to those who could not otherwise afford to buy coverage. Yet generous subsidies would increase the cost of the plan.

Pharmaceutical companies had opposed every serious attempt at universal coverage. They feared that government involvement would eventually lead to price controls. Obama wanted their support, but he also wanted them to close the donut hole (the gap in Medicare drug coverage between $2,250 and $5,100), a measure that could cost them eighty billion dollars over ten years. The drug companies would demand a quid pro quo. They wanted assurances that the government would not negotiate for lower Medicare prices or permit people to buy pharmaceuticals from other countries—two policies that Obama's liberal supporters strongly favored.

Small and independent businesses had opposed every attempt at universal coverage and were adamantly opposed to an employer mandate. The National Federation of Independent Business (NFIB) and the Chamber of Commerce had spent large sums of money to defeat the Clinton plan. Obama's plan was based on an employer mandate, so he could not hope to gain their support, but by providing subsidies and exemptions for small businesses he could possibly blunt some of their opposition. However, subsidies would add to the cost of the plan, and exemptions would add to the number of uninsured.

The American Medical Association (AMA) had opposed every previous attempt to enact national health insurance. Obama desperately wanted its support, but it also would exact a price. Congress had previously passed legislation that was scheduled to cut doctors' Medicare fees by 21 percent. Previous administrations had delayed similar reductions under this law, but the AMA wanted Obama to do more. It wanted him to repeal the requirement that limited physician fee increases. The AMA was also wary about any changes to the delivery and payment system that might negatively impact doctors' fees. Obama wanted to experiment with more cost-efficient payment structures such as bundled payments (i.e., paying for an entire episode of care rather than for each service rendered). But the value of cost-efficiency is in the eye of the beholder. Every dollar saved would be a dollar reduction in someone else's income. Hence, while many would pressure Obama to "bend the cost curve," and reduce the rate of growth of health spending, provider groups would oppose any change that could reduce their incomes.

The hospital associations had a similar perspective. They would support efficiency and cost reduction as long as it was not their revenue that was being reduced. Policies under consideration such as bundled payments, penalties for preventable incidents, a powerful public insurance plan, and a Medicare commission with enhanced powers to cut spending would all be matters of concern.

Even such liberal groups as the elderly and unions would have their misgivings. Obama would have to reduce the projected costs of the Medicare program to help pay for reform. Medicare recipients and the American Association of Retired Persons (AARP), ordinarily supporters of health care reform, would surely oppose any proposal that threatened to reduce their benefits. The unions would ordinarily be among the strongest supporters of national health care. However, many policymakers wanted to raise revenue for the program by taxing so-called "Cadillac" health plans that provided extensive health insurance benefits. Unions had fought for these plans through collective bargaining and would not want to give back benefits they may have secured by sacrificing wage increases.

## Political Opposition

In addition to the economy and interest group opposition, Obama would have to engage in an intense political struggle, some of it emanating from his own party. The Blue Dogs, a coalition of conservative Democrats mostly from the South, would oppose any large spending program that would add to the deficit. Antiabortion Democrats would abandon any proposal with a public insurance option or government subsidy that could be used to pay for abortions. On the other hand, Democratic liberals would insist on a public option and generous government subsidies to help people purchase insurance. Furthermore, they would rail against any compromise by Obama to limit abortion rights. Although Democrats generally favored Medicaid expansions to assist people who would be required to buy insurance, many state office holders would oppose any "unfunded mandates" and would want the federal government to assume the cost. Everyone wanted the Obama plan to bend the cost curve, but no one, Democrats included, wanted to reduce the income of medical providers or industries within their own congressional districts.

All of those obstacles paled in relation to Republican opposition. Obama could not expect conservative Republicans to support universal coverage or any large-scale, national health reform effort, particularly if it expanded the role of the federal government. However, he knew he would almost certainly need the support of some Republican moderates.

Obama remembered that in 1994, Republican Party leaders made a strategic decision to vote in a unanimous block against the Clinton health plan. Newt Gingrich and other party leaders believed if they defeated Clinton on health care, they could wound the president so badly that they would not only win the midterm election but might take over Congress for the first time in forty years. Their strategy was a stunning success, and Newt Gingrich became Speaker of the House.

Would Republicans again vote in a block to oppose his plan? Obama believed he could achieve a compromise with Republican moderates, but whether that was a reasonable expectation in early 2009 was not clear. What was becoming apparent, however, was that he did not anticipate the ferocity of the conservative opposition. In hindsight, we know that in the days before the Senate passed its version of the health bill in December 2009, Republican senators Sam Brownback (R-KS) and Jim DeMint (R-SC) participated in a public gathering to pray for defeat of the health care bill. As if there was not enough opposition to worry about, the president might even have to contend with supplications to God!

Altman and Shactman considered the magnitude of the task facing the new president: interest group pressure, political opposition, economic restraints, and intricacies involved in reforming a complex health care system. Was it possible for any president to navigate these shoals that had shipwrecked so many before them? *You couldn't possibly do it*, they thought, *without a complete understanding of the issues: health insurance markets, employer mandates, consumer demand for medical services, tax incentives, fee-for-service reimbursement, government subsidies... the list was extensive. And it was only part of the picture. You also had to understand the lessons of history. You had to know why so many efforts had failed in the past. There were so many pieces of this puzzle that you had to assemble, to fit together. It is such a long, complicated, and fascinating story,* they thought. *Maybe we should write a book!*

# ACKNOWLEDGMENTS

Acentury of history requires an enormous breadth of research and a herculean effort to distill it into a three-hundred-page narrative. Many of our topics involve settled history in which previous analysts and historians have devoted entire books to just one part of one of our chapters. Hence, we relied on many excellent texts as well as original sources and personal interviews. We have diligently tried to acknowledge all of our sources, but inevitably the insights and analyses of previous writers were bound to influence our thinking. We want to specifically acknowledge a few texts on which we heavily relied. In the Nixon chapter (and to a lesser extent elsewhere), we relied on *The Heart of Power* by David Blumenthal and James Morone. Haynes Johnson and David Broder's book *The System*, about the Clinton health plan, was an extraordinary example of historical journalism and we cited it frequently. For early history, we often consulted Paul Starr's Pulitzer Prize–winning book, *The Social Transformation of American Medicine*. The Medicare saga produced two outstanding books: Ted Marmor's *The Politics of Medicare* and Richard Harris's *A Sacred Trust*. Ted also met with us and was generous with his time and ideas.

We also benefitted from the work of David Smith's *Paying for Medicare: The Politics of Reform* and Rick Mayes and Robert Berenson's *Medicare's Prospective Payment and the Shaping of US Health Care*. We relied on Richard Himelfarb's book, *The Rise and Fall of the Medicare Catastrophic Coverage Act of 1988*. Finally, our Brandeis colleague Michael Doonan counseled us on the Health Insurance Portability and Accessibility Act and the State Children's Health Insurance Program. He also provided his excellent dissertation, *American Federalism and Contemporary Health Policy*. We can only hope that our research will be as valuable to future writers as theirs were to ours.

We also want to express our appreciation for those who agreed to share their insights and recollections in personal interviews. A list is provided in the end material at the back of the book. Our special thanks go to Chip Kahn, who was always helpful and who generously devoted his time for numerous interviews.

Our literary agent, Jason Ashlock of Movable Type Literary Group, offered us wise counsel and connected us with our publisher, Prometheus Books. We are grateful to Stuart's nephew Bennett Kleinberg who helped link us up with Jason and to Steve Rivkin for his advice and support for the project. Our final product reflects the efforts and expertise of the people at Prometheus, and we particularly thank Steven L. Mitchell, Ian Birnbaum, and Mariel Bard for their diligent work.

As academics, we were fortunate to have the assistance of some very able Brandeis University PhD students. We owe a debt of gratitude to Saleema Moore and Jeff Sussman, part of the next generation of thinkers who will confront the challenges of our complex health care system. We are both appreciative of Ann Cummings, who provided assistance and advice throughout the project.

On a more personal level, Stuart would like to thank his wife, Diane, and daughters Beth, Renee, and Heather for their love and support for so many years as he traveled frequently to Washington and asked them to pick up their lives several times and move across the country. Stuart will always carry a heartfelt appreciation for his mother, Florence, now departed, for her love of life and for prodding him to make Medicare a better program for its beneficiaries. Sustaining a two-year task with an uncertain reward is difficult, and David is thankful for the two people who have been most inspirational in his life: his wife, Ellen Wright, who, after reading drafts and redrafts ad nauseam, is still his wisest editor, loving companion, and best friend; and his son, Brian, who carries a heartfelt passion for social justice.

# PART 1

# The Hard Road to Success
## One Hundred Years
## of Past Failures

# CHAPTER 1

# NIXON COMES CLOSE
## OUR PLAN LOOKS LIKE A SLAM DUNK, BUT ENDS WITH JUST A DUNK

### Secret Meetings in the Church Basement

Stuart Altman steps out the rear door of the taxicab and glances up and down the sidewalk. Seeing no one he recognizes, he heads up the walkway toward the church. It would be unlikely to encounter a familiar face in this neighborhood, but just the same, he is cautious. It is June 1974, and Richard Nixon is president. Altman (the deputy assistant secretary for planning and evaluation—health), and two colleagues from the Department of Health, Education, and Welfare (HEW), are about to attend a secret meeting in the basement of the church. They know President Nixon would not be pleased if they were seen.

The Saint Mark's Episcopal Church sits on the corner of Third and A Street in Washington, DC, just behind the Library of Congress. Originally built in 1888 in the Neo-Romanesque style, the church has long served the Capitol Hill community. Altman is a Jewish boy from the Bronx, so he has not come to worship. He enters through the side door of the church and steps into the empty sanctuary. With no one else inside, an eerie quiet is broken only by his footsteps echoing off the stone walls and concrete balustrades. He walks down a steep staircase and enters a gathering room in the basement of the church known as "the pub."

"Good morning, Stuart," comes the greeting from Stan Jones, who arrived a few minutes earlier. Jones, a former divinity student, is a close friend of the church's rector, Jim Adams. The rector has kindly lent Jones this room where the participants can meet in secret. With all the intrigue, you might think of conspiracies from *The DaVinci Code* or *Angels and Demons*, but Jones is an aide to the liberal senator Edward M. Kennedy, and he is here to talk about health care legislation. Kennedy does not want anyone to know he is negotiating with the Nixon administration.

Two minutes later, a third member of the triumvirate enters the basement room. Bill Fullerton is an aide to Wilbur Mills, the Democratic representative from Arkansas and the powerful chairman of the House Ways and Means Committee. Everyone in the room knows that health reform will not happen without the support of Wilbur Mills.

There is such an easy camaraderie among the group that it seems odd to meet in secret. But in 1974, like today, there are widely divergent views about health care reform. All three factions advocate positions strongly favored by their own constituencies, and they do not want to alienate their supporters by appearing to compromise with their opponents. How did these three factions from different parties and different ends of the political spectrum come to meet secretly in the basement of a Washington, DC, church? We begin the story with a brief look at the players.

### Faction no. 1: Ted Kennedy

Universal health care was Ted Kennedy's issue. His brother, the slain president, championed the Medicare program but did not live to see it enacted by Lyndon Johnson in 1965. Ted Kennedy filed his first universal health care bill in 1971. It was based on a proposal by the Committee of 100 for National Health Insurance, a group Kennedy cochaired with Walter Reuther.

Reuther was head of the United Auto Workers (UAW) and had successfully negotiated many of the generous health benefits the autoworkers secured in the '50s. The big automakers could afford the concessions to labor because they had little competition in the '50s and simply added the cost of health benefits to the price of their cars. However, as the cost of providing health benefits increased, Reuther saw the wage gains of his workers becoming smaller. Early on, he understood the damage that runaway health costs could do to both American workers and industry. After withdrawing the UAW from the American Federation of Labor and Congress of Industrial Organizations (AFL-CIO), he formed the Committee of 100 for National Health Insurance. The members consisted of union activists, academics, medical professionals, and politicians—the most important of whom was Ted Kennedy. In 1969, the committee formulated its Health Security Plan. It was a universal health plan that combined all public and private health plans into one single-payer plan financed by federal taxes. The plan included a global budget and provided incentives for prepaid group practices (later called HMOs).

The proposal from the Committee of 100 became the basis for the Health Security Act that Kennedy filed after he became chair of the Subcommittee on Health in 1971. Although the bill never made headway, the effect that the committee and Kennedy had on Richard Nixon was significant. Always the cunning political observer, Nixon anticipated that Kennedy would win the Democratic Party's nomination and challenge him in the 1972 election. He did not want to cede the health reform issue to Kennedy. Hence, in 1971, goaded by public pressure from Kennedy and the committee, Nixon surprised his fellow Republicans by issuing his first proposal for comprehensive national health care reform.

From the start of his political career, Kennedy had aligned himself with big labor and other traditional, liberal Democratic constituencies. In concert with their positions, he advocated a single-payer health system in which the federal government provided everyone's health insurance and financed it largely with general revenues (taxes). Nixon, on the other hand, proposed an employer-based system that retained private health insurance. Liberal Democrats and labor unions believed the Democrats were likely to capture the White House in 1972, and they opposed Nixon's plan, figuring they could enact a single-payer system when they held power. Of course, they were proved wrong when Nixon easily won reelection.

The debate over national health reform continued through Nixon's second term, and Ted Kennedy faced a conundrum. Universal health insurance was, quintessentially, his issue. He cared about it deeply and wanted it to become a reality in the United States as it was in virtually all other developed nations. Yet he was realistic about the political opposition to his single-payer proposal. The health insurance lobby was strong, and its members would cease to exist or, at most, play a diminished administrative role if the government provided everyone's insurance. The American Medical Association (AMA) feared that government-provided insurance would eventually lead to regulation and price controls. Opponents branded Kennedy's plan "government-run health care" and claimed it would be the first step toward socialized medicine. Kennedy realized the opposition to single-payer was too powerful and feared he might become marginalized as Congress debated more moderate alternatives. He did not want to be left out, and he certainly did not want Nixon and the Republicans to get all the credit for national health insurance.

Hence, in early 1974, Kennedy met secretly with Wilbur Mills to create a more liberal version of the plan proposed by the Nixon Administration. In April they announced the Kennedy–Mills bill, surprising everyone, but disappointing Kennedy's liberal supporters. The bill was a modified single-payer that retained private health insurers, but mainly in the role of fiscal intermediaries. The proposal also required insured individuals to make substantial copayments. Liberals and big labor wanted a pure single-payer and opposed the bill, thinking they could wait out Nixon's second term. But Kennedy was determined to pass national health insurance and wanted to explore whether a bipartisan bill could be developed. At the same time, he was leery of further alienating his supporters, many of whom would be outraged if they knew he was negotiating away single-payer with Richard Nixon. That was why he sent Jones to meet secretly with Altman and Fullerton in the basement of the Washington, DC, church.

### Faction no. 2: Wilbur Mills

There may never again be a committee chairperson as powerful as Wilbur Mills. During Nixon's presidency, the structure and operation of Congress was much different than it is today. The major congressional committees were autonomous power centers that could push through or block any legislative initiative. The chairs of these committees, who by definition were always in the majority, dictated the procedures and ruled like kings. The Ways and Means Committee, chaired by Wilbur Mills, was the most powerful. Not only did it have undivided jurisdiction over important areas such as taxes and federal health policy, but it had no subcommittees. Mills did not have to delegate authority to subcommittee chairs, who would then have autonomy over their particular niches. Mills was also Chair of the Committee on Committees, and thus was able to delegate who got committee assignments throughout the House of Representatives. As a result, when Mills's Ways and Means Committee reported out a bill, it nearly always passed the full House. In the Ninety-Third Congress (1973–1974), thirty-nine of forty-five bills reported out by his committee passed the full House.[1]

Today's committee chairs would be envious of Wilbur Mills, and some of the blame can be visited on Richard Nixon. Partly as a reaction to Nixon's imperial view of presidential power, and his subsequent downfall from the Watergate scandal, a large congressional turnover occurred, replacing many of the old guard. The unusually large body of younger politicians sought to democratize the old power structure. The power of committee chairs was dispersed. Jurisdiction over large areas of policy became divided over several committees. The number of subcommittees grew exponentially, devolving much of the power to subcommittee chairs. Most importantly, seniority rules were relaxed, making it more difficult for a small clique of aging House members to cling to power.

These changes in the structure and operation of Congress may seem esoteric, but their impact on health reform legislation has been considerable. When Wilbur Mills was Chair of Ways and Means, decisions could be made by a few individuals. You could meet behind the scenes with a few powerful chairmen (and they were men), forge secret deals and alliances, and be nearly assured your bill would pass the full House. For the Clinton and Obama administrations, it was infinitely more difficult. The committee chairs could no longer deliver on promises without seeking wider support. Negotiating with a broad range of people, interests, and factions was a political necessity, and the ability to make backroom secret deals was limited.

Wilbur Mills occupied a central spot in the political spectrum. As a southern Democrat in the majority, he had the power to move democratic legislation through his committee and to block Republican initiatives. Not infrequently, however, he sided with conservative southern Democrats supporting the Republican side, particularly in matters that concerned race.

In 1971, Nixon sought Mills's help in his first effort at passing national health reform. He knew that Mills was interested in running for the presidency in 1972, and he suggested to John Ehrlichman, the assistant to the president for domestic affairs, that if they offered to let Mills get credit for the legislation, they might be able to win his support.[2] Apparently, Mills expressed interest, but his support never materialized and Nixon's 1971 plan died a quiet death. One reason may have been Mills's earlier experience with Lyndon Johnson and Medicare, when the actual cost turned out to be wildly higher than Johnson had projected and Mills decided he had been snookered.[3] Mills and other conservative members of Congress were wary of repeating that mistake with national health reform.

As the 1972 primary season approached, Kennedy was being coy about whether or not he would run, and Mills decided to enter the race for the

Democratic presidential nomination. Lee Goldman, Kennedy's staff director, knew Mills had no chance to win the party's nomination, but he saw an opportunity to use Mills's ambition to push national health reform. Goldman and Stan Jones had a tradition of beginning each morning with coffee in the Senate cafeteria. One morning Goldman suggested to Jones, "I'll bet you he [Mills] would go for a liaison with Kennedy on the assumption that maybe Kennedy will run and he'll be his vice presidential candidate."[4] Kennedy, an astute political player, slyly agreed with Goldman's idea, but he did not want to ask Mills directly. So Kennedy decided to use an intermediary, Wilbur Cohen, who was chairing a meeting of the Democratic Platform Committee in Mills's home state of Arkansas. During the meeting, Cohen casually suggested to Mills that he might try to work something out with Kennedy on health reform.

After returning to Washington, Mills shocked his aide, Bill Fullerton, by asking him to contact the liberal Kennedy and arrange a meeting. They met secretly about four or five times in Mills's famously huge office just off the House floor. Jones attended the meetings, but Mills would not let Fullerton attend. Apparently it would have been an affront to Mills if anyone thought he needed a staffer.[5] And he didn't. Mills knew nearly every detail of Medicare, Medicaid, and the tax code. As a result of the meetings, Mills and Kennedy put together a compromise plan. It never gained any traction but was an important forerunner to the Kennedy–Mills bill in 1974. It was also an early example of how Ted Kennedy would amass an impressive legislative record by compromising with some of his fiercest opponents. The Kennedy–Mills effort did become a plank in the 1972 Democratic platform, but it died along with the woeful presidential campaign of George McGovern.

Mills's primary results were dismal, never capturing more than 5 percent of the vote. He could not overcome his record on race with non-southern Democrats. Mills tried to explain that segregation was a "dead issue" and stated, "I voted as I did over the years [against civil rights] because it was necessary to vote that way if I was to stay in Congress."[6] Evidence uncovered in the Watergate investigation a few years later revealed that Mills had accepted an illegal campaign contribution of one hundred thousand dollars. The contribution came from a Texan who was amassing a fortune processing Medicaid and Medicare claims. The company was Electronic Data Systems and the Texan, Ross Perot, would later make his own run for president.

After Nixon's reelection, Mills's committee became the central focus for health reform legislation. The wily Mills agreed to cosponsor Nixon's 1974 health reform bill (HR 12684), but later met secretly with Kennedy and announced the Kennedy–Mills proposal. It was a significant compromise for Kennedy, who broke with his usual constituency in order to compromise and strike a deal. However, if there were to be further negotiations, the need for secrecy was clear. Each side knew there were many on the left and right who would do everything they could to scuttle the idea of a compromise between a conservative Republican president and the titular head of the liberal wing of the Democratic Party. Each side also knew they could not achieve their objective without the support of the House Ways and Means Committee and its all-powerful chairman, Wilbur Mills. It was this same Wilbur Mills who, with President Johnson in 1965, passed the Medicare and Medicaid programs—the most far-reaching pieces of health care legislation in American history. Sitting quietly in the middle of this political drama, and wielding enormous power, Wilbur Mills sent Bill Fullerton to meet secretly in the basement of the church.

## Faction # 3: Richard Nixon

Why did Richard Nixon propose national health insurance? Here is the man who earned his political stripes as an anticommunist conservative. He assisted Joe McCarthy in his prosecution of Alger Hiss. He won election to Congress by red baiting Helen Gahagan Douglas. He campaigned for the presidency by inventing the "Southern strategy;" appealing for law and order and exploiting fear and racism in the South. He opposed busing, nominated conservative Supreme Court justices, and took a hard line against war protestors.

Yet he was a study in contradictions. He opened American relations with China. He supported a negative income tax to fight poverty. He added disability benefits to Social Security. He created the Environmental Protection Agency, passed the Clean Air Act, created the National Oceanic and Atmospheric Administration, and left a legacy of environmental initiatives that have only been rolled back since he was president. Despite his free market Republican credentials, he instituted wage and price controls and enacted a series of government health care regulations and health planning initiatives that have been unequalled since his presidency.[7] In his second term, he was closer to enacting universal health care than any president until Obama.

On December 13, 1973, Nixon schedules a meeting of the Domestic Council on Health in the cabinet room of the White House. It is a rectangular room in the West Wing overlooking the rose garden. A long, elliptical mahogany table that seats twenty, a gift from President Nixon, dominates the impressive Georgian-style room. Two nineteenth-century empire-style chandeliers hang from the eighteen-foot-high ceiling. In the center of the east side sits the president's chair, the back of which is two inches higher than any of the others. Stuart Altman and many of the people who are running the country are sitting around the table. There is an air of skepticism and an undercurrent of discontent. What the hell is Nixon thinking? What is a conservative Republican doing promoting a plan for national health care? Why are we pushing a plan that is so liberal it could be coming from Teddy Kennedy?

Nixon walks into the room and brooks no discussion. He acknowledges that some are skeptical about supporting any program for national health insurance, but he assures them that they are going forward with a serious effort. "There is no question," he tells them, "that at some point in time, there will be a serious effort to push legislation through the Congress and we must have a proposal to counter it. You can't fight something with nothing."[8] Nixon has made up his mind and he does not want to hear from anyone. He tells Casper Weinberger, the secretary of HEW, to get it done quickly—to have it ready for the State of the Union.

As Altman gets up to leave the room, Casper Weinberger approaches him. "Stuart, you have two weeks to finish the plan you've been developing. Remember, the president wants it done. Don't let anyone derail the process." Altman knows there are many unresolved issues and much opposition. Without the clout of the president, he will never be able to get approval from the other cabinet departments. He also realizes he will have no Christmas vacation in 1973.

Historians venture a number of reasons why Nixon championed national health insurance. Some trace his personal interest to the anguish he suffered at the death of his two brothers and his family's struggle to provide them adequate care. More often, they attribute his efforts to political strategy. He compulsively worried about Ted Kennedy as a future presidential opponent and sought to co-opt the health care issue from the Democrats while, at the same time, claiming their proposals would result in socialized medicine. Some have theorized that he needed a grand gesture to deflect attention from Watergate, although he had floated comprehensive health reform proposals prior to the scandal.

Whatever his reasons were, and they were likely a combination of the above, his proposals were not in synch with many members of his cabinet— let alone the mainstream of the Republican Party. He certainly did not want to cause them additional anxiety by revealing he was negotiating with Ted Kennedy. So in the late spring of 1974, while Watergate was about to boil over, Richard Nixon instructed his secretary of HEW to try to make a behind-the-scenes deal with Kennedy and Mills; Casper Weinberger dispatched Stuart Altman and his team to meet in the basement of the Saint Marks Episcopal Church.

But these meetings occurred near the end of Nixon's presidency. Along the way, Nixon was responsible for many of the ideas and proposals that are still the driving influences in health care policy. His impact was so great that Blumenthal concludes his chapter on Nixon by stating, "All reformers stand in his shadow."[9] We get the first glimpse of this in 1970.

## How Richard Nixon Brought HMOs to Americans

In 1970, Paul Ellwood was the executive director of the American Rehabilitation Foundation. He had good reason to be disturbed about fee-for-service medical reimbursement, the almost universal means of payment for medical services. The faster his rehab hospitals returned their patients to health, the less they were paid. Conversely, those who kept their patients longer than necessary, perhaps because of poor treatment, medical errors, or simple greed, were rewarded with higher payments.

Ellwood was a strong advocate of prepaid group practices. If a group of doctors received a fixed annual payment in advance for each patient, it would behoove them to keep that patient as healthy as possible, and to provide preventive care in order to avoid an expensive illness or hospitalization. If the patient did become ill, the doctors' incentive was to provide the most efficient treatment, returning the patient to health in the shortest possible time, because the medical group would have already received all the reimbursement they were going to get. Moreover, the medical group would strive to treat the patient well, because a relapse or rehospitalization, besides being bad for the patient, was only going to require more medical services and cost the group more money. A group of doctors under such a system would have the incentive to manage their patients' care better and more efficiently than in fee-for-service medicine where unrelated, individual practitioners receive additional payments for each service or procedure they perform. The sicker the patient, the more money they make.

Although liberals liked prepaid group practices for their expanded services and cooperative nature, the Nixon administration saw them as a way to promote market competition. Ellwood already had a sympathetic ear in the new administration because Nixon and his health appointees were Californians and were familiar with Kaiser Permanente. At the time, Kaiser had a large presence in California and was one of the few prepaid group practices in the country. Nixon appointed a fellow Californian, Robert Finch, to be secretary of HEW. He had asked Finch earlier to be his vice president, but Finch declined and Nixon selected Spiro Agnew. Finch was a lifelong friend of Nixon, but his politics were decidedly more liberal than those of the president. Differences surfaced early on when Finch tried to appoint John Knowles as assistant secretary for health. The AMA wanted nothing to do with the liberal Knowles from Massachusetts General Hospital, and Finch had to back off, leaving the department with no senior health person. Finch appointed three moderate Republican Californians to HEW: Lewis Butler, John Veneman, and Leon Panetta. Without an assistant secretary, responsibility for the health care agenda fell to Lew Butler, a lawyer with limited knowledge of health care policy.

Ellwood met with Butler and Veneman on February 5, 1970. Aware of the administration's ideology, he presented his ideas as a model for more competitive markets. He convinced them that a national program to create prepaid group practices would be a significant improvement over the current system of fee-for-service reimbursement. Competition among these practices, Ellwood contended, would restrain the rapid growth in health care costs that had greatly accelerated since the passage of Medicare and Medicaid. It was at this meeting that the term Health Maintenance Organization was coined, and from then on, prepaid group practices were popularly referred to as HMOs.[10] A month after Ellwood's presentation, Finch proposed that Medicare and Medicaid contract with HMOs. That did not occur until the late '80s, but it was the first initiative in a long history of federal government support for HMOs.

We leave the Nixon story briefly for a quick primer on HMOs and examine why they remain an important but contentious element of health care policy.

## A Primer: Why is Managed Care So Contentious?

Paul Ellwood was correct. A prepaid or capitated annual payment for each insured person provides the incentive to treat patients more efficiently. Even as early as 1970, the problems generated by paying doctors and hospitals on a fee-for-service basis were well known. The medical community receives no reward for keeping people healthy. Quite the opposite: the more procedures health care providers perform, the more they are paid. Critics were concerned that capitation would provide a perverse incentive to provide too little care. Ellwood countered that a well-functioning market would provide patients with sufficient information to choose plans that provided the best care. Well-informed patients would not join plans that skimped or provided poor quality. In support of his arguments, Ellwood cited Kaiser Permanente and Group Health of Puget Sound, both of which provided excellent care.

If the market for prepaid health plans functioned as well as other competitive markets, few would have disputed Ellwood's theories. In practice, however, as capitated groups became more prevalent, some of them succumbed to the incentive to profit by providing less care. The press uncovered examples of patients who were denied care, and a negative public reaction followed that became known as the "managed care backlash." The extent of negative press was so strong that by the late '90s, the HMO movement abandoned many of its managed care principles. Although many organizations in 2009 are called HMOs, most operate more like traditional health insurers and continue fee-for-service reimbursement rather than capitation. As a result, they do little to control utilization and cost. This has reignited the debate over the failings of fee-for-service medicine.

Two kinds of questions characterize the debate. The first: "Do HMOs treat people more efficiently (less waste, fewer unneeded procedures and surgeries) or do they simply cut back on providing care?" It is a difficult question to answer. When hospitals began to discharge new mothers after one day, there was an uproar from patients and their families that they were being sent home too soon. Health plans had evidence that a one-day stay was sufficient for the vast majority of women who had had normal deliveries. Consumers did not agree and questioned the health plans' motives. Although the health plans may have been technically correct, they were forced by patient preferences and bad press to abandon the practice.

The efficiency-versus-cost question becomes more complex when a medical procedure provides a minimal benefit but incurs a large cost. This is particularly evident for life-threatening conditions. For example, should the health plan provide a $250,000 bone marrow transplant when there is very little or no evidence the treatment will be efficacious? American culture seems to demand unlimited amounts of medical service in the face of death. This is not necessarily the same in other cultures. In the US, over 27 percent of the country's annual medical expenditures are consumed in the last year of life.[11] This has prompted what has become an old joke in health policy conferences: "Most people in the world think that death is inevitable, but in the United States it is considered optional."

The second kind of question is "Should the process of receiving health care be managed, or should people be free to seek any provider or service they want?" The concept of managed care is to provide coordinated services according to evidence-based practice guidelines by a panel of medical providers who are responsible for adhering to those guidelines. Hence, tightly managed care employs their own closed panel of doctors, sometimes on salary, so they can evaluate and manage their performance. They often require gatekeepers, usually primary care physicians (PCPs), who refer patients to the proper provider in the least intensive setting. This requires contacting your PCP before going to the emergency room, or getting your PCP's referral before going to a specialist.

It is clear from the experience in the '90s that most Americans do not want their care to be tightly managed. They want the freedom to choose their own doctors and want to be able to see specialists without advance permission; they want to be able to take their children to the emergency room when they are running high fevers. Americans distrust insurance companies that limit their choices, suspicious that companies are trying to save money rather than appropriately managing patients' health care. Hence, while managed care has become pervasive in the United States in the twenty-first century, it has become largely unmanaged relative to the original concept. Only 20 percent of insured Americans under age sixty-five are enrolled in HMOs, down from 31 percent in 1996—a 35 percent reduction.[12] Most are enrolled in preferred provider organizations or PPOs (58 percent), or point of service plans or PSPs (8 percent), where they can choose their own doctors and hospitals.[13] Relatively few Americans under sixty-five are enrolled in capitated plans.

Today, there is a disconnect between the health policy community and the typical American consumer. Health policy analysts, in general, believe that the worst kind of care is the uncoordinated, independent practitioner model. It works outside any coordinated system of care, receives compensation on a fee-for-service basis, and often duplicates services and provides unnecessary procedures. They cite integrated systems of care such as the Geisinger Medical System in Danville, Pennsylvania, and the Mayo Clinic in Rochester, Minnesota. These organizations have demonstrated the ability to provide high quality care at lower costs. Whether the United States should change from fee-for-service medicine to these tightly managed integrated health systems was part of the debate in 2009.

In contrast, the average American consumer believes the best system is one that gives him independent, unfettered choice and complete freedom of action. Consumers do not trust private health insurers to manage their care. Most countries attempt to control their health costs through public regulation. They use global budgets, limiting or rationing the supply of services to their citizens who sometimes have to wait in long queues for such things as magnetic resonance imaging (MRIs) or elective procedures. If health costs continue to rise, Americans may someday have to choose whether they want their services regulated by private health plans or by the federal government.

## Back to Nixon and HMOs

About a year after Ellwood's meeting, on February 17, 1971, Edward Kaiser, the founder of Kaiser Permanente, came to the White House and met with John Ehrlichman. Kaiser's presentation, like Ellwood's, was received enthusiastically by Nixon's staff, and it convinced the president to support the development of HMOs.

Richard Nixon was concerned about health care costs. Federal spending for the Medicare and Medicaid programs had surpassed everyone's expectations. Their cost grew from 4.1 percent of the federal budget in 1965 to 11.3 percent by 1973.[14] HMOs seemed to have everything Nixon needed. The prepaid group practices described by Ellwood had cost-saving incentives. They appealed to Nixon and republican conservatives because they were a free market approach, and they preserved the private insurance market. Moreover, they did not require large government spending as in the case of liberal, Democratic reform proposals.

Democrats and liberals were also in favor of HMOs but for different reasons. The Kaiser Permanente model appealed to them. It was a nonprofit, community-rated system, which meant that everyone paid the same regardless of health status. The philosophy of taking care of its members was almost collectivist in notion. Liberal Democrats saw HMOs as a vehicle for expanding coverage and including treatments for such additional services as mental health, alcoholism, and substance abuse. They wanted these organizations to operate as nonprofits and employ their own salaried doctors like Kaiser Permanente.

Nixon, on the other hand, favored a more open market approach, allowing a variety of organizations including for-profit health plans. He wanted to include loosely affiliated groups of physicians (called independent practice associations) who could maintain their own private practices and see both HMO and fee-for-service patients. Nixon also wanted to limit the scope of the benefit package.

The administration launched a demonstration project with forty-five million dollars in grants and loans and $300 million in loan guarantees to spur the development of HMOs. Although the program was modest, the results were encouraging, and the administration sought to increase funding. Liberal Democrats, including Ted Kennedy, wanted to promote their own conception of HMOs and insisted on permanent legislative authority. Both sides managed to compromise, and they produced the Health Maintenance Organization Act of 1973. It permitted a variety of organizations to qualify for funding as Nixon wished, but most of the concessions went to the Democrats. HMOs were required to provide an expanded list of services. They had to admit anyone who applied (open enrollment) and were required to charge all applicants within a region the same premium (community rating).

The result was a historic piece of legislation. It required every company with twenty-five or more employees that offered health insurance to offer an HMO option if one existed in the area. Growth was slow in the early years of the legislation because the expanded benefits, open enrollment, and community rating often made HMOs uncompetitive with traditional health insurance. However, after several amendments eased these restrictions, the HMO concept gradually took hold and eventually changed the nature of health insurance in America. As of January 2009, HMOs (or one of the looser forms of managed care) insured 74.6 percent of privately insured Americans.[15] HMOs were to become the centerpiece of Clinton's failed health plan and the driving force behind the restructuring of health insurers and providers in the '90s.

By the time the HMO Act was adopted, the group of liberal, Republican Californians running HEW were mostly gone. Pete McCloskey, a seven-term Republican congressman who ran against Nixon for President in 1968, tells what happened.[16] At the 1968 Republican Convention, Nixon's chief opponents were Nelson Rockefeller and Ronald Reagan. Nixon had 650 pledged delegates, twenty-five short of the number he needed to win on the first ballot. It was crucial to stop southern Republicans from drifting to Ronald Reagan. On the second day of the convention, McCloskey attended a private hotel speech by Senator Strom Thurmond to southern Republicans. Thurmond urged them to stick with Nixon on the first ballot even though Reagan was more conservative. He relayed a promise by Nixon that he would not enforce the Civil Rights Act or the Voting Rights Act if he were elected. The South largely held, and Nixon won the nomination on the first ballot, but the promise had repercussions at HEW.

Secretary of HEW Robert Finch had appointed Leon Panetta as director of the Office of Civil Rights. Panetta thought he was doing his job enforcing the Civil Rights Act. In the spring of 1970, Finch and Butler were away and Veneman was acting as secretary. Bob Mardian, Nixon's general counsel for HEW, called Veneman and told him to fire Panetta. Mardian told Veneman, "Doesn't he understand Nixon promised the southern delegates he would stop enforcing the Civil Rights and Voting Rights Act?"

Finch and Veneman threatened to resign if Nixon fired Panetta, and Nixon backed off; but the handwriting was on the wall. Panetta resigned a few weeks later, returned to California, switched to the Democratic Party, and was elected to Congress for nine terms. As of 2009, he is director of the CIA under Obama and designated to be the next secretary of defense.

Finch resigned from HEW for personal reasons and became a White House advisor. Lewis Butler (McCloskey's former law partner) resigned in 1971 in protest over Nixon's invasion of Cambodia, and later became the founding board chairman of the Ploughshares Fund. Bob Mardian was indicted for his role in the Watergate cover-up.

Nixon's character and motives, like the man himself, remain elusive. Despite his campaign's "Southern Strategy," and his promise to Strom Thurmond, his overall record on civil rights was positive. He nationalized the Voting Rights Act and started bilingual education. Most importantly, he created affirmative action, one of the most consequential civil rights policies since emancipation.

Nixon replaced the "too left-leaning" Robert Finch with the liberal, Boston Republican Elliott Richardson, whose tenure was significant for health care policy. Richardson supported the expansion of HMOs and the 1973 act passed under his tenure. He also oversaw the creation of the National Health Insurance Partners Program. It was a genuine effort to enact national health insurance and a radical initiative for a Republican president.

## The Most Serious National Health Initiative Since Harry Truman

Richard Nixon's first proposal for national health insurance never even came to a committee vote in Congress. Yet the National Health Insurance Partners program stands as an important forerunner to his 1974 plan that was almost enacted. Nearly every comprehensive universal health plan in the ensuing years can find its roots in this proposal.

Nixon realized that health reform was going to be a major concern, and he knew that Ted Kennedy, his putative opponent in the next election, would be seizing the issue. In July of 1970, he asked Elliot Richardson to explore the alternatives for their own initiative. On February 18, 1971, Nixon sent a document addressed to the Congress of the United States entitled "Special Message to Congress Proposing a National Health Strategy."[17] The plan is worth examining because it reveals how the Nixon administration recognized and confronted many of the problems we still face today.

The Partners Program mandated employers to provide a minimum package of insurance benefits to all full-time workers. A government mandate for private employers was out of the mainstream of Republican thought, but it was a wise choice. Employer-paid premiums are not considered taxes. They are officially "off-budget," even though the government requires them. Hence, the administration could require employers to offer insurance to all full-time workers and avoid the stigma of raising taxes. For that reason, the employer mandate has been an attractive option for nearly all subsequent universal health plans.

The Partners Program also provided subsidized insurance to the poor that would largely replace Medicaid. The program would be free to those families earning less than five thousand dollars and then gradually phased in as incomes increased. However, subsidies were limited to families with children, similar to welfare. It left out single people, childless couples, and unemployed and part-time workers without children. Although the program proposed insurance pools for those who failed to qualify, the pools were not subsidized, so they likely would have been unaffordable to those at the lower end of the income scale.

Nixon's program had a reasonable benefit package but had substantial deductibles, coinsurance, and service limitations. Most services had a one-hundred-dollar deductible and 25 percent coinsurance. The subsidized program had less cost-sharing than the minimum employer benefit package, but limited coverage to thirty days of hospital care and eight doctor visits per year. Hence, the program was criticized for providing different levels of benefits to the rich and the poor. It included an annual catastrophic maximum of five thousand dollars per family. That was significant for the well-to-do but was a difficult plateau for those at lower income levels who did not qualify for fully subsidized care.

Although the program had shortcomings, it was comprehensive in scope and a radical proposal for a conservative, Republican administration. It is striking to consider how much of its structure and provisions are similar to plans proposed thirty-five years later. Employer mandates, subsidized insurance for the poor, cost sharing, insurance pools, and catastrophic insurance limits have been included in nearly all subsequent plans. In addition, Nixon proposed combining Medicare Parts A and B, requiring an HMO option, providing neighborhood health clinics in inner city and rural areas, granting loans for medical education, broadening the use of ancillary personnel such as physician assistants, and studying what could be done about malpractice insurance.

A final provision augured some of today's concerns about personal medical responsibility. Nixon stated, "Too many Americans eat too much, drink too much, work too hard, and exercise too little." He noted that those are personal issues, but also public issues because "the careful subsidize the careless, nonsmokers subsidize those who smoke, the physically fit subsidize the run-down and the overweight." He recommended establishing a private health education foundation to educate and raise awareness of these problems; quite an intrusive government proposal for a conservative, Republican president.

What happened to this amazingly forward-looking plan that Nixon proposed in February 1971? It went nowhere. Every stakeholder had its own idea about how to reform the health care system. Kennedy introduced his "Health

Security Plan" (Kennedy–Griffiths) based on Walter Reuther's proposal from the Committee of 100. It was too liberal for Republicans and southern Democrats. Kennedy called Nixon's plan a sellout to insurance companies.

The AMA opposed all other plans, putting forth its own proposal called Medicredit. It provided vouchers and tax credits to encourage individuals to buy insurance, but it was not nearly generous enough to approach universal coverage.

The insurance companies opposed Kennedy's single-payer because it would put them out of business. They opposed Medicredit because they were afraid the federal government's payment obligations would eventually encourage it to regulate prices. So they formulated their own proposal with Senator Russell Long, the chair of the Senate Finance Committee. Long proposed a catastrophic plan in which everyone would buy his or her own private insurance, and the federal government would supplement everyone's private policies with catastrophic coverage for annual medical expenses that exceeded two thousand dollars. Long did not support anyone else's bill, and none of the other major players supported Long.

Nixon's bill was too liberal for Republicans and not liberal enough for nonsouthern Democrats, who preferred to wait for the next election. By July of 1971, twenty-two health reform bills were filed. None were ever reported out of committee. Everyone supported health reform, but only if the particular bill would benefit his or her constituency. It was a perfect example of what would later become known in health policy circles as "Altman's Law":

> Nearly every major interest group favors universal coverage and health system reform, but, if the plan deviates from their preferred approach, they would rather retain the status quo.

Despite the outcome, the significance of Nixon's proposal should not be underestimated. A conservative, Republican president had proposed comprehensive national health insurance and an employer mandate. It failed to attain a vote in the Ninety-Second Congress, but the health care issue would return in Nixon's second term, and he would turn to Casper Weinberger and Stuart Altman to improve on his original plan.

## "Stuart, I Want a Top-to-Bottom Review"

Richard Nixon won the 1972 election by a landslide. Against a weak campaign by George McGovern, Nixon carried forty-nine states and 61 percent of the popular vote. Only Ted Kennedy's home state of Massachusetts voted for McGovern. Ironically, Kennedy, with his antiwar stance and health reform agenda, might have been a much stronger candidate. However, on the evening of July 18, 1969, Kennedy drove his Oldsmobile™ 88 off the Dike Bridge in Chappaquiddick. Kennedy swam to safety, but his young female passenger, Mary Jo Kopechne, drowned. Kennedy did not report the accident until the next day. He was eventually convicted of leaving the scene of a fatal accident and became mired in scandal. As a result, he declined to run against Nixon in 1972 even though polls showed he probably could have won the Democratic Party's nomination. Had Kennedy won the 1972 election, national health care would have been at the top of his domestic agenda. It would be the first of two automobile mishaps during the Nixon presidency and the first of three sex scandals since 1969 to alter the chances for national health care reform.

Richard Nixon was an activist president. He was a policy entrepreneur and a gambler, and he was rarely content with the status quo. So, when his second term began he wanted new initiatives and fresh ideas, and he requested resignations from his entire cabinet. Some people left the administration entirely while others simply moved from one department to another. Elliott Richardson moved from HEW to secretary of defense, and Casper Weinberger left his position as head of the Office of Management and Budget (OMB) to take command of HEW.

Stuart Altman and his colleagues who had remained in HEW were apprehensive. Casper Weinberger had eviscerated so many programs as head of OMB that he earned the nickname "Cap the Knife." Many in the department feared that Nixon had chosen Weinberger to eliminate social programs that were at the heart of HEW, but that was not the case. This was particularly true in health policy where Weinberger, acting on Nixon's instructions, strongly supported a comprehensive program that would allow the administration to regain the initiative in national health policy.

Nixon had reintroduced his National Health Insurance Partners program in 1972, but with little of his attention or support it never gained any traction. After the election, with the Watergate scandal growing, he needed an issue to show his administration was still capable of action. He sent a memo to Weinberger telling him to produce a "public–private plan that assured universal insurance, augmented private sector coverage, and used government to fill the gaps."[18]

Weinberger was not an expert in health policy and he turned to his deputy assistant secretary. "Stuart," he said, "I want a top-to-bottom review of all the health options that are available."

"Even single-payer?" Altman asked, concealing his surprise.

"Yes, even single-payer," Weinberger replied.

Altman and his team worked throughout 1973 to study and evaluate the potential alternatives. In particular, he relied on his key health insurance expert, Peter Fox, who had moved to Altman's staff from the budget office. This time they had the ear of the president. In his first term, Nixon was immersed in foreign policy, leading up to his famous visit to China in February of 1972. His chief aides had been Bob Haldeman and John Ehrlichman, who were known as the "Berlin Wall" because of their German heritage and their practice of tightly restricting any access to the president. Even cabinet secretaries had little or no access to Nixon. Haldeman and Ehrlichman had been classmates at UCLA. Both were devout Christian Scientists, and that likely dampened their enthusiasm for national health care. Ehrlichman's chief assistant in 1972–1973 was also a Christian Scientist by the name of Henry Paulson. Paulson later amassed a fortune as CEO of Goldman Sachs, became treasury secretary under George W. Bush, and engineered the financial bailouts in 2008. Another mutual friend and UCLA classmate was Mark Felt, the man who later became known as Deep Throat. Felt, who was Haldeman's fraternity brother, exposed the Watergate cover-up forcing Haldeman and Ehrlichman to resign on April 30, 1973, and eventually resulting in their imprisonment. With Haldeman and Ehrlichman gone, Cap Weinberger's access to Nixon was unprecedented. He became head of the Domestic Policy Council's Committee on Health and was a force in the administration. Nixon relied on Weinberger, and Weinberger relied on Altman. "I was thirty-six years old," says Altman, "and I have never had so much power—before or since."

In a memo dated April 16, 1973, Altman laid out the following options for a new attempt to enact national health insurance:[19]

- Resubmit the previous plan.
- Resubmit the previous plan with improvements.

- Switch to a catastrophic insurance plan such as Senator Long's.
- Combine the previous plan with a catastrophic plan.
- Formulate a new employer-based plan with an improved Medicaid program.
- Develop a proposal similar to the Federal Employees Health Benefits Program (FEHBP).

Altman and his team concluded that although the 1971 plan was surprisingly comprehensive for a Republican administration, it had severe deficiencies in two areas. First, it failed to cover large populations such as childless couples, low-income singles, and the childless unemployed. Second, the benefit package and cost-sharing requirements needed to be improved. The schedule of copayments and deductibles required excessive cost sharing, there was no coverage for outpatient prescription drugs, and the poor had different benefits than the nonpoor.

Altman, who was more liberal on social policy than the Republican administration, found himself in an enviable position. His president was concerned about Kennedy's bill, which had been resubmitted and was more expansive than the administration's proposal. His boss, Casper Weinberger, was pushing for a comprehensive bill and was dependent upon him for the details. It was one of those times when a staff member can become a policy entrepreneur and wield a disproportionate amount of power. Altman and Fox crafted what became known as the Comprehensive Health Insurance Plan (CHIP). It was a plan that many health policy advocates in the Obama administration would be happy to support. Yet Altman and Fox were able to sell it to a conservative administration as a plan that "retained the underlying principles of the 1971 plan,"[20] despite the fact that they had created a much more expansive proposal.

Before deciding on the final details, however, a number of issues remained controversial and had to be vetted and analyzed within the administration. Many of these issues are still the primary source of debate, almost forty years later. We leave the Nixon story again to examine some of these issues because they illustrate the difficult decisions that any administration must confront to enact national health reform.

## A Brief Primer on Selected Issues in National Health Insurance

### The Employer Mandate

Since Richard Nixon's first national health bill, the employer mandate has been the centerpiece of every serious proposal for universal coverage. Yet, it remains controversial. Although most large businesses already provide health benefits to their employees, many small businesses do not. In 2008, 96.5 percent of large businesses provided health benefits, but 43.2 percent of firms with less than fifty employees did not.[21] Often, small firms have thin profit margins and pay low wages, and the cost of insuring their employees represents a significant new expense. They fear that a health insurance mandate will significantly erode their profits, require them to lay off employees, or even go out of business. Hence, the NFIB and the Chamber of Commerce have consistently opposed plans with an employee mandate. Both were instrumental in helping to defeat the Clinton health plan. Republicans and economic conservatives generally oppose government mandates, and they avoid alienating small business, a usual source of support for the Republican Party. In contrast, large businesses, which already provide health benefits, often support a mandate to "level the playing field."

Economists generally agree that, in the long run, employees—not employers—pay for a mandate out of their wages. They claim the market for wages is based on total compensation, and workers who receive health benefits eventually earn that much less in salary than those with no benefits. However, they also recognize that those earning close to the minimum wage cannot be paid less and, in their cases, the cost of a mandate is borne by employers. This has the potential to reduce employment of low-wage workers. For that reason, low-wage industries and small firms are often exempted from employer mandates. Small businesses take little comfort when they are told not to worry because wages will adjust over the long run. They sometimes repeat John Maynard Keynes's reminder that "in the long run we're all dead."

Nevertheless, there are good reasons why an employer mandate remains the core of every universal plan. Most importantly, employer benefits are "off budget." The alternative is raising taxes, something extremely unattractive to politicians and taxpayers. Richard Nixon was not going to raise income or payroll taxes to pay for his health plan. Employer mandates also sustain the private health insurance industry. If the government provided everyone's insurance, the industry and its jobs would disappear or, at best, function simply as a fiscal intermediary administering claims for the government. Although some would be happy to see the health insurance industry disappear, others fear a government-run system even more.

Except for small firms, employment-based insurance incurs low administrative costs and spreads insurance risk effectively. People choose jobs for many reasons, but their health condition is rarely one of them. Hence, when a company insures its workers, there is likely to be a balance of good and bad health risks, and the resulting premiums are cost effective. That explains why a company has to offer insurance to all its workers and not just some. If only the sickest workers received benefits, insurance would not work—just as a casualty insurance company could not stay in business if it only insured houses next to the ocean. It also explains why small businesses—in which one or two unhealthy employees can change the average risk profile—often have to pay very high insurance premiums. For that reason, many employer mandate plans exempt very small firms.

## The Individual Mandate

There is an important difference between plans offering universal access and those offering universal coverage. The government can mandate that employers offer everyone health insurance for a price—even an affordable price—but many people will still not choose to purchase it. This presents two problems. First, those who choose not to purchase insurance may become "free riders." When they become ill, they go to hospitals for treatment. Hospitals are obligated to provide care to anyone who walks through their doors but often are not paid by those who lack insurance. Consequently, those of us who are not free riders pay for that care in the form of higher insurance premiums. The second problem is more subtle. It makes sense for the sickest people to choose the most insurance. After all, if you live in a flood plain you're apt to choose a policy with good flood insurance. But, if insurance companies only insure those who are likely to be flooded, insurance doesn't work. The same is true of health insurance. If everyone is insured, the risks are spread and insurance premiums are more cost effective. Hence, the question arises, should you not only offer everyone health insurance but mandate that everyone purchase it (as we do for auto insurance).

The Nixon administration was philosophically conservative and decided it did not want government to force people to buy health insurance. Economics and politics often clash.

## The Benefit Package

If you require employers and/or government to offer insurance, you have to specify a set of minimum benefits that qualifies as a genuine offer. If the package is comprehensive, it will also be expensive and require substantial taxes to cover the cost. Conversely, if the benefit package is narrow, people with low incomes may not be able to afford needed services that are not covered. In today's environment, every provider group lobbies the government to provide expanded benefits for its particular product or service. Pressure often comes from trade associations representing such specialties as chiropractic, acupuncture, vision, and hearing. It then becomes politically difficult to limit the size and nature of the benefit package. The scope of the benefit package is generally tied to the amount of cost sharing that individuals must assume.

## Cost Sharing

Cost sharing refers to the amount insured individuals must pay for medical services in addition to their annual insurance premiums. These additional expenses are usually in the form of deductibles, copayments, or coinsurance. As in the case of the benefit package, there is a tension between providing too much or too little. If you provide everyone with total coverage for everything (often called "first-dollar insurance"), they will demand excessive amounts of services. Why not? They don't have to pay anything. However, if they are subject to extensive cost sharing, they are likely to limit the use of preventive or other needed care, which could lead to more complicated illnesses at a later date.

The problem is finding the middle ground.

Both the deductibles and the coinsurance start low and increase with income. Today, cost sharing does not vary with income, and copayments are generally modest (often ten to twenty dollars). On the other hand, coinsurance, a percentage of the total bill, can be very expensive. The coinsurance requirements in Nixon's plan were relatively large by today's standards, but because of the protection afforded by the plan's maximum annual ceiling, the

Table 1.1
Proposed Cost Sharing Under the Comprehensive Health Insurance Plan

| Class | Annual Income | Annual Premium | Annual Per Person Deductible | Coinsurance Above Deductible | Maximum Annual Cost Sharing |
|-------|---------------|----------------|------------------------------|------------------------------|------------------------------|
| I.    | $    0 – 2,499 | $  0 | $  0 | 10% | 3% of Income |
| II.   | 2,500 – 4,999  | 0    | 50   | 15  | 6% of Income |
| III.  | 5,000 – 7,499  | 300  | 100  | 20  | 10% of Income |
| IV.   | 7,500 – 9,999  | 600  | 150  | 25  | 15% of Income |
| V.    | 10,000 - +     | 900  | 150  | 25  | $1,500.00 |

Source: Memorandum from Stuart Altman and Peter Fox to Casper Weinberger dated October 11, 1973.

cost sharing amounts could never exceed 15 percent of family (or individual) income.

Catastrophic insurance is an alternative to comprehensive benefits. It insures against very high medical expenses, but requires the consumer to pay for ordinary services. During Nixon's presidency, Senator Long proposed universal catastrophic insurance. Under his plan, no citizen would ever have to spend more than two thousand per year for health care expenses. Once he or she exceeded that amount, the government would pay the balance. Long's proposal was universal and was to be financed by increasing the social security tax. Catastrophic insurance, like fire insurance, is very efficient. Everyone has fire insurance, but only a very small proportion of homes burn down, so insurance is relatively inexpensive, but people are protected against a loss they cannot afford. Catastrophic health insurance protects people against the unaffordable cost of a serious illness, but they remain cost conscious about lesser medical expenses for which they have to pay.

The problem with catastrophic insurance occurs when individuals at the lower end of the income scale forego preventive services and necessary care, while richer people are apt to purchase supplementary insurance to fill in the gaps. The Nixon administration decided to have generous benefits, high cost sharing, and catastrophic protection. Altman's team wrote, "A fundamental principle that we have followed is that higher cost sharing with more comprehensive benefits is preferable to narrower coverage with lower cost sharing."[22]

## Subsidizing the Poor

Every proposal for universal insurance must provide subsidies for people who cannot afford insurance premiums. This is particularly important if there is an individual mandate. If subsidies are too small, insurance will be unaffordable or too burdensome. If subsidies are too large, many individuals and firms who might have stayed in the private market will take advantage of the public subsidy. In addition, generous subsidies can be a disincentive to work, because those who increase their income above the qualifying amount may become ineligible for the subsidy. Hence, in virtually all plans, subsidies are gradually phased out as income rises to minimize the disincentives.

A related issue is whether to provide categorical subsidies or universal subsidies. Categorical subsidies require you to fall within a specified group in order to qualify. Until the Obama plan, the Medicaid program provided categorical subsidies that varied by state. For example, in Alabama, only families with children could receive benefits, provided they met the designated income requirements (except for special cases such as blindness, disability, etc.). In Connecticut, childless adults who met the income requirement could still qualify for a limited benefit package. The 1971 Nixon plan did not provide benefits to unmarried individuals, childless couples, or unemployed people without children. The Altman team's CHIP proposal was much more inclusive. It was available to everyone except families earning over $7,500 who were offered insurance by their employers. Indeed, it would be generous by today's standards.

## Tax Deductible Health Benefits

Every universal plan has to subsidize premiums for low-income citizens, and it has to have a source of funds to cover the cost. Since 1943, the cost of health benefits has been a deductible expense for businesses and has been nontaxable income for workers. In 2008, the tax exclusion for health benefits cost the government $226 billion.[23] Every administration that has proposed universal coverage has considered using that attractive pot of money. In the Nixon administration, Casper Weinberger and the Council of Economic Advisers recommended ending the tax exclusion, but Nixon refused.

Health economists do not like the tax exclusion. It encourages employers to provide, and employees to purchase, more extensive coverage than they would otherwise demand (particularly first-dollar coverage). This reduces cost-conscious behavior and often results in people demanding more services than they need because they do not have to pay. Economists call such behavior *moral hazard*. The exclusion is also a regressive tax—it provides the most benefit to those with higher incomes. On average, higher income people receive more from the tax exclusion because they have coverage that is more expensive. In addition, the higher the income tax bracket, the more the tax deduction is worth. The uninsured and those not earning enough money to pay taxes derive no benefit at all.

Despite the fact that there are good economic reasons to end the exclusion, there are good political reasons not to. First, people do not like to lose any benefit they already have. Second, unions that have negotiated generous benefits in collective bargaining do not want to give the value of those benefits away, particularly if they have sacrificed wages to obtain them. A third reason is one that makes all financing for universal health care difficult: the 85 percent of the population that already has health benefits does not want to increase their taxes for the 15 percent of the population that is uninsured. The politically astute Richard Nixon, who frequently appealed to "the great silent majority," promised that he would not raise anyone's taxes to pay for his national health program. He would not be the last president to make that promise.

## The Comprehensive Health Insurance Program (CHIP)

The CHIP proposal, put together by Stuart Altman and Peter Fox under the direction of Casper Weinberger, was a comprehensive proposal. It remains a standard that has been used to measure subsequent attempts at universal coverage. Nixon introduced the program in a written message to Congress dated February 6, 1974. He described his program in much the same way as other presidents who would follow him: universal, comprehensive, and affordable health insurance that builds on the strength of existing public and private systems. He assured the Congress that citizens would still be able to choose their own doctor and he reassured everyone that no new taxes would be required. Eerily foreshadowing Bill Clinton, he wrote, "Every American who participates in the program will receive a health security card...honored by hospitals, nursing homes, emergency rooms, doctors, and clinics across the country."

An outline of the program is as follows:

1. Employer Mandate: All employers had to offer health insurance to their full-time employees. They had to pay a minimum of 65 percent of the premiums during the first three years and 75 percent thereafter. There would be transitional aid for small and low-wage employers.

2. Comprehensive Benefit Package: The benefit package included hospital expenses, doctor inpatient and outpatient, prescription drugs, lab tests and x-rays, medical devices, ambulance services, and other ancillary care. It had limited coverage for mental health services, alcohol and drug addiction, nursing home and home health care. For children, it included preventive care to age six and vision, hearing, and dental treatment to age thirteen. Exclusions for preexisting conditions were not allowed.

3. Government Subsidized Coverage (the Assisted Health Insurance Plan–AHIP): Every citizen not covered by employers or Medicare was eligible for AHIP. This included people who were unemployed, self-employed, disabled, low-income, or high-risk. There were no categorical exclusions. Premiums were free for any family earning less than five thousand dollars and were phased out as income increased. It replaced Medicaid for most services and had uniform national federal benefits and eligibility requirements. As previously discussed, the plan included substantial cost sharing by today's standards (see table 1 on page 51), but also had an annual catastrophic maximum expense of fifteen hundred dollars per family so that no citizen would ever have to pay more than 15 percent of his or her income in any year.

4. Regulation: The plan recommended continued wage and price controls for medical care (which Nixon instituted in 1971). It required employers to offer an HMO option, provided one was available. It created Professional Standards Review Organizations (PSROs) to review utilization and quality of services, Certificates of Need (CON) to obtain permission to build new facilities, and state oversight of insurers and providers to assure fair practices and prices. It also recommended prospective reimbursement for hospitals.[24]

Nixon described the plan as one that would preserve private enterprise and not "place the entire health care system under the dominion of social planners in Washington."[25] Yet the plan included a menu of regulatory provisions that arguably represented the most extensive government intervention in the nation's health system before or since. We examine Nixon's policies on regulation and cost control in chapter 9.

## Alcohol, Sex, and Burglary: Health Reform Fails Again

Nixon thought his administration had created a centrist plan that could be enacted by the Ninety-Third Congress. It was more conservative than Kennedy's bill that called for a single-payer system financed through general revenues. Yet it had conservative appeal because it retained private insurance, individual choice of doctors and hospitals, and required no new taxes. Although the bill expanded the role of government, its conservative opponents could not resurrect their traditional cries of socialized medicine because the author of the bill was Richard Nixon, a certified anticommunist.

In February 1974, Wilbur Mills and Bob Packwood (R-OR) agreed to cosponsor the bill. Although there was little organized opposition, there was not much support. Liberals, labor, and nonsouthern Democrats supported Kennedy. Many Republicans wondered why the Nixon administration was advancing such an expansive proposal.

Kennedy realized he could not get a bill through Congress that eliminated private insurance companies. Fearing he would be left out, he began again to meet secretly with Wilbur Mills. Kennedy was willing to compromise, but he wanted to keep the support of big labor, so he invited leaders of the large unions to a private meeting in his Senate office. Kennedy aides Paul Kirk and Stan Jones attended the meeting, and Jones walked them through a written summary of the compromise proposal. The union leaders adamantly opposed the compromise. They told Kennedy if he went through with it, "they would call him a traitor all over the country."[26]

Kennedy was flabbergasted because the only significant thing he was giving up from his single-payer proposal was a continued but reduced role for insurance companies. Kennedy explained to them that the votes simply were not there for single-payer. He took out a congressional directory and went through the names of senators who would oppose single-payer. "What are you going to do about him?" he asked rhetorically. "Is he going to be back [after the 1976 election]? The election isn't going to change anything. This is the best deal you guys are ever going to get."[27]

The union leaders were furious. They sat in stone-faced silence until Kennedy stood up and said, "Well, you're just going to have to call me a traitor."[28] Kennedy opened the back door of the office and the union leaders filed out.

Surprising nearly everyone, Kennedy and Mills announced their bill on April second. It was a single-payer health insurance system supported by an employer mandate. Unlike Nixon's bill, however, the Social Security Administration would collect the employment-based payments and would negotiate directly with insurance companies as a single-payer. Private insurers could still offer supplemental (gap) insurance to cover coinsurance and deductibles, and they would act as fiscal intermediaries, administering the claims and payments between the government and medical providers. Significantly, employee payments would vary by income, the higher earners paying a higher percentage of their incomes. Kennedy agreed to the substantial cost sharing in Nixon's plan—anathema to his liberal supporters—but his catastrophic provision reduced the out-of-pocket maximum annual expense from fifteen hundred dollars to one thousand dollars per family. It was an early example of Kennedy's ability to forge health care compromises with his opponents, something he proved better able to do than any other legislator of his generation.

Not surprisingly, the Kennedy–Mills proposal was attacked from both the Left and Right. The AMA immediately labeled it a socialized plan, and the NFIB said it was the first step toward socialized medicine.[29] The AFL-CIO would not accept the continued role of private insurance companies or the large copayments and deductibles. Labeling the proposal a sellout of its principles, it opposed the plan and decided to wait for the next election. Nevertheless, Kennedy–Mills was a true compromise. It convinced many observers that national health insurance was going to happen in the Ninety-Third Congress, and only the specific details needed to be hammered out. Most importantly, it persuaded the Nixon administration that a compromise solution was possible, and thus laid the groundwork for future negotiations.

In retrospect, it appears the big unions cared little about universal health care. At the time they were powerful organizations, and they had extracted generous health benefits from America's large industries. Their workers would be no better off, and might be worse off, as a result of national health reform. Hence, they took the position that they wanted everything or nothing, knowing all along that everything was not possible. Stan Jones says, "They kicked the legs out of health reform."[30]

Important as Kennedy was personally, the power in the Senate over health care legislation resided in the Senate Finance Committee. The committee chairman, Russell Long, was the Democratic senator from Louisiana. He was an expert on taxation and was cautious about spending. Long exercised so much power in the Senate that the *Wall Street Journal* once referred to him as "the fourth branch of government."[31]

Long had proposed his catastrophic plan, as mentioned earlier. His former aide James Mongan recalls Long's reaction to Kennedy's bill. "Kennedy talks about this huge thing. It will break the bank. It'll bust the budget—it's bullshit, basically."[32] One might note that in 1969, Kennedy had ousted Long from the powerful position of party whip.

Mongan, and Long's powerful aide Jay Constantine, realized that a catastrophic proposal would do little for the poor and would never gain any traction. "How are they going to pay the first two thousand dollars?" they asked. Together, they drafted a proposal that combined catastrophic insurance with a federalized Medicaid program. They convinced Long and Abraham Ribicoff (the Republican senator from Connecticut who succeeded Prescott Bush) to support the proposal, and it became the Long–Ribicoff bill. Constantine was so convinced of Finance Committee support for his bill that he never took Nixon's effort seriously. Mongan recalls him saying, "It's all bullshit. It's only going to be Long–Ribicoff. We got the votes in committee, and we know what's going to happen."[33]

By late in the spring of 1974, optimism about health reform was in the air. It seemed nearly everyone wanted national health care, but similar to the 1971 effort, everyone was still supporting their own bills. That was when Stuart Altman found himself on a chairlift in Albuquerque, New Mexico, with Kennedy's aide Stan Jones. Altman and Jones were attending a meeting of the National Governors Association. With some spare time away from the indoor sessions and long, political speeches, they decided to take a ski lift to the top of Sandia Peak. Gazing out from the spiritual setting high above the forested hills, with the city of Albuquerque spread out in the distance, the two men thought they solved the problem of bringing universal health care to America.

Altman and Jones's idea was to bring Kennedy's, Nixon's, and Mills's people together and craft a compromise between Nixon's CHIP proposal and Kennedy–Mills. Upon returning to Washington, they got all three principals to agree to a meeting. There was just one problem: neither the Nixon administration nor the Kennedy people wanted their constituents to know that they were willing to compromise further with the other side. After all, both had gone out on a political limb trying to enact national health care. Kennedy had courageously gone against his longtime base of organized labor. Labor leaders had already expressed their opposition to Kennedy–Mills and would be furious if they thought Kennedy was open to further compromise. Nixon had confounded members of his own cabinet, as well as his Council of Economic Advisors, by proposing the CHIP plan. Already appearing weak because of Watergate, he was not anxious to be seen compromising with Kennedy. And so Stan Jones went to see his pastor at Saint Mark's to arrange the secret meetings in the church's basement.

It would make a good ending to the story if the secret church meetings in June resulted in a successful compromise, but it was not to be. The Nixon administration needed Kennedy to support an employer mandate in which employers purchased coverage from private insurance companies. Kennedy had already been told by the unions that "they were ready to dump him because he had moved so far to the right on health insurance;" and he just couldn't do it.[34] Neither side felt they could agree to the concessions necessary to make a deal. Years later, "asked about his greatest regret as a legislator, Ted Kennedy would usually cite his refusal to cut a deal with Richard Nixon on health care."[35]

In June and early July there was much action but little progress. A retrospective editorial in the *New York Times* on August 23 summarized the situation: "Organized labor's 'all or nothing' position has been as directly responsible for scuttling an effective compromise as have the opposite pressures of the conservative medical societies and those bent on keeping the private insurance sector in virtually complete control. As long as Congress permits itself to remain the prisoner of these warring extremes, the nation will be deprived of adequate and humane protection."[36]

Thirty-five years later, the Obama administration's political difficulties were eerily familiar. In 2009, liberals threatened to oppose health reform if there was no "public insurance option." Conservatives were unwilling to support any measure that increased the role of government, even if such increased role was confined to mandating private insurance.

By the middle of July, the Nixon administration was in disarray because of Watergate. On July 16, Alexander Butterfield, a former Nixon aide and another UCLA classmate of Bob Haldeman, testified before the Senate Watergate Committee and revealed that all of Nixon's conversations in the Oval Office had been secretly tape-recorded. Nixon refused to turn over the tapes, claiming executive privilege. However, on July 24, the Supreme Court ruled against him, and recordings that incriminated the president in the Watergate cover-up were released to the public. Nixon resigned on August 8, and Gerald Ford became the thirty-eighth US president.

Ford had never been a supporter of health reform, having voted against the Medicare program in 1965. However, the administration needed to show it could move beyond Watergate, and Melvin Laird, a close advisor to Ford, urged him to support national health care reform.[37] In his first speech to a joint session of Congress on August 12, Ford stated that national health care was one of his two top legislative goals.

Meanwhile, as Nixon was struggling through his final days, Wilbur Mills had decided to fashion his own compromise. Perhaps he was trying to repeat his greatest legislative success in 1965 when he was able to secure passage of Lyndon Johnson's Medicare program by proposing his "three-layer cake strategy" (a story we recount in a later chapter). He had directed his aide Bill Fullerton to craft a compromise weaving together the important elements of CHIP, Kennedy–Mills, and Long–Ribicoff. Fullerton had been working behind the scenes with Altman as the Watergate crisis came to a head. After Ford's address to Congress, Mills told Fullerton to finish the health plan "over the weekend."[38] Fullerton, in consultation with Altman, put together what became known as "the Committee Print."

The compromise was much closer to CHIP than Kennedy–Mills. It included Nixon's employer mandate and retained the role of private insurance. The benefit package was similar to Nixon's, but cost sharing requirements were eased. The one specific instruction Mills gave to Fullerton was to include catastrophic protection that would be financed through a payroll tax. That requirement was not ideological. Payroll tax financing, which had been used to fund the social security program, allowed Mills's Ways and Means Committee to retain jurisdiction.

President Ford supported the compromise, and Mills was initially optimistic he could get the bill through his committee. Throughout his long tenure as committee chair, Mills refused to report out major legislation unless his committee gave him a clear majority. Ways and Means began debating provisions of the Committee Print on August 20, but Mills found himself with only a 12–11 majority. The southern Democrats and all but three Republicans were opposed. The next day, on August 21, the committee voted on financing provisions. Lobbyists for the AMA floated a proposal to replace the employer mandate and payroll tax funding with tax incentives to buy insurance, a provision that would have destroyed any chance of a deal. When Mills could only defeat their measure by one vote, he adjourned the meeting. Mills had a vicious exchange with William Green (D-PA), and angrily told the liberal Democrats that this was the best they were going to get. He castigated Republicans for not supporting their own proposal. He told them he would bring the bill back after the summer recess, and they should think hard before opposing their president.

But the bill was never brought back. On October 8, Mills was found drunk in his car with a local stripper named Fannie Fox. Hoping to avoid scandal, Ms. Fox ran from the car and jumped into the Washington tidal basin, forever giving her the nickname, the "Tidal Basin Bombshell." Mills managed to be reelected in November, but in December he was seen again with Fox who was performing in a Boston strip joint. With his alcoholism public and his stature diminished, Mills's power evaporated, and he eventually retired from Congress in 1976.

The failure to enact national health reform was summarized in a *New York Times* article on August 27. The headline read, A LEGISLATIVE GOAL THAT HAS NO FOES STALLED BY DIFFERENCES IN APPROACH.[39] The article went on to say, "National Health Insurance doesn't seem to have an enemy in town. The president, all Congressional leaders of both parties, most Senators and Representatives, and nearly every special interest group, whether conservative or liberal, support the concept."[40] The problem was that everyone still supported his or her own concept. At least fourteen bills had been filed, and they varied enormously. Labor supported a one-hundred-billion-dollars-a-year federal program that would pay for nearly everything. Organized medicine supported a bill in which out-of-pocket costs for individuals would quadruple. Some wanted the federal government to become the single-payer and collect premiums through social security taxes. Others wanted to preserve the private insurance market. No less than thirteen of the twenty-five members of the Ways and Means Committee were sponsors of their own bills. Mills himself had cosponsored Nixon's CHIP proposal before meeting with Kennedy and sponsoring Kennedy–Mills. The failure of Nixon's health reform again illustrates Altman's Law.

Many of the same issues that made health reform difficult to enact in the '70s would reappear in the Clinton administration in the '90s and in the Obama administration in 2009. Despite the flexibility of their leaders, the extreme wings and special interests of both parties held fast to their ideological positions. Nixon, despite his public posturing, was above-all a pragmatist. For Kennedy, even though he was a committed liberal, the plight of the uninsured always trumped ideology. For a brief instant, it appeared that the center might hold and the major political players could finally overcome the opposition from both extremes. But Nixon resigned because of Watergate. Kennedy was weakened from the Kopechne affair. Mills was disgraced by the Fannie Fox incidents. President Ford's overriding domestic concern was not health reform but inflation. As a policy solution, he told members of his administration to wear WIN buttons—an acronym for "Whip Inflation Now." Stuart Altman's attempt to find a compromise solution faded into obscurity, and he left government to return to academia, eventually becoming dean of the Heller School for Social Policy at Brandeis University. There would not be another significant attempt at national health reform until Bill Clinton, more than twenty years later.

# CHAPTER 2

# CLINTON CHOOSES WRONG
## THE COLOSSAL DEFEAT
## OF MANAGED COMPETITION

### The Fateful Decision

"**I**t was as if some alien force propelled my hand in the air. It was certainly against my better judgment," Stuart Altman recalls, "but before I could retract my arm, the president-elect had noticed."

"Yes, Stuart?" Bill Clinton asked, and Altman's brief tenure on the Clinton health team was about to come to an end.

It was January 11, 1993, and people were seated two-deep around the long table in the basement of the Little Rock Governor's Mansion. Hillary was sitting next to Bill. Al Gore, George Stephanopoulos, Bob Rubin, Ira Magaziner, and other members of the Clinton transition team were on hand. Ken Thorpe was presenting the budget for the health care plan hammered together by the Health Policy Group, and Judy Feder, the group's director, was worried. The cost of the proposal was $270 billion over the first five years,[1] and she knew that Clinton was deeply concerned about balancing the budget. Furthermore, the health transition team was on shaky ground. Rumors had been circulating that Ira Magaziner, a close friend of the Clintons, was secretly formulating an alternative proposal. Magaziner favored "managed competition," a more complex and less traditional approach than the Feder group's proposal. Altman had previously asked Feder to find out if the rumors were true, but Magaziner denied them. The night before the meeting, Feder had confided her worries to Jay Rockefeller, the Democratic senator from West Virginia. Rockefeller advised her to be honest about the cost projections. "Of course, I was wrong," Rockefeller later told Haynes Johnson and David Broder.[2] "She got crushed. They were furious at her. Clinton personally was furious at her because he couldn't do what he wanted."[3] Indeed, when Ken Thorpe presented the budget numbers, Bill Clinton was distressed. The overriding theme of his successful presidential campaign was that "it's the economy, stupid," and that remained his chief concern. How was he going to balance the budget if he had to spend $270 billion on health care?

The answer he wanted to hear came from David Cutler. Cutler was a young economist on leave from Harvard who was a member of the economics transition team. He was enthusiastic about the potential of managed competition to control health costs and had been working with Ira Magaziner. Cutler argued that the transition team was thinking too traditionally. He told the president-elect that there was an alternative way to accomplish everything he wanted without any additional cost. That was when Stuart raised his hand. "I understand their plan," Altman said, "and it is a radical departure. It would necessitate a major restructuring of the entire health care system."

"All of it?" Hillary Clinton asked.

"Yes, a total restructuring. Everyone would have to change the way they choose their doctors and hospitals. I don't think the country is willing to undergo that amount of change."

Some historians have called the January 11 meeting disastrous.[4] It certainly ended in disagreement. Bill Clinton finally wound up the meeting and assured the group that they would work it out back in Washington. As they prepared to leave, Clinton put his arm around Stuart Altman. "You're a great American," the president-elect told him, but unbeknownst to Stuart, his role in the Clinton administration had just ended.

As Stuart and the transition team members waited outside in the van to return to the airport, other insiders stayed behind to talk. It may have been at that moment that Clinton finalized the fateful decision to go with Ira Magaziner, Hillary, and managed competition. Most historians think the unofficial decision was made well before, and there are indications as early as December that, despite his denials, Ira knew he was going to be the policy director for the health reform effort.[5] Even Judy Feder, in retrospect, believes that the transition team was just a placeholder for Ira and the first lady.[6]

Two weeks later, on January 25, President Clinton publicly announced his Health Policy Task Force led by Hillary Clinton and Ira Magaziner. Altman thought about the past two months and his life on the transition team. "It was the most all-consuming effort I've ever experienced. There was this brand new office building on Twelfth Street that was still empty. We literally occupied it, cramming in desks, furniture, and phones wherever we could fit them. I shared this crowded space with three other people, and it was a zoo. All day there was a constant stream of stakeholders and constituent groups that wanted to influence the process. We would start at 8:00 a.m. and meet with these people all day, and then we would have to write our reports at night. Staffers brought in sandwiches and pizza, so we rarely left the building. It was like the outside world didn't exist, and, after a while, you began to think that the whole world revolved around your little group. I made a habit of leaving at midnight and going back to my hotel, but many people worked through the night."

He had taken a two-month leave from Brandeis University, hoping to help enact a health plan that would insure every American—the same goal he failed to achieve twenty years earlier under Richard Nixon. Altman believed that the best strategy to pass universal coverage was to build on the current system; to minimize the amount of change and reduce the numbers of winners and losers who would lobby against each other. He and the rest of the team had been led to believe that the president felt likewise, and they were giving him what he wanted. Despite their efforts, however, Clinton made the critical decision to embrace managed competition, a choice that would lead to widespread opposition and near certain failure. To understand why, and what implications it has for current policy, we must first go back to 1990 and the campaign of Harris Wofford.

## The Wofford Campaign—
## Health Care Reform Takes Center Stage

"If a criminal has the right to a lawyer, I think working Americans should have the right to a doctor."[7] With that phrase as his campaign theme, Harris Wofford managed one of the greatest upsets in recent political history. It is hard to imagine a less likely scenario than the Pennsylvania Senate election in 1990 in which Wofford defeated Dick Thornburgh.

Everyone assumed Thornburgh would win. He had been a popular two-term governor who was first elected in 1978 and then reelected after shepherding Pennsylvanians through the Three Mile Island nuclear disaster. Interestingly, Thornburgh won the 1978 Republican primary against Arlen

Specter. Specter had originally been a Democrat, but decided his electoral chances would improve if he switched parties; a strategy he would repeat over thirty years later in 2009. After his two terms as governor, Thornburgh served as US attorney general under Presidents Reagan and Bush, resigning in 1991 to run against Wofford. With 100 percent name recognition and notoriety as a cabinet officer, no one gave Thornburgh's opponent a chance.

Why would they? Wofford was appointed to the Senate just six months earlier when the popular Republican senator John Heinz was killed in a plane crash. Pennsylvania governor Bill Casey wanted to appoint Lee Iacocca, former chairman of Chrysler, to fill the job, but Iacocca declined. The soft-spoken Wofford, cofounder of the Peace Corps and former president of Bryn Mawr College, was an unlikely candidate. Mary McGrory once described him as "a disciple of Gandhi and Martin Luther King [Jr.] who was too liberal for the Kennedy White House."[8] It had been thirty years since Pennsylvania elected a Democrat to the Senate, and Wofford began the campaign forty-five points down in the polls, a seemingly insurmountable deficit.

Nevertheless, the economy was in the midst of a severe recession, and people were losing their jobs and their health care. Wofford hammered away at the health care issue, and it resonated with worried Pennsylvanians. In a stunning upset, he carried the state by ten percentage points. The national media touted health care as the emerging issue in the upcoming presidential campaign, as if they just discovered the problems of rising health costs and the number of uninsured. But they hadn't. The underlying problems in the US health care system had been percolating for years, just below the boiling point. The Pennsylvania election may have crystallized the issue for the news media, but the Wofford campaign was merely the result, and not the cause, of a ragingly expensive health care system that was becoming unsustainable.

What had changed to propel health care to the top of the policy agenda? After all, the two underlying problems in the American health care system in 1990 were the same ones that existed under Nixon in 1973 and still confronted Obama in 2009. It cost too much and was too hard for many people to get. By the time Clinton was elected, a decade of rising costs and a weakening economy was bringing pressure to bear on all sectors of the economy: consumers, business, and government.

## Consumers

Consumers felt rising health care costs where it hurt the most: right in the pocketbook. National health expenditures rose from $253 billion in 1980 to $714 billion in 1990, an annual rate of increase of almost 11 percent.[9] In personal terms, the average American spent $1,100 on health in 1980 and $2,814 in 1990.[10] In the second half of the '80s, when the economy was strong, anxiety about health costs remained just under the surface. As the country entered a steep recession in 1991, that was no longer the case.

In 1991, the US economy grew at only 1.9 percent (adjusted for inflation), and in 1992 it actually declined by .2 percent.[11] As the economy turned down, Americans began losing their jobs. Unemployment rose from 5.6 percent in 1990 to 6.8 percent in 1991 and to 7.5 percent in 1992.[12] The unemployment rate would not reach those levels again until the Obama administration in 2009.

In 1990, 72.2 percent of working-age Americans received their health insurance from employers. As people lost their jobs, they also lost their health insurance. By 1992, 17.8 percent, or more than one in six, working-age Americans were uninsured.[13] Unlike previous cycles, the recession of '91 did not only affect the poor. Among working age people earning 200–399 percent of the federal poverty level, 14 percent had no health insurance in 1992.[14]

Harris Wofford's remarkable victory crystallized what many Americans already knew about health insurance. Those that didn't have any couldn't afford it, and those that did were afraid they were going to lose it. And this time, consumers were not alone. Business and government had finally reached the point where they agreed something had to be done.

## Business

Traditionally, American business had opposed comprehensive health reform. Many feared government mandates, and they were reluctant to support universal coverage if they were going to be the ones burdened with the cost. Nevertheless, by 1990, rising health costs were a major concern for many firms. The rising cost of health benefits for current workers was reducing company profits. When firms tried to pass the increased costs on to employees, either through smaller wage increases or reduced benefits, they faced pitched battles with unions, sometimes resulting in strikes. The problem was compounded for traditional American manufacturers such as the automobile and steel industries. They had granted generous retiree health benefits when they dominated their markets at a time when there was little foreign competition. Most of their benefits to retired workers were unfunded, and they had huge obligations coming due.[15] Congressional testimony from leaders of the American automobile industry in May 1989 typified industry concerns and was an early warning of the financial meltdown these companies would face twenty years later. Lee Iacocca, the chairman of Chrysler, testified that the company's health care spending rose from $432 million in 1985 to $702 million in 1988.[16] That amounted to $700 per vehicle, double the health care expense incurred by French and German manufacturers and triple that of Japan.[17] Iacocca stated, "American industry cannot compete effectively with the rest of the world unless something is done about the great imbalance between health care costs in the United States and national health care systems in almost every other country. That is why a national health insurance program is being discussed widely for the first time since the late '70s."[18] Perhaps Iacocca would not have declined the opportunity to run for Wofford's seat if he had realized how well his concerns would resonate.

## Government

Government was also suffering the effects of rising health costs. Federal and State governments provided approximately 40 percent of national health expenditures. This was up from about 25 percent before Medicare and Medicaid were enacted. With public sector health costs increasing over 11 percent a year in 1989 and 1990, the system was placing a huge burden on federal and state budgets. There was a general consensus in government that something had to be done.

What distinguished the health care debate at the beginning of 1992 was that all three sectors of the economy—consumers, business, and government—appeared to be on the same page. Everyone seemed to agree that comprehensive reform was needed.

## Bill Clinton and Managed Competition

Bill Clinton no doubt had his shortcomings, but most would agree that he was politically astute. He quickly seized on the health care issue, making it a fixture in his stump speeches. After all, health care reform was quintessentially a Democratic Party issue, and President Bush was paying it scant attention in his own reelection campaign. Not coincidentally, Clinton hired James Carville and Paul Begala, the masterminds of Wofford's victory, to direct his own campaign strategy. After engineering Clinton's victory, Carville was voted campaign manager of the year by the American Association of Political Consultants. Aside from his marriage to the archconservative strategist Mary Matalin, he is best known for his phrase, "It's the economy, stupid." Most people do not realize the phrase originated in the Wofford campaign. Instead, they attribute it to the now-famous memo Carville tacked to the wall of the Clinton "war room:"[19]

1. Change vs. more of the same.
2. The economy, stupid.
3. Don't forget health care.

At the beginning of the campaign Clinton appeared to have three choices for reforming the US health care system: single-payer, play-or-pay, or tax credits.[20] Each had its advantages and shortcomings.

### Single-payer

In a universal single-payer system, one single entity (the government) pays for all covered health care expenses for all its citizens. The Medicare program is a single-payer system for people sixty-five years of age and older. Hence, a universal single-payer system is like Medicare for everyone. The system is financed by taxation, likely a payroll tax similar to Medicare and Social Security. Everyone can choose his or her own doctor or hospital, and the government pays for all covered services, just as in Medicare. The financing is straightforward and administrative costs are low, as they are in Medicare.

Opponents often deride single-payer as government-run health care. This is not an accurate description. It is government *financed* health care, but all of the players—doctors, nurses, hospitals, drug companies, medical device companies, and so on—remain private. Only the insurance companies are forced out of the private market or left with a much-diminished role. Yet, this is the key point for supporters. Administrative costs of private insurance (including marketing) can comprise about 30 percent of premiums. A single-payer system could save billions of dollars in administrative expense.

Although a single-payer appears to be simple and attractive on the surface, it presents several problems that need to be overcome. In order to pay for everyone's insurance, a payroll tax of roughly 7 to 10 percent is necessary, depending on the breadth of coverage. In recent times, a tax increase of that magnitude has been politically impossible.

In addition, there is no cost or budgetary control if the government simply pays what providers bill. Hence, single-payer systems need to administer (i.e., fix) prices in order to control costs (all Medicare prices are fixed except for prescription drugs). Administered pricing systems can successfully control costs, but they are complex and bureaucratic. For example, the cost of providing medical services varies across different regions of the country. The government has to pay providers more in higher cost areas and less where costs are low. However, the process of adjusting rates is both complicated and controversial, and political power often bears on decision making. In the case of Medicare reimbursement, there are often political disagreements about rate setting differentials in urban versus rural areas. Furthermore, political power often plays a role in deciding what services are reimbursed. Those who favor free markets oppose single-payer systems, preferring the market—not government—to set prices. Doctors, hospitals, and other medical providers often oppose single-payer because their incomes becomes dependent on government-set prices. Currently hospitals are paid less than their costs by Medicare, and they have to make up the difference by charging much higher rates to private payers (a practice known as *cost shifting*). Another serious problem is that single-payer largely replaces private insurance companies. Hence, the health insurance industry would be virtually wiped out, and most of its employees would lose their jobs.

### Play-or-Pay

In a play-or-pay system, universal health care is financed by an employer mandate. Employers must either provide a minimum package of health insurance to their workers or pay into a public fund that will purchase or provide insurance. It is the least disruptive type of universal reform because it builds on the current, employment-based system. One hundred and fifty-six million Americans received health insurance from their employers in 2009.[21] Play-or-pay does not alter the way most people already get insurance or choose their doctors. Opposition comes chiefly from small and low-wage businesses. Although nearly all large companies already provide health benefits to their workers, many small and low-wage businesses do not. Hence, for them, play-or-pay represents a new and costly mandate, and it could cause them to hire fewer employees. They also fear that the initial cost might increase over time. Despite the fact that most play-or-pay proposals include a protective cap on small business contributions (usually about 7 to 10 percent of payroll), many small firms fear that once the system is established, the government could raise the cap in the future. In their basic form, play or pay systems do little to control cost. Hence, some proposals include government-administered prices, a global budget, or both. Similar to single-payer, such government control is anathema to those who advocate competitive markets.

## Tax Incentive Plans

Tax incentive plans reduce the number of uninsured by providing tax credits or vouchers to make private health insurance more affordable. These plans are often combined with insurance market reforms that, on the margin, make health insurance easier and less expensive to purchase, especially in the small group and individual markets. Tax incentive plans do not disrupt current systems of financing and delivery of care. However, they are difficult to target and tend to provide tax credits to many people who already pay for their own health insurance. As a result, they require extensive new federal spending if they are to actually provide near-universal coverage. Because of the cost, most tax incentive plans in the past, including those proposed by George W. Bush, provided only limited subsidies and only incremental improvements in coverage. Additionally, people with little or no income, who are required to pay little or no tax, do not benefit from tax credits. To the extent personal tax credits may reduce the incentive of employers to provide coverage and, hence, force more people into the individual insurance market, they could cause reductions in the number of insureds that offset some of the gains.

## Clinton Seeks a Middle Road

Which option was Bill Clinton going to choose? Clinton had been head of the Democratic Leadership Council (DLC), a conservative-leaning branch of the party that favored fiscal responsibility. They often called themselves "New Democrats," shunning the party image of big government and tax-and-spend liberals. Hence, he opposed the single-payer option early on, unwilling to embrace a system in which the government takes over all financing and pays for it through higher taxes. He also disdained the tax incentive approach because he was committed to universal coverage and cost control—a combination not readily achieved by that option. That left play-or-pay, which Clinton appeared to support in the beginning, although he specified few details other than promising universal coverage. With no specific plan to defend, he soon came under attack from the Republicans. They preferred tax credits and identified him with play-or-pay, which they claimed would be government-run, hugely expensive, and detrimental to employment.

Clinton's top priority was balancing the budget ("It's the economy, stupid"), and he wanted to distance himself from the mounting criticism of expensive, government-run health care. As a result, he demanded two key conditions for health care reform—conditions that, at first glance, appeared to satisfy his political requirements, but eventually played a large part in the effort's failure. First, he insisted the reform must be budget neutral or, at the very least, paid for by a "minor" tax such as a cigarette tax. Second, he sought a middle road for reform that would satisfy both the Right and the Left. He wanted to stress private market competition to attract conservatives and universal insurance coverage to appeal to liberals. Where could he find a health reform proposal that would do both?

## The Jackson Hole Group and Managed Competition

The Grand Teton Mountains in Wyoming would not be the obvious place to look for groundbreaking health research. Nevertheless, in Jackson Hole, Dr. Paul Ellwood had been bringing health policy experts and industry leaders to his mountain home to talk about the American health care system. This was the same Paul Ellwood who encouraged the Nixon administration to support HMOs. Ellwood was concerned about government's increasing role in health care. He feared that the inexorable increase in costs was going to make health care unaffordable to many Americans, and, as a result, the system would eventually collapse and be taken over by the government. One of the experts he brought to Jackson Hole was Alain Enthoven, a tall, lanky professor from Stanford University who had been an assistant secretary in the Defense Department from 1961 to 1969. In 1976, Enthoven had been teaching economics at Stanford when President Carter's HEW secretary, Joseph Califano, asked him to consult on health care reform. Enthoven developed the "Consumer Choice Health Plan" based on a theory he called managed competition. The Carter administration never advanced the plan, but Enthoven kept pushing it, and it became the basis of the discussions at Ellwood's ranch. As the group developed their reform theories, they brought in additional policy experts. One was Lynn Etheredge, who had worked on national health care proposals in the Nixon and Ford administrations. Etheredge, a quick-thinking analyst and savvy Washington insider, produced policy papers and coined the name, "The Jackson Hole Group."[22]

Etheredge and Ellwood completed four papers in August 1991 and began to circulate them throughout the health policy community. This, of course, was right after Wofford's victory, a time when health policy had high visibility on both the political agenda and in the national media. Even before the papers were completed, Michael Weinstein of the *New York Times* became familiar with the group's work and began to support it on the *Times* editorial page. The *Times* made an editorial decision to take a strong position on health care reform. Weinstein became the advocate-in-chief for managed competition, publishing twenty-six editorials, from May 1991 through the end of 1992, that either endorsed the plan or criticized competing proposals.[23]

Thanks in part to the *Times*, and to some lobbying by people affiliated with the Jackson Hole Group, members of Congress became familiar with the concept of managed competition. One of those interested congressmen was Jim Cooper of Tennessee, who was the first to introduce legislation based on the plan. Cooper's health policy aide at the time was Atul Gawande, a young Harvard Medical School student. Gawande left Cooper to join the Clinton campaign and became the director of health and social policy.[24] After the election, both Gawande and Etheredge became part of the Clinton transition team.

## What is Managed Competition?

Managed competition is a concept in which capitated (also called prepaid) health plans compete against each other in a structured marketplace. As we know from the previous chapter, a capitated plan is one that receives a prepaid annual sum for each enrollee. In return, the plan has to provide all the health services the person needs, whether or not the prepaid sum exceeds the cost of care. Theoretically, this gives the plan the incentive to maintain and manage the health of its enrollees in the most efficient possible manner. In managed competition, employers are mandated to pay a portion of the insurance premium for all employees, but they do not choose the specific insurance plan. Instead, they submit their portion of the capitated payment to intermediaries (called health insurance purchasing cooperatives or HIPCs) who "manage" the competition among plans. Employees choose from a menu of plans offered through the HIPCs, but their employee benefit is limited to the cost of the least expensive plan (that satisfies a standard minimum benefit package). If the employee wants a more expensive plan, he or she has to pay the difference. Each competing health plan is required to have open enrollment, community rating (everyone in the same plan pays the same amount regardless of their age or health status), standardized policies, standard quality and customer satisfaction reporting, and regulated marketing practices. Theoretically, with such standardization, plans have to compete on price and quality and not on selecting the youngest and healthiest enrollees. Employees' choices are "managed" by the HIPCs, which "risk adjusts" the amount received by the plan. Hence, employees (and their employers) pay the same amount for similar plans, but the HIPC adjusts the payments to the health plan according to the risk profile of the enrollees. For example, even though different-aged individuals would pay the same insurance premium, the HIPC would pay the health plans more for an older person and less for a younger person. If the risk adjustment was accurate, the plan would be indifferent about whom to enroll and would not have the incentive to discriminate against older or sicker individuals.

## Clinton Makes a Critical Choice

Managed competition appeared to be the answer Bill Clinton was seeking. It was potentially the elusive middle road that could satisfy both the Left and the Right and could come reasonably close to budget neutrality. At least, that was what its supporters told him. Magaziner was insistent that managed competition could squeeze so much waste out of the current system that it would pay for itself, even with all the expanded coverage.

In the beginning, Clinton appeared to vacillate between the more traditional play-or-pay approach and the new theory of managed competition. In a speech given to Merck employees on September 27, shortly before the election, he appeared to endorse managed competition. Nevertheless, after the election, he appointed a transition team headed by Judy Feder that included Stuart Altman and Ken Thorpe. All three preferred a more traditional approach. In the end, it was Clinton's determination to balance the budget that made the difference. When Judy Feder and her transition team advised him of the cost, he blamed the messenger, leaving Feder "feeling devastated (and) treated abominably."[25] Despite the fact that managed competition had never been tried in the marketplace, and, in fact, was virtually unheard of more than a year before, Clinton was persuaded by Magaziner and his optimistic assurances. It was a severe miscalculation.

## A Mainframe Kind of Guy in a PC Kind of World

There is no question Ira Magaziner had a brilliant analytical mind. As an undergraduate at Brown University, Magaziner and a fellow student, Elliott Maxwell, wrote a paper that completely redesigned the Brown curriculum by eliminating the traditional grading system. The plan remains in effect today.[26] Magaziner was valedictorian of his class in 1969, and his speech was featured in a *Time* magazine article on student leaders—one of which, coincidentally, was Hillary Clinton (then Hillary Rodham).[27] Magaziner did not meet Hillary at that time, but he met Bill Clinton a short time later when they were both Rhodes scholars.

Magaziner's effort to create the Clinton health plan was gargantuan. It took over six months and, at one time, employed more than six hundred people. Jay Rockefeller quipped, "I don't think that there's been this kind of effort since they planned the invasion of Normandy."[28] The final draft was 1,342 pages. Magaziner was widely criticized because the plan was achingly complex and impossible to explain to average citizens. It was so prescriptive that it usurped any role for Congress, creating resentment instead of "buy-in" among the lawmakers who would actually have to vote on the plan. Critics described Magaziner as a "mainframe kind of guy in a PC kind of world,"[29] and the *New York Times* called him "the tone deaf architect of the ill-fated Clinton health plan."[30]

Magaziner's plan had a huge influence on Obama's effort fifteen years later, but largely because it indicated what to avoid. Some of the problems with Magaziner's proposal can be attributed to Clinton's insistence to pay for most of the plan by reducing other health care costs. Hence, the plan had to include budget cuts, premium caps, and regional spending limits. Otherwise the Congressional Budget Office would not consider the plan budget neutral. This created strong opposition from many stakeholders who feared they would be worse off if the plan was approved. Much of the problem, however, was the wrenching change required by Magaziner's plan. It largely reorganized the delivery system, creating competition among integrated health plans in a market managed by the HIPCs, which were nonprofit, quasipublic health alliances. That changed the way most individuals received their health care. When people realized they might not only have to change their insurance companies, but also their doctors, many began to fear they might be worse off. It was the kind of change Altman's transition team had warned against, and the kind Obama was careful to avoid.

Obama, taking cues from Clinton's failure, carefully stayed away from delivery system changes. As a result, he was able to garner support from doctors, hospitals, nurses, insurance companies, and drug companies, almost all of whom opposed the Clinton plan. He also was able to reassure the 85 percent of Americans who already had insurance that they could keep the coverage and the doctors they already had.

Although Magaziner's plan was not politically realistic, it did constitute an impressive piece of work. Regardless of whether one agrees with the policy, one has to admire how the intricacies of the plan meshed together. This was a redesign of much of the American health care system—a system that would be the sixth largest economy in the world—and one would be hard pressed to pose any question that Magaziner's reform plan did not address.

In addition, there were a number of similarities with the plan Obama initially proposed. They included universal coverage, an employer mandate, competition among insurance plans (Obama's with a "public option" and insurance exchange), insurance pools, and strict regulation of insurance underwriting. Obama also gave limited support to the concept of integrated health plans and to plans that received capitated payments as opposed to fee-for-service reimbursement—an echo of Magaziner's strategy. However, he only provided demonstration funding within Medicare and was careful not to mandate any changes of that nature in his actual proposal.

Originally, Clinton wanted to have his health bill ready for Congress in his first one hundred days. He knew from past history that he would never have more power than right after his election—the period often referred to as the "honeymoon" for newly elected presidents. Since Franklin Roosevelt's famous accomplishments in his first one hundred days, every president has sought to emulate his success. Lyndon Johnson began his efforts to enact Medicare immediately upon gaining office. George W. Bush spoke of "spending his political capital." Clinton wanted to send his health reform bill to Congress at the peak of his power and not give anyone time to organize opposition or to pick apart the details of his plan. However, managed competition was a huge change from the status quo. Translating it into legislation would be a lengthy and complex endeavor under any circumstances. But, with Ira Magaziner leading the effort, it was bound to be constructed in minute and drawn out detail.

Learning from Clinton's mistakes, Obama outlined a far less ambitious plan to reform the system and made an all-out effort to force a congressional vote within his first year in office. Furthermore, rather than writing the bill in the executive branch, he stated only broad outlines of what he wanted, encouraging congressional committees to seek consensus on a bill. Ultimately, however, both presidents were concerned about the same hurdle: getting sixty senators to support a plan in order to avoid a filibuster. As an alternative, they both considered a congressional maneuver known as reconciliation.

## The Byrd is the Word

Robert Carlyle Byrd was the oldest serving member in Senate history. He was first elected to the Senate in 1959. In 2009 he was ninety-two years old and third in succession for the presidency behind Joe Biden and Nancy Pelosi. At the time of Clinton's inauguration, Byrd was seventy-five years old and had been in the Senate for thirty-four years. He had written a four-volume history of the US Senate and was generally regarded as the leading expert on Senate rules. Had it not been for this man known as "the guardian of Senate procedure," Bill Clinton's health plan may have been enacted and Barack Obama's may have failed.

Clinton realized how difficult it would be to get his health reform proposal approved by the Senate because of the increased use of the filibuster. According to Senate rules, a member can speak on any issue for as long as he or she chooses. Hence, any senator can prevent a vote on a bill by speaking interminably. Under a procedure called cloture, however, senators can vote to end a filibuster by a three-fifths vote. Throughout most of American history, the filibuster was rarely employed. When it was, it was for issues of national significance. Most commonly, southern senators used the filibuster to block civil rights legislation. In fact, Byrd filibustered the 1964 Civil Rights Act for fourteen hours, an action for which he later expressed regret. As late as the '60s there were never more than seven filibusters per year. Since 2000, however, there have never been less than forty-nine filibusters per year. The widespread use of the filibuster now means that sixty Senate votes are often needed to pass legislation, and many bills can be blocked by a determined minority.

Senate rules provide for one important exception to the filibuster. Bills relating to the budget can be debated according to a procedure called reconciliation. Under this process, a maximum of twenty hours of debate is allowed, so bills cannot be filibustered. Hence, if a bill is submitted under reconciliation, only a simple majority of fifty votes, not a three-fifths vote of sixty, is enough to ensure passage. Bill Clinton wanted to include his health reform proposal under reconciliation.

The impediment was the Byrd Rule. It specified that only matters directly affecting the budget could be included in reconciliation.[31] Although Byrd was not necessarily opposed to the health care initiative, he insisted that limiting debate on such a broad measure would be contrary to Senate tradition and would not be allowed under the Byrd Rule. Despite personal urging from Majority Leader George Mitchell and President Clinton himself, Byrd could not be moved. With strong partisan opposition in the Senate, Clinton realized he would need sixty votes to enact health care reform.

In 2009, the Obama administration considered the same strategy. By that time, the historic use of the Byrd Rule had changed. Originally, its only intended use was to reduce government spending (or increase revenues) in order to comply with annual budget resolutions. However, George W. Bush used reconciliation to cut taxes without covering the cost by reduced spending, and he was able to do so without violating the Byrd Rule. As a result, Obama felt entitled to use reconciliation for health reform, accepting the fact that every provision in the bill would have to affect spending or revenues. If he only needed fifty votes instead of sixty, it would allow him to exclude policies that he might otherwise need to gain Republican votes. Even fifty Senate votes is a substantial hurdle for any industry-changing proposal that creates winners and losers. Those stakeholders who are negatively impacted will lobby their congressional representatives to oppose the legislation. The lobbying effort by tobacco states during the Clinton reform effort provides a good example of how vote trading affects policy.

The original designers of the Clinton health plan decided to raise the cigarette tax to finance part of their plan.[32] After all, it was a health plan, and smoking tobacco is unhealthy. Increasing the price of cigarettes has proven to be an effective method of reducing the number of smokers, and reducing the number of smokers reduces the health costs caused by smoking-related illnesses. It was a win–win solution for financing the cost of health reform.

The problem, of course, was that tobacco growers, and those whose jobs and incomes were tied to tobacco, lobbied their representatives to oppose the tax. There were twenty-nine tobacco-state Democrats in the House, and they all knew Clinton could not pass health care reform without their votes. The Ways and Means subcommittee had set the tax at $1.25 per pack. When Sam Gibbons (D-FL), the Ways and Means chair, had to negotiate with L. F. Payne (D-VA) and William Jefferson (D-LA) on behalf of the tobacco states, he knew he could not afford to lose their votes. Gibbons was forced to agree to freeze the cigarette tax at forty-five cents per pack and to phase it in gradually. In order to make up for the lost revenue, he delayed the start of long-term care benefits. That prompted John Rother from AARP to say, "It's just amazing, even to someone who's fairly cynical, that people would make a conscious decision to screw the elderly and the disabled in order to help tobacco."[33] It turned out that the tobacco tax was not the only thing Jefferson froze. In 2005, FBI agents found ninety thousand dollars in Jefferson's freezer and he was subsequently convicted on eleven counts of corruption.

The tobacco story illustrates the difficulties of enacting large-scale reform. The best policy is not necessarily the best politics, and without compromise on the politics, there is no opportunity to change policies. As a result, major reforms, if they are enacted at all, are often watered down. That is one reason why Obama chose to minimize the amount of change in his proposal while Bill Clinton and Ira Magaziner pushed ahead with their proposal based on managed competition.

## Bob Reischauer and the Congressional Budget Office

Ira Magaziner's assurances that managed competition would save more money than it would cost may have satisfied the president, but it did not satisfy Robert Reischauer. Reischauer was the director of the Congressional Budget Office (CBO), an agency created by Congress to estimate the cost of proposed legislation. From its inception in 1975 under the direction of Alice Rivlin, the CBO had been fiercely independent. When it estimated the cost of pending legislation, it routinely incurred either the anger of the bills' supporters or the wrath of its opponents.

Reischauer told us how members of Congress and senior administration officials would scream at him if they did not agree with CBO projections. When the CBO attributed an additional cost to an Israeli loan guarantee because of a small risk of default, leaders of Congress called him and screamed, "You asshole, we're going to fire you" (something they could not easily do).[34]

There may be no other appointed office where the director wields so much power because of the impact of his decisions but takes so much grief for performing his job. "To be the CBO director, you have to have the hide of a rhinoceros," joked Reischauer. Despite his imposing height (well over six feet), he is disarmingly unassuming and soft-spoken, and he has a boyish smile and a sense of humor that endears him even to his adversaries.

His equanimity was severely tested, however, during the Clinton health initiative. In February 1994, the CBO was preparing to score the Clinton health plan. The budget numbers were crucial to the administration, not only because of the president's insistence on budget neutrality, but also because of conservative opposition to the cost of the plan. One of the major points of contention concerned the employer mandate. A requirement for employers to purchase health insurance for employees had never been considered a tax. However, under managed competition employers would not directly purchase the benefit, but remit the cost of each worker's health insurance to a "health alliance (HIPC)." The CBO had to decide whether the health alliances were actually government agencies and whether an employer's mandated contribution was an employee benefit or a tax. If it was a tax, the revenue collected would be a tax increase, and the payments from the alliances to the health plans would be an on-budget expense.

Reischauer was lobbied heavily from both sides, parrying calls from Majority Leader Mitchell and Senator Kennedy as well as from opponents of reform. Two days before his testimony to the Ways and Means Committee, he ran into John Kasich (R-OH), who was the ranking minority member of the House Budget Committee. Reischauer reported to us that Kasich put his arm on Reischauer's shoulder and said, "You know, Bob, you're in one hell of a position, and I realize that you're really a good guy and have been shooting straight. But, I know what you have to do. And I know there's going to be a resolution in the Republican caucus to dismiss you because you're going to come out and say, 'These aren't governmental resources. This is off-budget.' And I want you to know that I'm going to do everything I can to defend you."[35]

Nothing of the kind happened because Reischauer (having nothing to do with Kasich) came down on the other side of the issue. The CBO concluded the Clinton plan would cost $133 billion more than administration estimated. Although Reischauer called the employer payments "government receipts" rather than a tax, the CBO included the payments on the federal budget.

Before his testimony, Reischauer told his staff that the CBO budget could be decimated as a result of their decision, and their jobs could be lost.[36] He asked them to take a secret vote on whether they wanted to stick with their estimates, even at the risk of losing their jobs. They voted unanimously 'yes,' and Reischauer delivered the testimony. The *Washington Post* called his testimony "A ruling from the most powerful umpire in Washington, a man who braves political pressures daily and calls them as he sees them.... Though nearly every lawmaker on Capitol Hill has taken shots at Reischauer publicly for one reason or another, in private, most describe him as that rarest of creatures in an intensely political town: an honest man."[37]

The CBO scored many versions of the Clinton plan, and their estimates were a crucial element in the plan's failure. Reischauer and his team could not accept Magaziner's arguments that the efficiencies of managed competition would pay for the cost of the plan. In order for the CBO to score the plan as budget neutral, the administration had to impose regional caps on insurance premiums and institute a global budget. Alain Enthoven's original concept of managed competition morphed into "managed competition within a budget." The altered plan could satisfy the CBO, but it would cause dramatically increased opposition, even alienating its original founders.

## The Pitfalls of Managed Competition within a Budget

One of the most critical decisions Clinton made was attempting to provide universal coverage and reduce costs at the same time. In speeches he gave across the country, Stuart Altman explained it this way: "You have to realize that one person's cost is another person's income. Clinton was going to cover about forty million additional people, add a Medicare drug benefit, mental health parity, and long-term care. In order to do this in a manner that was anywhere close to budget neutral, he would have to reduce other health costs by tens of millions of dollars per year. You tell that to the people and the businesses that are going to be the target of those cuts, and see if they're going to support you."

Health reform is hard enough to enact without trying to cut costs at the same time. Massachusetts learned that lesson well. In 2006, it passed a universal health plan, deciding to expand coverage first and deal with costs later. At the time of this writing, 97.5 percent of Massachusetts residents were insured. After the plan was successfully implemented, the state planned to consider policies to contain costs. Theoretically, political support would be greater because so many citizens would have become insured. The proposal put forth by Clinton's transition team on January 11 had largely avoided any cost control. It would have increased government health care spending by about 10 percent. But for Clinton, it was a nonstarter. His first priority was balancing the budget. Where was he going to find $270 billion?

Ira Magaziner (with the help of Paul Starr, Walter Zelman, and others), forced by the decision of the CBO, altered the original theory of managed competition and created managed competition within a budget. Under his plan, a National Health Board would set a global budget, placing a ceiling on the amount the federal government could spend on health care for the fiscal year. The budget would be broken down by state, and the purchasing alliances would negotiate prices with the health plans, but they would have to keep within the budget. In areas where competition was insufficient or unable to meet budgetary requirements, the government would simply set prices.

Magaziner continued to argue that managed competition alone would squeeze out so many inefficiencies that it would pay for universal coverage without the need to resort to the budget and price controls. Clinton publicly asserted that the controls would not be necessary. The system would rely on competition, he stated, but the budget and price controls would serve as a backup, just in case. However, industries that had achieved success by competing for revenues in the marketplace were not about to have those revenues subject to a global budget.

Hence, doctors, hospitals, and their trade organizations that previously supported the concept of health reform began to back away. Many were not willing to support a plan in which their reimbursement could be reduced arbitrarily to meet a government-devised budget.

Large insurance companies, especially those experienced with prepaid plans, did not oppose the Clinton plan. In general, they believed the new market structure would disadvantage the smaller companies and work to their advantage. The smaller insurance companies, which did not offer prepaid plans and wrote insurance primarily for individuals and small groups, saw the Clinton plan as a dire threat. In fact, had the Clinton plan passed, many would have ceased to exist. Consequently, their trade association, the Health Insurance Association of America (HIAA), which supported health reform at the outset, strongly opposed the plan. The association sponsored a series of television commercials that is now considered the most successful issue-advertising campaign in history.

## Harry and Louise

The television screen is completely black except for white letters spelling *Sometime in the Future*.[38] It then flashes to a middle-aged couple, Harry and Louise, sitting together at their kitchen table. The dialogue begins:

> Announcer: Times are changing, and not all for the better. The government
>     may force us to pick from a few health care plans designed by government bureaucrats.
> Louise: Having choices we don't like is no choice at all.
> Harry: If they choose...
> Louise: We lose.

It was not that the ads were angry or mean or outrageous. Actually, they were kind of homey and soft-spoken. They were just enough to raise people's doubts, to make them a little bit worried. And that was mostly what Bill Gradison and Chip Kahn originally intended. They never dreamed the campaign would be so powerful.

Bill Gradison had assumed command of the HIAA in February, just after Clinton's inauguration. Two months earlier, the organization had done an about-face by publicly supporting the concepts of universal health care and an employer mandate. Gradison was a person who could potentially work with the Democratic administration. He had been a nine-term Republican congressman from Cincinnati and had a reputation for seeking compromise. His executive vice president, Chip Kahn, described him as a "classic moderate."[39] Gradison recruited Kahn from the House Ways and Means Committee, where he had been the chief health care counsel. Both men were Washington insiders.

The HIAA had serious problems. Five of the largest insurance companies in the country had withdrawn from the trade organization in the past year. They were left with mostly small- and medium-size companies, many of which specialized in the small group and individual markets. They no longer had as members the large integrated managed care plans—the kind of plans central to the Clinton health plan. In fact, if the Clinton plan was enacted in its present form, many of these companies would not survive.

Both Gradison and Kahn assumed that Congress would pass some kind of health reform. They were reluctant to oppose the president publicly because there were bound to be prolonged negotiations over the health plan, and they wanted to retain a seat at the bargaining table. So, early in the spring while the Clinton task force was designing the plan, they arranged several meetings with Ira Magaziner. The meetings did not go well. Gradison and Kahn knew there was a large gap to bridge, but they felt that Magaziner never even listened. "It was just clear that Ira Magaziner turned off his hearing aid," Kahn told us. With Ira, "it was our way or the highway."[40]

Gradison tried again in May, sending a letter directly to Hillary. He asked her to stop bashing the insurance companies and requested a meeting. However, no meeting was forthcoming and the administration found that blaming insurance companies resonated with the public—a strategy that would later appeal to Obama. The HIAA responded with a $3.5 million advertising campaign that supported health reform but raised questions about the Clinton plan. "There's got to be a better way," the ads stated; a phrase that would later be repeated by Harry and Louise.

Meanwhile, Chip Kahn was being squeezed. The CEOs of his member companies wanted him to be more aggressive. The Clinton plan could put them out of business. He had to please his members and an increasingly wary executive board, but he also had to please Gradison, who was an inside player and was never enthusiastic about advertising. Kahn was also reluctant to go out on a limb when passage of some kind of plan seemed nearly certain. "I realized we had to do something," he told us. "I became convinced that to get a chair at the table, we had to make ourselves known."[41]

Kahn hired the advertising firm of Goddard Claussen, and he began to work with Ben Goddard to develop the right message. It was tricky. He did not want to be anti–health reform, but he wanted to raise doubts about the Clinton plan. Meanwhile, Gradison had been giving speeches around the country, telling audiences that families would decide the fate of health care reform as they talked about it sitting around their kitchen tables. Kahn liked the image and he and Goddard tried it out in focus groups, where the response was positive. Goddard hired Harry Johnson and Louise Clark to play the characters, all three unsuspecting that the ads would make them famous.

If Kahn and Gradison's motivations sound too innocent, they probably were. The gap between Clinton's health plan and the needs of the HIAA was probably too large for compromise. The HIAA may have sincerely wanted health reform, but they would have fought to the death to defeat anything like the Clinton plan, and they probably knew it all along.

For one thing, the HIAA could not live with community rating, particularly since they insured many individuals and small groups and were subject to adverse selection (mostly sick people choosing to buy individual policies). They also opposed premium caps, since their rates for some individuals and groups would have to be quite high to counteract the selection risk. Finally, Clinton wanted the government to certify each plan before it could join a health alliance. The large national plans would undoubtedly receive certification, but the small plans in the HIAA would be at risk.

Gradison and Kahn made several more attempts to negotiate with the administration. They agreed to halt the Harry and Louise ads before Clinton's major health policy address to Congress in September 1993. When they did not receive a positive response, however, they resumed the ads in the fall. Later, they reached a temporary accord with Dan Rostenkowski, the chair of the House Ways and Means Committee. When Rosty resigned, however, his successor, Sam Gibbons, ignored the deal. By the time the committees debated the bills in the summer of 1994, the advertising campaign had had a devastating effect.

The HIAA spent over fifteen million dollars on the Harry and Louise campaign. It was not a large amount, but Ben Goddard spent the money wisely. He ran many ads on CNN, which, at the time, had little cable news competition and reached the opinion leader demographic that Kahn was targeting. Then, in November 1994, Hillary inadvertently gave the campaign a major boost when she lambasted the Harry and Louise ads in a speech before the American Academy of Pediatrics. Her remarks and the ad video appeared on every network news show, and Harry and Louise became a household name to television viewers across the country. The media became so caught up by the campaign that the HIAA would hold press conferences announcing each new iteration of the ad, and the evening news shows would send their reporters to cover the event. Kahn told us the ad campaign generated an additional twenty million dollars in contributions. In all, the HIAA spent fifty million dollars to defeat the plan. Jay Rockefeller called it "the single most destructive campaign I've seen in over thirty years."[42]

For Ben Goddard, the campaign was a trifecta. First, he initiated the genre. Lobbying by television began with Harry and Louise and made Ben Goddard famous. Second, he sold Goddard Claussen at the height of their notoriety for a very large amount of money. And, third, Ben Goddard married the actress Louise Caire Clark.

Although the Harry and Louise ads have been criticized for the way they changed public opinion about Clinton's health reform, the HIAA had good reasons to oppose the plan. It is worth pausing to understand some of the genuine problems in an industry that is often much maligned.

## Not All Insurance Companies Are Evil

We usually insure against an event that has a small chance of occurring but is unaffordable or catastrophic when it does occur. For example, very few of our homes burn down, but the cost of losing our home is often unaffordable, so we purchase fire insurance. Similarly, the chance of dying when we are middle-aged and healthy is small, but many of us buy life insurance because our families may not be financially secure if they suddenly lose a working parent.

These examples of insurance, however, depend upon symmetric information. If you could wait until your house catches fire and then buy fire insurance you could save a lot of money, and that is what most people would do. However, the fire insurance companies would go broke. Similarly, if you could wait until you are diagnosed with cancer before buying life insurance (or health insurance), nobody would buy until they got sick. Then, of course, the life and health insurance companies would also go broke.

When you apply for health insurance, there is an asymmetry of information. You know whether you are healthy but your insurer does not. Hence, your insurance company excludes preexisting conditions. Everyone hates that, but the insurance company has to do it.

If health insurance works so badly, you might ask, why not get rid of it? Start a single-payer system like Canada or Great Britain. However, the reason those problems do not exist in those systems is not because insurance does not work—it is because everyone has to be insured. If insurance coverage was mandated in the United States (like automobile insurance), there would not have to be rules to protect companies from people selecting to buy insurance only when they were ill (the technical term is *adverse selection*).

During negotiations on the Obama health plan, the health insurance industry agreed to end exclusions for preexisting conditions and to sell insurance to all prospective buyers (called *guaranteed issue*) if the plan mandated that everyone had to have insurance. However, when Congress amended the Finance Committee bill to reduce the penalty for individuals who did not comply with the mandate, several large health insurance companies reversed their position, opposing the bill unless it had a stricter individual mandate.

The insurance industry's understanding with Obama also included modified community rating.[43] In a pure, community rated system, everyone pays the same amount regardless of his or her age (or medical condition). If everyone has to buy insurance, the companies can set an "average rate" that will cover their risk of insuring both young and old people. However, if insurance is not mandated, fewer young people will buy insurance, because, at the same rate, it is obviously a better deal for older people than for younger people (the "average rate" is above what young people would pay and below what old people would pay). As young people drop out, the insurance pool is left with a disproportionate number of older people and the companies would have to raise the average rate. This would cause more young people to drop out, and the cycle could continue until you get what insurance people call a "death spiral." People hate the fact that insurance companies charge higher premiums to older people. However, community rating only works well if insurance coverage is mandated.

An additional problem occurs because of moral hazard, a term we discussed in chapter 1. Unlike most kinds of insurance, health insurance does not only cover catastrophic events, but also ordinary health procedures that people expect to undergo at regular intervals. The fact that people do not have to pay—or have to pay very little—for these services results in people using more services than they need. Why not? The services are virtually free. Hence, insurance plans employ utilization review in order to control costs. People hate utilization review. They want MRIs to diagnose pain, they want to go to specialists without consulting their primary care doctors, and they want to go to the emergency room when their children are ill. Everyone wants insurance to cost less, but no one wants their use of services to be constrained.

Why have private insurance companies, you might ask, if there is moral hazard and utilization review? Wouldn't it be better to have single-payer where health care executives do not try to ration your care? Unfortunately, a single-payer system would confront the exact same problems. In order to constrain costs or keep within a government budget, the government program would have to perform the same kind of utilization review as private insurance companies.

Some people might rather have the government control utilization instead of private companies, but that is not at all clear. For example, the Obama administration proposed a policy called *comparative effectiveness*. In short, an independent agency would conduct research by medical professionals and would decide what drugs or treatment regimens were the most effective for a given condition in comparison with alternative drugs or treatments. This seemed to be a reasonable, scientifically based policy, but it was lambasted by opponents as government rationing. It became the source of claims that there would be government "death panels," denying treatments that were not favored by the government. Although it is true that Americans distrust insurance companies and claim that they ration care, it is also true that they distrust the government at least as much.

This discussion is not meant to take sides against single-payer or to support private insurance companies. Some private insurance companies have not been model citizens. There are egregious examples of abuses of power, denials of care, and unforgivable horror stories that ruined the lives of many patients. However, there are over 175 million people with private insurance. Most of them, when they are polled, dislike insurance companies in general but like their insurance companies in particular. Even an abuse rate of one-half of one percent would yield a volume of horror stories. That is not to forgive transgressions, but it makes no more sense to call all insurance companies evil as it does to call all banks, lawyers, oil companies, or cable television companies evil. They are us. And insurance companies exist in a market that requires them to institute policies that we do not always like. Otherwise, they cannot survive. Fortunately, there are ways to restructure and regulate the insurance market so that it works better for everyone. Alternatively, we can replace private insurance with government insurance that will confront many of the same problems, but possibly with a better result. In either case, as much as people like to vilify private insurance companies and criticize government bureaucracy, they have to have one or the other (or both), and there are no obvious villains or easy solutions.

Although the insurance industry and the Harry and Louise campaign helped change public opinion, it was not the primary culprit in the failure of the Clinton health plan. It may have been one of the triggers, but it was certainly not the smoking gun. The problem was the plan itself: by its nature, it was going to be a nearly impossible sell. And even one of the smoothest salesmen of his generation could not figure out how to do it.

### Clinton Sells the Plan

It is 9:00 p.m. on September 22, 1993, and Harris Wofford escorts President Clinton into the House chamber. This is the day Bill Clinton will introduce his long-awaited health care proposal to a joint session of Congress.

Originally, the plan was to be ready within the first one hundred days. However, the budget battle had intervened along with lengthy confirmation battles and the issue of gays in the military. Through it all, Ira Magaziner's huge, six hundred–person task force had labored for months on the mammoth 1,342-page proposal, and even now, it still isn't ready. But Bill Clinton is. Resplendent before the crowded House chamber, he acknowledges the thunderous applause and prepares to give the most important speech of his presidency. Glancing at the teleprompters on either side of the podium, he is thunderstruck to see that the wrong speech is queued on the monitors.

It is hard to imagine what must have gone through the president's mind as he stood before a joint session of Congress and tens of millions of television viewers without his prepared speech. Certainly he could have explained there were "technical difficulties" and postponed his address for a few minutes. Another speaker might have felt panicky, or might have soldiered on, perhaps somewhat haltingly. But Bill Clinton was a self-confident and consummate orator. Furthermore, as a compulsive policy wonk, he was familiar with the minutest details of the health care reform proposal. Never wavering, he began to deliver as good a speech as any in his presidency.[44] After seven minutes, the teleprompters were reloaded and the correct text was in front of him, but you would not have known the difference, and neither did anyone else. The speech was hailed by his supporters and even lauded by many of his opponents. Single-handedly, he turned the polls back in his favor, and at that time, at that moment, nearly everyone believed that national health reform was inevitable; maybe not the Clinton plan per se, but at least some version of national health reform.

The delays through the spring and summer months had fueled the opposition. The impact of Harry and Louise, the lobbying from vested interests, and the outright opposition of Republican political opponents had eroded public support for reform. It had not helped that there was no concrete plan to defend. Worse still, what was there was nearly impossible to explain to a casual television audience. Yet the president, by the sheer force of his bully pulpit and his extraordinary communication skills, had turned it around. As long as the president could speak in generalities and platitudes and assure people that providing health security to everyone would enhance the greatness of America, he could advance his cause. However, when the debate progressed to the actual details of the plan, when it became obvious who would win and who would lose—who would receive the benefits and who would pay the cost—the opposition to his plan became intense.

The Democrats had majorities in both houses of Congress. In the Senate, their advantage was 57–43, and in the House 258–176. In order to get sixty votes in the Senate and a majority in the house, Clinton realized he would have to hold virtually all of the liberals and moderates in his party, and he would have to attract enough moderate Republicans to make up for losses among Democratic conservatives. He thought that managed competition could satisfy moderates from both sides. The Jackson Hole Group's conception of competing managed care plans was a procompetitive theory. Universal coverage through an employer mandate was appealing to most moderates and liberals, although many on the party's left wing preferred single-payer.

Clinton may have been able to cobble together a majority if it were not for the requirement of budget neutrality, a precondition that forced him to alter his plan. Once managed competition became managed competition within a budget, it became a different political animal. As discussed previously, it contained a global budget, price controls, large, government-run health alliances in every state, and a powerful National Health Board. The tools Clinton needed to satisfy Bob Reischauer and the CBO would cost him vital support in both industry and government. Even Alain Enthoven, the inventor of managed competition, opposed the Clinton model and published a scathing article entitled "A Single-Payer System in Jackson Hole Clothing."[45]

When the actual 1,342-page version of the Clinton health plan was finally completed in the fall of 1993, the action moved from the executive branch to the Congress. Each of the relevant committees in the House and Senate would attempt to report out a bill. Then, the reported bills (if there were more than one) within each chamber would be merged and brought before the full chamber floor for debate, followed by a vote. If passed, the House and Senate versions would be reconciled prior to a final vote in both chambers.

Throughout the winter, spring, and early summer of 1994, the committee chairs attempted to assemble bills that would attract a majority of members. The conventional wisdom was that some version of reform was inevitable. A number of bills would be reported out of committee and brought to the floor. A compromise would eventually be reached. It was just a matter of time for the process to work its way through. However, there was at least one person who was convinced that the conventional wisdom was dead wrong.

## Newt Gingrich and Republican Opposition

Right from the beginning, Newt Gingrich recognized the potential damage to the president and the Democratic Party if their most important domestic initiative could be defeated. Gingrich seized the opportunity and propelled his party to a congressional majority for the first time in over forty years.

During Richard Nixon's tenure, both political parties accommodated candidates with a wide range of perspectives. Although the Democrats were dominated by northeastern liberals, the southern conservatives were always a force within the party. Republicans, even through the Reagan years, had liberals from the northeast like Nelson Rockefeller and Lowell Weicker and many moderates from the Midwest and other areas of the country. In 1993, however, a sea change was taking place within the Republican Party. Although mild-mannered Bob Michel was the minority leader, the real power came from the party whip; an ambitious, no-holds-barred politician who coveted Michel's position to become the next Speaker of the House.

Newt Gingich was elected to Congress in 1978 and subsequently won reelection ten times. His temperament more closely resembled the angry outbursts of a British backbencher in the House of Commons than the relatively staid and traditionally polite behavior in the US Congress. Gingrich made his name by tearing down liberals and railing against any misdeeds he could identify. He condemned Dan Crane and Gerry Studds in the congressional page sex scandal in 1983. In 1988 he earned his stripes in the party by helping to lead the ethics charges against Democratic Speaker Jim Wright over a book deal. Partly as a result, Gingrich became the House Republican whip in 1989, succeeding Dick Cheney, who became secretary of defense. A few years later Gingrich faced ethical questions about his own $4.5 million book deal with HarperCollins. In 1990, he led the charges against Democrats in the House banking scandal. Gingrich called it "the largest institutional scandal in the history of the US House."[46] Never mind the fact that Gingrich himself had thirty overdrafts at the House bank.[47] He was vociferous in leading the impeachment charges against President Clinton. However, he has since admitted to conducting an extra-marital affair with a former congressional aide during the impeachment saga.[48]

These actions are relevant because Gingrich was instrumental in changing the tone and nature of congressional proceedings. For the first time in many years, it became acceptable to demonize personally those with whom one disagreed. More importantly, it became acceptable, in matters of national significance, to oppose legislation not on its merits, but simply to deny an accomplishment to the opposing political party. Gingrich accomplished this when he led all-out opposition to the Clinton health reform effort, and it set an important precedent. The next time health reform was on the national agenda in 2009, the republican leadership decided to oppose the Obama plan regardless of its substance.

During congressional negotiations over Clinton's health initiative in 1994, a small group of Republican and Democratic moderates attempted to create a bipartisan health reform bill. They became known as the "mainstream coalition" and included Republican moderates John Chafee, David Durenberger, and John Danforth. However, at the same time they were seeking a solution to the Gingrich-led Republicans, and conservative strategists such as William Kristol were insisting that fellow Republicans not even talk about a health care plan, much less negotiate with Democrats.[49] No health plan at all was the preferred strategy, even compared to a sound, well-constructed bill.

A prime example in the House occurred in the Energy and Commerce Committee, one of the three House committees with jurisdiction over health reform.[50] John Dingell, the committee chair, approached Carlos Moorhead, the ranking minority member, to try to work out a compromise bill. Dingell quoted Moorhead's response as follows: "John, there's no way you're going to get a single vote on this [Republican] side of the aisle. You will not only not get a vote here, but we've been instructed that if we participate in that undertaking at all, those of us who do will lose our seniority and will not be ranking minority members within the Republican Party."[51]

John Dingell was the second most senior member of Congress next to Robert Byrd. He succeeded his father in Michigan's Fifteenth Congressional District in 1955. Dingell's father supported universal health insurance under FDR. Since 1955, he has introduced his father's universal health bill at the beginning of each new Congress. In 1994, facing a veritable Republican boycott and disagreements among Democratic members, Dingell was unable to secure enough votes to report a health care bill out of his own committee.

On the Senate side, Bob Dole had always been supportive of health reform. He was the ranking minority member of the Senate Finance Committee, one of three Senate committees with jurisdiction over health reform. Many observers thought a compromise between Dole and Finance Committee Chair Daniel Patrick Moynahan would produce a bill that would reach the Senate floor. Dole had supported Republican health reform bills earlier and was coauthor of the Dole–Packwood proposal. Dole–Packwood provided federal subsidies, on a sliding income scale, for low-income families to purchase private health insurance. It had neither employer nor individual mandates, but it required guaranteed insurance issue, and it limited exclusions for preexisting conditions. Taken together, these provisions would not have put a significant dent in the number of uninsured but would have been a challenging proposition for health insurers.

Despite its weaknesses, forty of the forty-four Republican senators endorsed Dole–Packwood. Nevertheless, Bob Dole had a major problem: he wanted to be the next president of the United States. By the late summer of 1994, it was evident that "no bill" was the Republican strategy. Dole was in danger of wandering off the reservation. Conservatives had already attacked his senior aide, Sheila Burke, calling her a liberal Democrat, and it became clear to Dole that if he pursued any compromise on health care reform it would end his chances of securing the Republican presidential nomination. Bob Bennett, the Republican senator from Utah, best summarized the remarkable movement of the Gingrich-led Republicans to a position of absolute opposition by the late summer of 1994: "All the cosponsors of Dole–Packwood were prepared to vote against Dole–Packwood," Bennett said, "including Dole and Packwood!"[52]

Newt Gingrich had successfully plotted his opposition to Clinton from the start, long before the president realized that the political ground had shifted beneath him. Clinton had always believed a compromise was possible and was unprepared for absolute Republican opposition regardless of the substance of his effort. His two-year losing battle gave a huge victory to Gingrich and his allies.

It was not simply a matter of defeat on the floor of the House or Senate. It was worse. No health reform bill ever even reached the floor of either chamber for a vote. Who could have watched Harris Wofford in 1990 or Bill Clinton in September of 1993 and suspected that such a colossal turnabout could have occurred?

The resounding defeat further weakened the president and gave Gingrich and the Republicans momentum for the 1994 midterm election. It was a disaster for the Democrats. They lost fifty-four seats in the House and ten in the Senate, yielding Republican majorities in both chambers. Forty-one Democratic incumbents lost their seats while not one sitting Republican was defeated.

Newt Gingrich became the Speaker of the House. He seized the moment and enacted much of what he called "The Contract with America." However, he overreached in his subsequent battles with President Clinton, taking a public relations beating for shutting down the government over a budget dispute. On January 21, 1997, he was reprimanded by a 395–28 vote in the House and fined $300,000 for ethical violations. It was the first time a Speaker of the House had ever been disciplined for ethical wrongdoing. He resigned on January 3, 1999, following a Republican defeat in the 1998 congressional election. As of this writing, Gingrich is a leading contender for the 2012 Republican presidential nomination.

## The Plan's the Thing

The ultimate blame for Clinton's failure to pass health reform does not lie with Newt Gingrich. Neither does it lie with Harry and Louise or Bob Reischauer or Robert Byrd. No doubt, each of them played a role, but the chief reason for failure was the plan itself. It is worthwhile to review its shortcomings, because they had a significant effect on future attempts at reform.

Too much change and too much government were the factors that caused widespread opposition. Altman and the transition team wanted to avoid changes for the 175 million Americans who already had health insurance. In contrast, the Clinton Plan, with its alliances and competing health plans, would result in changes for both patients and industry. Employees who already had insurance would likely have to choose different health plans and, thus, different doctors and hospitals. Large employers who were purchasing health benefits directly would have to purchase through alliances instead. Small employers who were not providing health benefits would have an added expense that many considered unaffordable. Many small insurance companies would be forced out of business, and independent insurance agents would no longer be necessary. Many doctors and hospitals would have to realign themselves with integrated health plans. There was something for nearly everyone to oppose. It is no simple matter to convince 85 percent of the population and most of the health care industry to change so that 15 percent can get access to insurance.

Every National Health proposal, with the possible exception of Richard Nixon's, has been vilified by opponents as "government-run" health care or the beginning of socialized medicine. Minimizing government involvement is a good strategy to avoid such political opposition. The Clinton Plan, however, was easy to attack because it increased government regulation and created new government entities. It included an employer mandate, a government-defined benefit package, fifty state-based health alliances, a national health board, insurance premium caps, and a global budget. For those in industry and politics who were leery about the increasing role of government, the plan was a huge target.

## Could It Have Been Different?

Much has been written about the failure of Clinton's health reform effort. Most analyses have focused on mistakes made during his presidency and on the many obstacles enumerated in the paragraphs above. We contend that the president sealed his fate even before he was inaugurated, although this certainly was not evident until after the long battle was over. All indications are that Bill Clinton had made up his mind well before the fateful transition team meeting on January 11. He was going to choose managed competition over the much simpler play-or-pay. He was going to strive for budget neutrality despite the transition team's estimates, or their lack of enthusiasm for cost control. When Stuart Altman objected to the complexity of the plan and the amount of change it would require, he could have stood on his head in the governor's mansion and it would not have made a difference.

Could Bill Clinton have succeeded with a different strategy? It would have been exceedingly difficult, but we will never know for sure. There were numerous obstacles in addition to the substance of the plan.

A major problem was leadership. Bill Clinton won the election, but only with 43 percent of the vote. He might have been able to claim a mandate for his platform early in his presidency, but by the time his health bill reached the Congress he was weakened by numerous scandals.

The congressional leadership was also weak, and the Democratic Party was divided. In the House, Speaker Tom Foley was not a strong leader. John Dingell, the chair of the Energy and Commerce Committee, had a 27–17 majority and could not report out a bill. Dan Rostenkowski was the strongest leader in the House, but he was indicted on May 31, 2004 and resigned his chairmanship of the Ways and Means Committee. The Senate had a strong leader in George Mitchell, who may have sacrificed a seat on the Supreme Court in order to champion health care reform. However, the chair of the key Senate Finance Committee, Daniel Patrick Moynihan, was focused on welfare reform and largely disinterested in health. The Democratic leadership in both houses could not satisfy the liberals and still hold the Blue Dog Democrats, who were fiscally conservative and generally did not favor an expanded government role in health care. And, of course, regardless of the bill's provisions, there would be no votes coming from the Republican minority.

The problem was not that stakeholders opposed health reform. Large insurance, small insurance, doctors, hospitals, large employers, small employers, drug companies, labor unions—every interest group wanted to benefit from an increased number of insured customers. In the beginning, nearly every group supported the concept of universal coverage and health care reform. But, when it came time to apportion the burden, no one wanted to pay a price. They met repeatedly with the transition team, the task force, the leaders from the administration and Congress, and they all were willing to support a plan from which they could benefit. But, in the end, they all succumbed to Altman's Law:

"Nearly every major interest group favors universal coverage and health system reform, but, if the plan deviates from their preferred approach, they would rather retain the status quo."

You might have thought that this was something the Clintons and their advisors would be well aware of. Certainly Stuart Altman was. He had learned it twenty years earlier with Richard Nixon, and now wondered if he would have to go through it again with Barack Obama.

# CHAPTER 3

# THE PAST FORESHADOWS
# THE PRESENT
## EARLY ATTEMPTS WITH LITTLE SUCCESS

### A Plot by the Kaiser and the Bolsheviks

Long before Bill Clinton and Richard Nixon, there were other failed attempts to enact national health insurance in the United States. Germany instituted health insurance for industrial workers in 1883, and England insured low-income workers in 1911. In the early 1900s, progressive social reformers in the United States watched what was happening in Europe and tried to secure similar protection for American workers. The American Association for Labor Legislation (AALL) was organized in 1905 and fought a successful battle for workman's compensation. National Health Insurance was next on their agenda, and they won the support of Theodore Roosevelt, who ran for president in 1912, but he lost the election to Woodrow Wilson.

The AALL released its first comprehensive proposal in 1915 to insure low-income workers and their dependents.[1] Portending many future battles for health insurance, interest group politics was largely responsible for defeating the issue. For a short time, however, the interest groups were on the opposite side of where they are today. Ironically, the AMA originally supported the effort but the American Federation of Labor (AF of L) was opposed.[2]

Samuel Gompers, the President of the AF of L and the most powerful labor leader of the time, argued that unions, and not government, should supply worker benefits.[3] Government health insurance, he contended, would replace the need for unions to secure workers' rights and benefits.[4] In fact, Gompers opposed all government protections, including the minimum wage, unemployment insurance, old-age pensions, and the eight-hour day.[5] Not all of labor supported Gompers's reasoning, and few people today would give back those government protections. Nevertheless, given the decline of labor unions in the United States, one might ponder how much stronger unions would be today if they were the sole providers of those benefits.

As support for the AALL's proposal began to grow, the AMA reversed its position. Reformers, even in 1915, wanted to replace fee-for-service doctor's fees with capitation and wanted to transition from individual, uncoordinated physicians to group practices.[6] The AMA saw both of these recommendations as threats to physicians' incomes and autonomy. Thus began its long and vitriolic opposition, not only to these specific policies that many still recommend but also to any form of national health insurance.

The AALL estimated the cost of their program would be 4 percent of wages.[7] Similar to many recent proposals, employers and employees would share the cost (although government would contribute 20 percent). Business interests did not like the mandated cost and feared it would escalate beyond the original estimates. Thus, the National Association of Manufacturers and other business interests began their long opposition to employer-based health benefits and national health insurance.

Insurance companies also provided significant opposition. At the time, industrial life insurance was sold to workers throughout the manufacturing sector. It provided death benefits that paid funeral expenses and helped cover the cost of terminal illnesses. It was a large part of insurance company profits, but was incredibly inefficient, requiring agents to go out and physically collect about twenty-five cents per week from each individual worker.[8] The AALL proposal included funeral benefits and thus threatened to reduce insurance company profits. Hence, another special interest began their long opposition to national health insurance.

Many across the political spectrum were familiar with European programs and recognized the need to provide health insurance to workers. Yet business, labor, organized medicine, and the insurance industry all found specific reasons to oppose the AALL initiative. If any part of the proposal threatened their interests, they would prefer the status quo. It was Altman's Law twenty years before Stuart Altman was born.

The final nail in the coffin of the AALL's efforts also resonates with familiarity. The United States entered World War I in 1917. Opponents denounced national health insurance, first initiated by Kaiser Wilhelm, as part of a German plot to take over the free world. Then, following the Bolshevik revolution in Russia, postwar America became virulently anticommunist. Opponents claimed that national health insurance was the tool of social-ists and communists—rhetoric that still reverberates today in the halls of Congress.

## FDR and the Missing Piece of the New Deal

After suffering its initial defeat, the issue of national health insurance did not resurface for another generation—a cycle that would repeat itself for nearly a century. It was not until 1934 that Franklin Roosevelt considered a national health proposal as part of his New Deal legislation. FDR appointed the Advisory Committee on Economic Security to consider old-age pen-sions, unemployment insurance, and health insurance. In the wake of the Depression, pension and unemployment benefits were much more pressing than health. Although FDR supported the concept of national health insur-ance, he faced strong political opposition from interest groups and the Con-gress. Fearing that opposition to a health care proposal would endanger his Social Security legislation, he had the Advisory Committee issue its report without any proposal for health insurance.

As the battle for Social Security continued, FDR quietly kept the health issue alive. He instructed Henry Perkins, the head of the Committee on Economic Security, to prepare recommendations in secret for a system of national health insurance. Perkins delivered his recommendations in June, but the president, not wanting to risk losing the battle for Social Security, did not release the secret report. We now know that the report recommended state-run programs subsidized by the federal government.[9] Participation by each state would be voluntary, but within any state that chose to participate, all workers of "small and moderate means" (and, at the option of the state, their employers) would be required to pay a proportion of earnings into a common fund. In return, the workers and their families would receive health insurance benefits that would vary by state but would meet minimum fed-eral standards (including, at least, coverage for hospital and physician fees). The federal government would provide subsidies to states based on the number of insured residents but with an initial global budget of sixty mil-lion dollars per year.

The report was particularly deferential to both states' rights and the autonomy of the medical profession, two hurdles that still exist today. Nevertheless, FDR understood that his opponents were unlikely to be appeased and kept the existence of the report secret until after Social Security was enacted in August. Then, characteristic of his presidential machinations, he made no public mention of the report, avoiding any negative political fallout, but kept the issue alive by quietly forwarding it to the Social Security Board for further study.

The main opposition had come from the AMA. It actively opposed any government involvement in medicine as well as any form of public or private health insurance. Furthermore, it was concerned about doctors' incomes. With many people unable to afford medical services because of the Depression, the reduced demand had lowered doctors' incomes. Rather than support health insurance or other ways to expand services, Walter Bierring, the incoming president of the AMA in 1934, recommended closing half of the country's medical schools, thus dividing revenues among fewer doctors.[10] In the same year, the Council on Medical Education warned about an over-supply of doctors, causing medical school admissions to decline for the following six years.[11] Clearly, the medical establishment was focused more on doctor's incomes than making health services more widely accessible.

Republican conservatives and southern Democrats were also opposed to national health legislation. Labor unions had abandoned their opposition during the Depression, but in 1934 they were focused on unemployment insurance and Social Security, and not national health care.

FDR was a consummate politician. Despite his support for a national health program, he was not willing to pursue it at the risk of political defeat. He was acutely aware of his opposition, and, rather than initiate a stormy fight with vested interests, he waited until the political winds were more to his advantage. As careful as he was engineering the United States' entry into World War II, he was even more cautious with national health insurance. Three times during his presidency he brought the issue to the fore. The first two times, he withdrew his support to avoid a fight and protect the rest of his agenda, but he kept the issue alive within the executive branch. The third time, he died before the legislation was filed.

His second attempt occurred three years after the first. In the intervening time, he had created another commission and study group to make recommendations for national health insurance. Their proposal was similar to the one in the 1935, and the president convened a major conference in July of 1938 to present their recommendations. Enthused by the conference, FDR initially indicated he would make national health an issue in the 1938 midterm elections. However, political opposition soon convinced him otherwise.

Although Democrats had large majorities in both houses of Congress, conservatives and southern Democrats formed a bloc that was strongly opposed. In an attempt to isolate the supporters of national health insurance, the AMA reversed its opposition to private insurance and supported every other health care expansion except a national health insurance program. FDR, trying to change the political balance, actually campaigned against conservatives in his own party including Walter George, the senator from Georgia. Despite the president's efforts, conservatives and southern Democrats gained greater power in the 1938 elections, and Walter George became chair of the powerful Senate Finance Committee. Again biding his time, the president quietly forwarded the national health proposal to Congress in January 1939 with no endorsement or recommendation. For a second time, he had advanced and then withdrew his support for national health insurance.

In February, Robert Wagner, the liberal senator from New York, submitted a bill incorporating the recommendations made by Roosevelt's committee. FDR did not endorse the effort, and it was easily defeated by political opponents and the AMA. Then, in September, Germany invaded Poland, Britain and France entered the war, and FDR focused on building up America's defense. The scenario of 1917 had repeated itself—first when interest groups prevailed and then when war intervened.

World War II was the catalyst for FDR's most important health policy legacy, but, ironically, it was not what the president envisioned. In 1942, with the demand from war production threatening to cause inflation, he instituted wage and price controls. Employers were competing for scarce labor and, since they could not raise wages, many started offering health insurance benefits to attract workers. FDR's War Labor Board ruled that employer-provided health insurance benefits did not count as wages. If they weren't wages, it followed that they shouldn't be taxed. In October 1943, the Internal Revenue Service (IRS) reached that very conclusion, formally deciding that the cost of health insurance benefits was a deductible expense for employers and was not taxable income for employees. That decision would have far-reaching consequences. FDR, the father of Social Security and the first presidential advocate for a system of publicly provided health insurance, had inadvertently provided a strong, government-supported financial incentive for the growth of the private insurance market.

Roosevelt initiated one more attempt before his death. With the war seemingly approaching a favorable end, FDR recommended "cradle to grave" social insurance in his 1943 State of the Union address.[12] Then, the following June, Robert Wagner introduced the Wagner–Murray–Dingell bill for national health insurance. The proponents knew that the bill had no chance of passing. However, it put the issue back on the national agenda. For the first time the bill departed from previous state-run proposals and recommended a universal, compulsory federal program financed by employer and employee payroll taxes. It was the forerunner to every serious universal health proposal that has been made since. FDR never directly endorsed the Wagner bill, but in 1944 he campaigned for an "economic bill of rights" that included national health. Then, in his State of the Union address in January 1945, he called for a comprehensive bill including health insurance, disability protection, and hospital construction. The president finally seemed prepared to take on the AMA and complete the long-awaited last chapter of the New Deal. But on April 12, 1945, FDR died suddenly of a cerebral hemorrhage. The ball was in Harry Truman's court.

## Truman Takes Up the Cause
## (When WMD Meant Wagner–Murray–Dingell)

Unlike Franklin Roosevelt, Harry Truman was passionate about national health care. Whereas FDR was cautious and politically practical, Truman was ardent, committed, and aggressive. Even in the face of opposition and near-certain defeat, Truman tried to rally the country behind his program. Five months after taking office and less than a month after the war ended, he affirmed his support for FDR's health care agenda. Then, two months later, in November 1945, he delivered a special message to Congress. In that message Harry Truman became the first president to support a single-payer, comprehensive, and compulsory program of national health insurance. He believed that every American should have access to adequate health services, and unlike FDR and his predecessors, he was not willing to accept a separate system for the poor. His words reflect an agenda that is still supported by liberals:

> Everyone should have ready access to all necessary medical, hospital and related services. I recommend solving the basic problem by distributing the

costs through expansion of our existing compulsory social insurance system. This is not socialized medicine. Everyone who carries fire insurance knows how the law of averages is made to work so as to spread the risk, and to benefit the insured who actually suffers the loss. If instead of the costs of sickness being paid only by those who get sick, all the people—sick and well—were required to pay premiums into an insurance fund, the pool of funds thus created would enable all who do fall sick to be adequately served without overburdening anyone. That is the principle upon which all forms of insurance are based....I repeat—what I am recommending is not socialized medicine. Socialized medicine means that all doctors work as employees of government. The American people want no such system. No such system is here proposed.[13]

The proposal was comprehensive and included federal aid for hospital construction; programs for public, maternal, and child health; federal aid for research and education; and protection against disability.

Truman not only expected cries of socialism but also anticipated opposition from the medical establishment. Hoping to blunt opposition, he promised to "pay most doctors more than the best they have received in peacetime years." He also promised that doctors' participation would be voluntary, and his program would require neither organizational reform nor restrictions on doctors' or patients' freedom of choice.

Despite his assurances, the reaction to his proposal was vitriolic. Senator Murray (D-MT), the chair of the Committee on Education and Labor, incorporated Truman's recommendations in the Wagner–Murray–Dingell bill (WMD), filed in April of 1946. In the first hearing, Murray became involved in a confrontation with the conservative senator Robert Taft, who interrupted the chairman, stating "I consider it socialism. It is to my mind the most socialistic measure this Congress has ever had before it."[14] After a heated exchange with Murray, Taft threatened a Republican boycott of the hearings and walked out.

The AMA was no less strident, claiming "Truman's health insurance plan would make doctors slaves,"[15] and they called Truman's White House staffers "followers of the Moscow party line."[16] They organized a lobbying and public relations campaign to oppose the bill and recommended the expansion of private insurance with subsidies for the poor. They were supported by the American Hospital Association (AHA), the American Bar Association, the Catholic and Protestant Hospital Associations and the

National Grange, all of whom opposed Truman's efforts.[17] Even parts of Truman's own health administration opposed the bill, fearing it would diminish funds for their own particular programs.

The bill never had a chance. It failed to get a hearing in the House and died in the Senate. However, before the session was over, Congress separately passed the first part of Truman's proposal, the Hill–Burton bill for hospital construction. It was an easy bill to pass, giving state legislators the power to distribute federal funds in their districts to build new hospitals. However, as we shall see in the next chapter, it had far-reaching effects.

Senator Murray promised to refile WMD after the midterm elections in 1946, but the vote went against the Democrats. The Republicans gained control of both houses of Congress, and Taft became the chair of Education and Labor. In 1947, anticommunist sentiment was spreading throughout the country, and national health legislation had no chance of passing the Congress. Nevertheless, the feisty president was undaunted and submitted yet another proposal for national health care. It never got a hearing.

In the famous presidential campaign of 1948, in which Truman came from far behind to beat Dewey, the president campaigned against the Republican "do-nothing Congress." With the Progressive Henry Wallace running against him on the left, Truman seized upon the issue of national health, hammering the Republican Congress for ignoring his previous proposals.

Following his unexpected victory, he submitted his health plan in April of 1949. However, interest group opposition had not abated. The AMA, panicked by Truman's unexpected victory, launched the largest and most expensive lobbying campaign in American history. An oft-quoted AMA pamphlet read, "Would socialized medicine lead to socialization of other phases of American life? Lenin thought so. He declared 'Socialized medicine is the keystone to the arch of the socialist state.'"[18] There is no evidence that Lenin ever said this. However, the repeated warnings about socialized medicine became so ingrained over time that the president of the Association of American Physicians and Surgeons repeated the fabricated quote during the 2000 presidential campaign.[19]

In addition to opposition from the AMA, Congress remained an impenetrable obstacle. Nearly all Republicans remained opposed. Southern Democrats were already angry with Truman because of his civil rights agenda, and in 1949, the thought of federally directed health benefits for all southern citizens, including blacks, was unacceptable. Within the Congress there were alternative proposals, some truly seeking alternative strategies and others proposed simply as roadblocks to more liberal plans. Thus, Taft submitted a bill granting subsidies to states to provide medical services to the poor. Senators Hill and Aiken proposed federal aid to help states subsidize private insurance for the poor. And Richard Nixon, already thinking about the presidency, submitted a proposal with the liberal Republican Jacob Javits for a system of private insurance with federal subsidies that would vary with income. Despite the various proposals, the defeat of health legislation in 1949 was not primarily a result of competing proposals. In fact, it could barely be called a defeat as Truman's proposal never got out of committee. Interest group opposition was just too powerful, and the anticommunist attitude was pushing the country to the right. Even the feisty president became less aggressive in his support. Then, in February 1950, Joe McCarthy began his anticommunist crusade; and on June 25, America entered the Korean War. If the slightest chance to enact national health care ever existed, it was clearly gone.

Nevertheless, there was a silver lining. Oscar Ewing, the first secretary of HEW, convinced Truman to pursue a more incremental goal. If Congress would not support health insurance for everyone, maybe it would support it for one sympathetic group: elderly Americans over the age of sixty-four. In April 1952 Senators Murray and Humphrey (D-MN) and Representatives Dingell and Celler (D-NY) filed a new health bill. As expected, the initiative was largely ignored, and no congressional action was taken. However, the battle for Medicare had begun.

## The Past Frames the Future

The issues that confronted Barack Obama, Richard Nixon, and Bill Clinton were not new. In fact, by the time of Obama's presidency many were nearly a century old, and they illustrate the importance of understanding the present by studying the past.

As early as 1915, the AALL proposed financing health insurance with employer and employee payroll deductions, earning the everlasting opposition of business. Even the earliest reformers recommended capitation in place of fee-for-service medicine and suggested coordinated groups of physicians in place of individual practitioners. FDR confronted the issue of states' rights versus federal control in 1935, and every serious health bill since has dealt with that issue—one that was filled with racial overtones until after Lyndon Johnson and the civil rights movement. FDR tried to placate the medical establishment by guaranteeing doctor and patient freedom of choice and promising that government would not interfere with the delivery system or the professional autonomy of physicians. Despite his efforts, he never earned their support and, to a large extent, neither did those who followed. FDR's proposal even contained a global budget, a policy option that haunted the Clinton effort.

Harry Truman was the first president to insist on a universal system for both the rich and the poor. He also was the first president to support a single-payer and a mandate for every citizen to participate in order to broaden the pool for health insurance.

Altman's Law was evident as early as 1917. Interest group politics, particularly the strength of the AMA, organized business, and insurance companies, was instrumental in blocking legislation throughout the twentieth century. And every battle for national health reform has pitted liberal Democrats who advocate expansion of government-financed insurance against Republicans and conservatives who favor the private market and tax credits. All of these present-day issues and political obstacles had their roots deep in the American past.

Perhaps the most important legacy to emerge from these past events was the way they framed the future. The tax advantage conferred on employer-provided health benefits under FDR sowed the seeds for the emergence of private health insurance; and the failure to enact a public program enabled those seeds to blossom. One should not underestimate the impact of the tax advantage. In 1940, less than ten million Americans had health insurance. By 1950, that number had exploded to 76.6 million. Suddenly, over half the American population had private health insurance, and enrollment was growing rapidly. Any new proposal for national health would have to change a system that was already entrenched. By the time Truman left office, the framework of the American health care system had been constructed, and its foundation was private health insurance.

The emerging private system achieved much success in expanding insurance and providing comprehensive health benefits to its enrollees. Health technology was much less sophisticated than today and costs were lower. Hence, insurance premiums were widely affordable. Nearly all large employers offered health benefits, and by 1960, 68 percent of Americans had private health insurance.[20] Nevertheless, many doubts about the tax exclusion began to surface.

As we discussed in chapter 1, economists generally agree that the tax exclusion made the net cost of health insurance artificially low, and insurance insulated consumers from the real cost of health care services. As a result, health spending began to skyrocket. Between 1948 and 1958, per capita spending increased by 82 percent. Although out-of-pocket spending rose by a more modest 48 percent, payments by insurance companies increased by 442 percent.

Arguments remain for and against the tax credit, and we address them in a later chapter. But in the '50s, with most of the population insured, the revenue lost from the federal tax exclusion grew rapidly. In 1953, the IRS changed its mind and repealed the tax exclusion. By that time, however, it was too entrenched. Citizens had become accustomed to the tax break, and unions had traded wage increases for health benefits in collective bargaining. President Eisenhower easily persuaded Congress to reverse the IRS ruling, solidifying the tax advantage in the Revenue Act of 1954.

It soon became apparent that the nascent system of employer-provided health benefits had some problems. It worked for middle- and upper-class citizens who purchased private health policies and for those who received health benefits from employers. However, the elderly, the poor, the sick, and the unemployed often could not afford or could not buy private insurance, so a need developed for government assistance. Health care costs continued to increase, and tens of millions of Americans became uninsured and unable to afford care. In response, the United States developed a patchwork of separate programs rather than a coordinated, universal system, insuring people in separate groups. Thus, the elderly got Medicare and the poor got Medicaid. There were separate programs for children and for individual diseases such as kidney failure and AIDS. And the uninsured, who didn't fit into any group, relied on charity and federal requirements that hospitals provide care to those who could not pay. Historical events forced the country to insure its citizens piece by piece. It is to these piecemeal parts of America's health care system that we turn next.

## PART 2

# EXPANDING HEALTH COVERAGE PIECE BY PIECE

# CHAPTER 4

# THE HILL-BURTON PROGRAM
## HOW AMERICA'S UNINSURED POOR GOT A RIGHT TO FREE HOSPITAL CARE

### What Was the Right Number?

Stuart Altman had no idea what the number should be. In the entire history of the country, the government had never given the uninsured poor any legal right to receive medical care. But in 1970, patients began suing HEW. They claimed hospitals that had received grants from the twenty-four-year-old Hill–Burton program were obligated to give them free care.

If that was the case, Altman asked himself, how much free care should hospitals have to provide? Should it depend on the size of the Hill–Burton grant? The size of the hospital? The needs of the community? The financial strength of the hospital? There simply was no precedent. Altman had just joined HEW. Elliott Richardson, the secretary of HEW, was his boss, and he wanted to know the number.

Altman worked closely with Scott Fleming, who had also recently joined HEW from Kaiser Permanante. Fleming had given up a lucrative and prestigious position as a senior vice president to join the Nixon administration and help shape federal health policy. In a bureaucratic moment that could only happen in government, Fleming arrived in Washington and thought someone already had his job. As it turned out, Altman's title was deputy assistant secretary for planning and evaluation/health, and Fleming's was deputy assistant secretary for health/planning and evaluation. Despite the overlap, they developed a good working relationship and collaborated on a number of important initiatives including the Health Maintenance Organization Act of 1973 and the Health Planning and Resource Act of 1974.

With the help of the legal office at HEW, Altman and Fleming examined the data and recommended a requirement of 5 percent. Any hospital that accepted grant money under the Hill–Burton program had to provide free care at a minimum annual rate of 5 percent of its total yearly operating costs, or 25 percent of its net profit—whichever was less. Richardson approved their recommendation and published the decision as a draft regulation on April 18, 1972. In actuality, hospitals provided uncompensated care (free care + bad debt) in amounts between 5.1 and 6.4 percent of costs every year from 1980 through 2007.[1] But that was not the case in the early '70s, and the AHA went ballistic! How were nonprofit hospitals going to afford to give that much free care? HEW received more than two thousand letters opposing the draft regulations.[2] An AHA survey showed that only 14 percent of hospitals in the country presently met that requirement.[3] The AHA claimed that 93 percent of hospitals would have to raise prices by more than 4 percent to finance that much charity care.[4]

After intense lobbying from the AHA and its members, Richardson asked Altman and Fleming to review their analysis and see if a lower number was more appropriate. After their review, Richardson issued new regulations requiring Hill–Burton hospitals to provide annual charity care equal to 3 percent of their yearly operating costs or 10 percent of the amount of their grant—whichever was less—and to file an annual report. Alternatively, they could simply agree not to refuse any indigent patient who requested care. The new regulation was issued on July 22, 1972, and affected 6,300 federally financed hospitals and health care institutions.[5] Over the years, this federal requirement would rank just behind Medicare and Medicaid as the largest source of subsidized care to low-income patients. But in 1972, for the first time, American hospitals had a legal obligation to provide medical care for individuals who were unable to pay.

## The Hill–Burton Act of 1946

In 1945, many areas of the country lacked adequate hospital facilities. The Depression and then the war resulted in a dearth of new construction. Many existing facilities were old and obsolete, and 40 percent of US counties had no hospitals at all. Most hospitals were public or nonprofit institutions, and it was difficult for them to raise funds for construction. In the last year of FDR's administration, Senators Lister Hill (D-AL) and Harold Burton

(R-OH) filed a bill to provide federal grants for hospital construction. It made no mention of providing services to the poor.

FDR died on April 12, 1945, and the war ended in August. In November, the new president, Harry Truman, unveiled his universal health care program. Truman's proposal included a program for hospital construction, but he did not have sufficient support in Congress for his comprehensive plan. Meanwhile, the Hill–Burton bill, an incremental federal aid program popular with both political parties and the AHA, was moving through the Congress.

The congressional debate in October 1945 contained many of the political divisions that still exist today. The Democratic liberals, led by Robert Wagner and James Murray, wanted to broaden Hill–Burton to a system of national health insurance financed by Social Security. In May, they had introduced the Wagner–Murray bill (later becoming Wagner–Murray–Dingell), the same bill that is still introduced at the beginning of each congressional session by Dingell's son, John Dingell Jr. (D-MI). However, their attempt garnered little support.

Senator Murray was upset because Hill–Burton gave so much power to the states. Although the federal government was providing the funds, it would have no discretion on how the money was distributed. Funding would be allocated to the states strictly by a formula, and the states would award the individual grants for hospital construction. Murray complained that state management of hospitals had a poor history and it was wiser to institute more federal control.

Republicans, led by presidential hopeful William Howard Taft, wanted to maximize state control and minimize intrusion by the federal government. Taft called Truman's national health insurance plan socialism, but he supported the incremental Hill–Burton program as long as the states maintained control. He also supported inclusion of the "Federal Hospital Council," a body of industry and consumer experts who would have to approve the oversight decisions of the responsible federal authority—at the time, the surgeon general. Murray and the liberals opposed the council because it would further weaken federal control.

Republicans and conservatives carried the day. Burton left the Senate, accepting Truman's appointment to the Supreme Court, and Hill "tended to give Taft anything he wanted."[6] Taft devised the formula for allocating federal funds. It correctly favored rural, southern, and poorer states—the places that hospital construction was most needed. It also required the community to raise matching funds, as the bill would provide grants for no more than one-third of project costs. Murray argued that poor communities would not be able to raise the matching funds. Furthermore, he contended, poor communities would not be able to earn sufficient revenues to operate and maintain their facilities. He argued that the Social Security Act should be amended to pay for hospital care for the poor. Otherwise, hospitals built with Hill–Burton funds could not sustain themselves in poor communities where many of the patients could not afford to pay. What was the point of constructing hospitals in communities that would not be able to afford to operate them?

Taft agreed, stating, "The very places hospitals are most needed are the places they cannot operate without getting assistance for operation and maintenance."[7] The conservative Taft was not about to support federal health insurance, but he was amenable to a compromise with liberal advocates. It may not have seemed very much to the liberals at the time, but two important concessions were written into the bill.

The first became known as the *community service obligation*. Hospitals constructed with Hill–Burton funds could not discriminate on account of race, creed, or color. The second became known as the *uncompensated care obligation*. Hospitals constructed with Hill–Burton funds had to devote "a reasonable amount of services" to people who were unable to pay.

Although the two concessions were granted, no funds were appropriated to provide assistance for the operation and maintenance of hospitals, and "reasonable amount of services" was never defined. Notwithstanding the vague requirements, the Hospital Survey and Construction Act, popularly known as Hill–Burton, became law on August 13, 1946.

## Intended and Unintended Consequences

Hill–Burton spurred a renaissance in hospital construction. By 1968, it had assisted in financing 9,200 new medical facilities and 416,000 new inpatient beds.[8] When expenditures for the initial program ended in 1975, Hill–Burton had assisted in financing almost one-third of all hospital projects in the country.[9] Many rural areas had access to hospital care for the first time.[10] Eventually, the law was extended to provide loans and to help finance nursing homes and rehabilitation centers. By the year 2000, more than $4.6

billion in grants and $1.5 billion in loans had helped build facilities in over four thousand communities.[11] As a program to increase the number of health facilities, Hill–Burton was spectacularly successful.

Nevertheless, it had a number of shortcomings. Hill–Burton grants required communities to raise matching funds and to show that projects would be financially viable. As a consequence, many poor communities, often the places that most needed new health facilities, could not qualify. Hence, the formula developed by Senator Taft successfully allocated funds to the states most in need, but, within those states, most of the funds went to middle class communities. Of the billions of dollars in Hill–Burton grants, few ever reached poor or nonwhite communities.

Southern black communities had an additional problem. The community service obligation secured by liberals forbade discrimination on account of race. In 1946, the South was racially segregated, and southern senators were not about to vote for a federal program that would integrate their hospitals. Yet southern Democratic votes were needed to pass Hill–Burton through the Senate. To secure their votes, Lister Hill added a provision to the bill allowing "separate but equal facilities."[12] The practical effect was that black people in the South could not access Hill–Burton hospitals until 1963 when separate but equal public facilities were ruled unconstitutional.

The uncompensated care requirement was also a problem. The government simply ignored it. The bill specified that the surgeon general and the Federal Hospital Council (mentioned earlier) would issue specific regulations regarding the details of the program. However, the Council, largely made up of hospital industry representatives, had no interest in enforcing the free care obligation, and no action was taken.

By 1970, billions of dollars of federal money had been granted and allocated to medically underserved states with the express statutory intention "to furnish adequate hospital, clinic, or similar services to all their people." In addition, those facilities had to make available "a reasonable volume of services to persons unable to pay." Yet, hardly any facilities were built in the poorest, neediest communities, racial discrimination in the South excluded blacks from those facilities, and the free care requirement was completely ignored. Completely ignored, that is, except by one person in Washington, a young attorney by the name of Marilyn Rose.

## Marilyn Rose—One Person Can Make a Difference

Marilyn Rose received her Bachelor of Arts degree from Brandeis University in 1956. From there she attended Harvard Law School, graduating cum laude in 1959. After working in national labor relations, she joined HEW, becoming the acting chief of the Health Civil Rights Branch from 1966 to 1968.[13] During her work at HEW she discovered the community service and uncompensated care obligations in the Hill–Burton Act. Realizing their potential to provide access to hospital care for the uninsured poor, she wrote an internal memorandum explaining how they could be utilized. Her memo was ignored.

In 1968, she left HEW and transferred to the Department of Labor. In the course of her work, she met the director of the National Legal Program on Health Problems of the Poor (currently, the National Health Law Program or Nhelp).[14] Rose joined Nhelp, relocating to Los Angeles in October 1969.[15]

The '60s were the heyday of civil rights enforcement and the war on poverty. Throughout the decade numerous public service law firms organized to help the poor and disadvantaged, and the government created a number of agencies to enforce civil rights legislation. Among those was the Office of Economic Opportunity (OEO), created by Lyndon Johnson in 1964 and directed by Sargent Shriver. OEO coordinated such programs as Head Start, the Job Corps, and VISTA (Volunteers in Service to America). The Nhelp was funded by OEO.

Marilyn Rose took on the enforcement deficiencies of the Hill–Burton plan as a cause célèbre. Within five months of joining Nhelp, she published two papers arguing that Hill–Burton hospitals had a statutory obligation to provide free care.[16] Moreover, she contended that individuals who were denied such care had standing to take legal action and could do so through class action lawsuits.[17] No enforcement of the free care clause had occurred since the law was passed in 1946. However, Rose published her interest in representing individuals who had been denied care and then traveled around the country looking for potential test cases.[18] As a result she became the attorney of record in several lawsuits, including the groundbreaking case of *Cook v. Ochsner Foundation Hospital.*

In July 1970, Rose represented eight plaintiffs in metropolitan New Orleans who had been denied care at ten Ochsner Foundation Hospitals. She brought suit claiming the hospitals, which had accepted Hill–Burton grants, had an obligation to provide free care. The hospitals claimed the individual plaintiffs had no right to bring a legal action, but the court disagreed and granted them standing. Before the case was decided, claimants in at least three similar cases were given standing, including a case that Rose won on appeal in Colorado.

Although HEW had never issued any enforcement action on Hill–Burton, it filed an amicus brief in support of Rose in Colorado and announced it was drafting regulations for standards of enforcement.[19] At the time, the courts had not mandated a response from HEW, but Secretary Richardson apparently agreed with the initial court decisions. The extent of President Nixon's support is not known. But suddenly, after twenty-five years of inaction, HEW decided to require Hill–Burton hospitals to provide a minimum amount of free care. But how much should they be required to provide? Marilyn Rose had almost single-handedly pushed the HEW secretary to address the question. And that was when Richardson turned to Stuart Altman, Scott Fleming, and their colleagues for the answer.

## A Rose-Colored Legal Trail

Marilyn Rose not only pursued her own cases, but she provided training sessions at Nhelp conventions for other poverty attorneys with similar interests. As the cases were adjudicated, they kept extending the obligations of hospitals and granting broader individual rights to patients. In *Corum v. Beth Israel Medical Center*, the court ruled that hospitals must give prospective patients a written determination of eligibility for free care before rendering service. Otherwise, if people were not told in advance whether they had an obligation to pay, poor people, fearing the cost and/or legal collection efforts, might be deterred from seeking care. HEW incorporated the decision into their pending regulations.

When the Cook case was finally adjudicated, Rose argued that Ochsner's denial of service to Medicaid patients, who made up 11 percent of the population of metropolitan New Orleans, "constituted discrimination in violation of the community service obligation."[20] HEW again amended its regulations to require Hill–Burton hospitals to participate in the Medicaid program.

In 1974, the Nixon administration folded Hill–Burton into the National Health Planning and Resources Act. The Hill–Burton court decisions and the HEW regulatory response incited Congress to demand stronger enforcement. Title 16 of The Public Health Service Act of 1975 specified that HEW would become the primary enforcement authority, replacing the states, and that it would be responsible for monitoring hospital compliance.[21]

Two later court decisions resulted in still more stringent regulations. In *Lugo v. Simon*, HEW entered into a consent decree to develop new regulations that would set forth a specific program to monitor compliance of Hill–Burton hospitals. The department agreed to make copies of the proposed regulations available for public comment and to mail copies to a list of nine hundred names provided by the attorney for the plaintiff, Marilyn Rose.

Finally, the *Newsom v. Vanderbilt* case marked the high point for poverty law advocates. Callie Mae Newsom overstayed her Medicaid coverage because of a complicated pregnancy. Never informing her of her Hill–Burton eligibility, the hospital sued and turned her case over to a collection agency that eventually garnished her wages. In his judicial decision, Judge Morton cited two articles authored by Rose.[22] According to Morton's decision, each individual, indigent patient had a "constitutionally protected right" to receive care under the Hill–Burton Act and, therefore, Callie Mae Newsom had due process rights that the hospital had violated.

With the Newsom decision, the initial understanding of the Hill–Burton law had been completely reversed. What began as the hospital's obligation to provide a reasonable amount of care to an undefined class of people had become an individual's constitutional right to receive care—what James Blumstein called "a privately financed mini-Medicaid program."[23] Judge Morton was prepared to issue a mandate to HEW to change its regulations, but the department promised that new regulations were already being formulated in response to the Lugo and Newsom decisions. The new regulations, adopted in 1979, not only required hospitals to meet the 3 percent (or 10 percent of grant) standard, but to create an affirmative action program to seek out uncompensated care if they fell below the required level. Hospitals also had to provide patients with written notice of eligibility criteria for Hill–Burton free care and written reasons for any denial of care. Furthermore, any patient denied care had the right to appeal.

## Irony of Ironies

Of all the Hill–Burton court decisions that favored indigent plaintiffs, none were appealed. HEW accepted the rulings of the district courts and issued stricter regulations in response. But after Judge Morton's decision in Newsom, Vanderbilt University filed an appeal. The Sixth Circuit Court of Appeals reversed much of Morton's decision. The court stated that although individual patients were eligible to be considered for free care, no individual had any entitlement to free care. Furthermore, without any entitlement, no individual had to be granted due process.

In his *Iowa Law Review* article, James Blumstein summarized the court's analysis of the legislative history this way: Congress clearly never intended Hill–Burton hospitals to meet the country's total need for uncompensated care. Hence, services had to be allocated to only a portion of those who were eligible. The statute stated neither how services should be allocated nor granted any right to individuals to receive services. Nor did the 1975 Public Health Service Act. All indigent patients were eligible for consideration as a class, but it was up to the discretion of the hospital to allocate services. The hospital had an obligation to meet the free care requirements of the total class, but no individual patient had a right to legal redress.[24]   ·

The decision of the sixth circuit court of appeals nullified many of the legal rights Rose and her colleagues had fought for over the past decade. Ironically, however, it had no effect on the 1979 Hill–Burton regulations. One reason was the action was brought in 1978, before the new regulations were promulgated. A second reason was the appeal concerned the right of Callie Mae Newsom, as an individual, to sue for denial of free care. Despite the fact that the appeals court ruled against her, the HEW regulations were not a matter that was before the court.

HEW issued new regulations on May 18, 1979. The AHA, which had been watching the obligations of its member hospitals grow over the decade of adverse decisions, filed a lawsuit on June 27 to invalidate the new regulations. Challenging a federal agency's rulemaking process, however, is much different than appealing a class action lawsuit. Courts rarely interfere with government agencies that make rules, in accordance with a law called the Administrative Procedures Act. To invalidate the rules, the court would have to find them "arbitrary, capricious, an abuse of discretion, or otherwise not in accordance with law."[25] The AHA lost its case.

Despite the Newsom reversal and the AHA challenge, the 1979 regulations remained in effect.

## A Watershed for the Poor

Ask almost anyone who has heard of Hill–Burton, and they will tell you it was a program for hospital construction. Indeed it was, and a very successful program at that. Initially, it preserved much of the status quo, allowing states to administer the program at their own discretion. However, the legislation became a milestone granting indigent patients, for the first time in American history, the right to receive hospital care.

Despite the Sixth Circuit Court's reversal, there is no question that the statute required hospitals to provide free care to a class of people. That, in itself, had the potential to be groundbreaking. The irony is that no one might have ever enforced the free care provision if Marilyn Rose had not instituted litigation—and, yet, the basis of the lawsuits that brought about the HEW enforcement was invalidated by the Court of Appeals. Had the defendant hospitals or the AHA or HEW brought or joined in an earlier appeal of the district court decisions, the inaction by the government might never have been challenged.

But in 1970, the Nixon administration was interested in expanding access to health care.[26] As we know, Nixon twice tried to enact national health insurance. He appointed Robert Finch and then Elliott Richardson, both liberal Republicans, to head HEW. Richardson was under no compulsion to file an amicus brief in support of Marilyn Rose in Colorado. Nor was he forced to consider issuing regulations to Hill–Burton in 1971. Had Richardson not acted, it is certainly possible that other kinds of challenges to the law might have occurred, and the federal government might have eventually issued and enforced regulations. However, given the fact that the issue was ignored for twenty-four years, it seems at least as likely that no action would ever have been taken.

Elliott Richardson had a like-minded staff at HEW that supported increased access to health care. When he decided to issue Hill–Burton regulations, he asked his staff for recommendations. As we know, they recommended that each Hill–Burton hospital be required to devote a specific amount of free care to indigent patients. Stuart Altman never reconsidered the matter. "I remember it was a difficult thing to decide," he recalls, "because there was no precedent. We made the recommendation, which was eventually scaled back a little, but afterwards, I never gave it much thought. In fact, until we started writing this book, I had essentially forgotten about it. But Hill–Burton was truly a watershed. It provided free care to millions of poor, uninsured citizens who had no place else to go. And many people believe it was the basis for EMTALA, the Emergency Medical Treatment and Active Labor Act of 1986. That law obligates hospitals to treat and stabilize anyone who arrives in an emergent condition without regard to their ability to pay. Looking back at all the policy issues I've been involved with over the years this, perhaps, might have been the most important!"

# CHAPTER 5

# THE THREE-LAYER CAKE
## LYNDON JOHNSON, WILBUR MILLS, AND THE EPIC BATTLE TO ENACT MEDICARE

### Bargaining with the Devil: The American Medical Association, Medicare, and the Tobacco Industry

The chief impediment blocking Medicare was Wilbur Mills. Health legislation first had to be reported out of the Ways and Means Committee before it could reach the House floor. Chairman Mills and his committee had defeated previous attempts in 1959, 1960, 1961, and 1962. The AMA had mounted huge lobbying and grass roots campaigns to help defeat the bills. Nevertheless, Medicare remained a high priority on John F. Kennedy's domestic agenda, and he thought he had his best chance in 1963.

After the 1962 midterm elections, Ways and Means had fifteen Democrats and ten Republicans. All ten Republicans were opposed, as were two southern Democrats: Sidney Herlock of Florida and John C. Watts of Kentucky. Committee members were evenly divided 12–12, and Chairman Mills represented the thirteenth vote.

Kennedy worked hard during 1963 to gain Mills's support. On October 3, he traveled to Little Rock to dedicate the Greer's Ferry Dam in Mills's congressional district. Rumors abounded that Mills had reached an accommodation with the president on Medicare. His committee began hearings on the Medicare bill (then called King–Anderson) in November, but they were interrupted by Kennedy's assassination.

Mills always sought a clear majority from his committee, and he made it clear that he would not be the deciding thirteenth vote to report Medicare out of Ways and Means. By the time the hearings resumed in January, however, a significant development had taken place. John Watts had changed his mind on Medicare and promised Mills his proxy.[1] That constituted the important thirteenth vote in the committee, and Mills's vote could make it 14–11.

The AMA was apoplectic and willing to go to extraordinary lengths to prevent the bill's passage. It so happened that the surgeon general's report on smoking was released on January 11, 1964. Its conclusions were unambiguous: "Average smokers had a nine- to ten-fold risk of developing lung cancer compared to nonsmokers; and heavy smokers had at least a twenty-fold risk."[2] On February 7, the AMA suggested the surgeon general's report was "inconclusive" and announced it had accepted ten million dollars from six tobacco companies to study the problem.[3] There was an outcry from its members, but the Association published a folder called "Smoking: Facts You Should Know." The folder acknowledged that some researchers warned against the health hazards of smoking. Then, it said:

> Some equally competent physicians and research personnel are less sure of the effect of cigarette smoking on health. They believe the increase in these diseases can be explained by other factors in our complex environment. They advise, "Smoke if you feel you should, but be moderate."[4]

The AMA's position on smoking and health was not coincidental. Frank Thompson, a Democratic congressman from New Jersey said, "The AMA has made a deal with the tobacco industry...to get tobacco-state congressmen to vote against Medicare. It's an outrage."[5]

On June 23, one day before the Ways and Means Committee vote on Medicare (King–Anderson), John Watts told Mills he was taking back his proxy and voting against the bill. The Democrats, rather than having another defeat go on the record, withdrew the bill. The principal crop in John Watts's congressional district in western Kentucky was tobacco. The AMA had protected his most important industry by questioning the health hazards of smoking. Medicare would have to wait for another day.

## Those Who Need It Can't Get It

Dwight Eisenhower succeeded Harry Truman in 1952, and any serious attempt to enact national health reform ceased. Just because it disappeared from the congressional agenda, however, did not mean that the underlying problems had gone away. The cost of medical care was rising rapidly. National health expenditures doubled between 1953 and 1963 as technological advances increased the number of conditions that were treatable by medical science.

The elderly were hit hardest. As people age, their incomes decline and their medical expenses rise. In 1958, medical expenses for elderly Americans (over the age of sixty-five) were more than double those under sixty-five. However, the median income for an elderly two-person family was only $2,530 versus $5,315 for the nonelderly. For the single elderly it was even worse: $1,055 versus $2,570.[6]

Those who had private health insurance tended to be wealthier and healthier, but those who needed medical services the most were the poorest and sickest. Only 38 percent of the nonworking elderly had any health insurance in 1958 (and it was often inadequate), and only 37 percent of those who described themselves in poor health were insured.[7] With two-thirds of the elderly having incomes under one thousand dollars, one serious illness could cause financial hardship, indebtedness, and the loss of homes and other assets they had worked all their lives to obtain.

Those who could not afford health insurance often went to public hospitals for treatment. As their numbers swelled and as the cost of hospital care rose, public hospitals needed government support for the free care they provided. Their demands for funds overwhelmed some community and state budgets. As a result, a political constituency began to form for a program targeted at the poor.

Among the elderly, it was not only the poor who lacked insurance. Many in the middle class either could not afford it or could not get it at all. Since the latter part of the '40s, insurance markets had changed. Before that time, nonprofit Blue Cross plans underwrote virtually all health insurance policies, and those policies were community rated.

As we discussed in chapter 2, a community rate is an average across an entire population. Hence, young people pay more relative to their average expected cost and old people pay less. Similarly, individuals with a history of illness pay the same as those who have been well, even though their expected costs are higher. The Blue Cross system acted as a form of social insurance in which younger, healthier people, in effect, subsidized older and sicker people who otherwise might not have been able to afford insurance. State governments permitted Blue Cross to limit the number of plans in each geographic area, and the national Blue Cross office required plans to community rate. If all insurance is community rated, the system can work.[8] Toward the latter part of the '40s, however, commercial (for-profit) insurance companies began to compete with a different rating method.

The commercial insurers set their premiums by "experience rating." They considered a person or group's age and past health history and charged a premium based on their expected cost. Hence, an older person or a person with past health problems would be expected to cost more than a young, healthy person and would have to pay a higher premium. Conversely, younger, healthier people, whose expected costs were lower, would be charged less. Offering lower prices, the commercial insurers began to draw the younger, healthier, and lower-cost customers away from the community-rated Blue Cross plans. At the same time, they avoided higher risk customers by target marketing and by charging higher experience-rated premiums.

The ability to select customers with low risk was particularly effective in health insurance markets because most health spending was concentrated in just a few people. For example, in 2004, 1 percent of people in the United States accounted for nearly a quarter of spending on health care services and 10 percent accounted for 64 percent.[9] Indeed, the half of the population with the lowest health expenditures accounted for only 3 percent of national spending on health services.[10] If some insurers could attract that healthy half of the population and avoid those at the expensive end, they could keep their premiums low and dominate the market.

As a result, the commercial insurers became very profitable and Blue Cross plans watched their enrollment plummet (and their premiums rise because their average patient was older and sicker). By 1952, commercial enrollment exceeded that of Blue Cross,[11] and by 1958 Blue Cross was forty million dollars in the red.[12] By 1963, commercial plans held 60 percent of the privately insured market.[13] Community rated plans could not compete, and by the late '50s most Blues were forced to switch to experience rating. Blue Cross executives deplored the change because it violated one of their core principles. Despite their regrets, however, the market had changed and there was no turning back.

Except in states that prohibit it, most health insurance is now experience rated. This is considered fair and appropriate by those in the insurance industry and others who believe that basic insurance principles require premiums to be set in relation to each person's expected cost. That is the way most insurance works. For example, if you own a house that sits on a cliff overlooking the ocean, your house is more apt to sustain damages from weather and tides, and you will pay a higher insurance premium than someone who lives in a rural, suburban subdivision. Of course, people who live in the subdivision would not want to pay the average insurance premium for all houses, including the ones on the cliff. They would say, "If people want to live on the cliff, they should pay the extra insurance themselves." However, this reasoning is anathema to those who believe that health insurance is a social good—something everyone should be able to afford. Liberals contend that experience-rated markets fail to provide affordable insurance to older and less healthy people. They favor a social insurance system in which government collects taxes and provides benefits without regard to age, sex, or medical history. Alternatively, many across the political spectrum will accept a middle ground in which government limits rating differences based on those attributes and also limits the ability of insurance companies to deny or rescind coverage. These kinds of insurance regulations were an important part of the Obama health plan.

By the time Congress debated Medicare in the late '50s, most health insurance was experience rated. This was problematic for older and sicker people unless they were part of a large employment group. Otherwise many who were elderly or unhealthy—those that needed health insurance the most—either could not afford it or could not get it at all. Hence, the debate about health insurance in 1958 was not about providing health insurance as a human right. It was about the financial problems of the elderly facing economic distress as a result of illness. It was about children having to provide financial support for their parents, many of whom were impoverished by the cost of health care. In 1958, health insurance for older parents and grandparents was an economic issue that was gaining political traction.

## The Fight for Medicare Begins

Congress began hearings on health insurance for the elderly in 1958. The Democrats realized how difficult it would be to enact any health reform under the Eisenhower administration. After all, they failed to pass anything under Truman when they controlled the White House and both houses of Congress. Hence, they formulated a conservative, almost austere, proposal for the elderly, a narrowly defined but seemingly deserving group.

The Forand bill, introduced by Congressman Aime Forand (D-RI) in 1958, provided severely limited benefits: sixty days of hospitalization per year (including surgeon's fees), 120 days of nursing home care per year, and inpatient lab and x-ray. The government would pay for the program by increasing the social security tax one-quarter of 1 percent for both employers and employees on the first $4,800 of income. Democrats thought that the limited benefit package would make the bill acceptable to opponents. They excluded reimbursement for doctors (except inpatient surgical fees), hoping to blunt opposition from the AMA.

The Forand bill also limited eligibility to those elderly who had paid enough during their working lives to qualify for social security. That left out a sizeable minority of the elderly, many of whom were domestic or farm workers. Democrats calculated, however, that social security recipients were a sympathetic group who would not be perceived as lazy or undeserving. In addition, their medical debts were becoming a burden on their children, causing many families, even those in the middle class, to favor government support.

Despite the limited nature of the bill, the Ways and Means Committee rejected it on March 31, 1960, by a vote of 17–8, and it never reached the House floor. President Eisenhower threatened to veto any similar legislation, which he called "a definite step toward socialized medicine."[14]

Presidential politics, however, kept the issue very much alive. Richard Nixon was planning his 1960 campaign, and he knew both his Democratic opponents and Nelson Rockefeller, a presumed Republican opponent, supported a Forand-type bill. Nixon couldn't change Eisenhower's position but urged other Republicans to take a more positive approach. Meanwhile, Sam Rayburn, the Speaker of the House, was trying to help his favorite candidate, Lyndon Johnson. Rayburn and Johnson lobbied Wilbur Mills, trying to convince him to support a bill.

Wilbur Mills was not about to report out a bill without a secure majority in the full House. Neither was he going to change his long-held opposition to Medicare and risk alienating the southern Democrats who comprised the base of his political support. Yet he could not ignore the pressure to respond to the hotly politicized issue. The wily chairman authored the Kerr–Mills bill. It provided federal grants to states to provide health benefits for the needy aged. It permitted a more generous benefit package—much broader than the Democratic proposals—but let each state decide its own standards and benefits within broad limits. State participation was voluntary, and states had to finance 35 to 50 percent of the total cost.

The bill fulfilled Mills's objectives to respond to the issue without increasing federal jurisdiction, especially in the South. An attempt to liberalize Kerr–Mills failed in the Senate when sixteen out of nineteen southern Democrats opposed an amendment by John Kennedy. After that, Congress passed the bill easily with solid support from Republicans and southern Democrats. Regardless, few states had the resources to participate with matching funds. After three years, 90 percent of the funding went to only five participating states, and eighteen states did not participate at all. Eisenhower signed the bill without comment. Nixon called it "most inadequate."[15] Kennedy vowed to support only a bill that was federally financed through social security. When Kennedy won the 1960 election, Medicare remained high on his agenda. The AMA, which had originally opposed Kerr–Mills, executed a quick about-face. Concerned about the new Democratic administration, the AMA supported Kerr–Mills as a way to head off Medicare.

## Health, Race, and Politics

The various proposals submitted to the 1960 Congress illustrated political differences that would affect health policy for many years. The overarching difference was the role of the federal government. Conservative Republicans generally opposed any increase in the size and role of the federal government—particularly when it might interfere with the private sector. This was particularly true in health care where there were virtually no federal programs prior to the '40s. Even as late as 1960, the major federal health programs, except for Hill–Burton, focused only on American Indians, the military, and public health hospitals.

Conservative opposition to federal programs drew strong support from doctors and hospitals that viewed their industry solely through a professional paradigm. The AMA opposed any political encroachment into the practice of medicine. It feared that once government helped pay for medical care, it would dictate how care was provided and how much doctors were paid. In fact, its resistance was so absolute that the AMA opposed compulsory vaccinations against smallpox and diphtheria!

Conservative Republicans also received crucial support from southern

Democrats whose primary concern was race. Southerners believed that any federally administered program would force them to integrate hospitals and other health care facilities that were still segregated throughout the South. The thought of white patients sharing wards or even hospital rooms with black patients was anathema to the "Jim Crow" culture that persisted in the '60s. The combined political strength of conservative Republicans and southern Democrats had defeated virtually every attempt by Democrats and liberal Republicans to increase access to health care or health insurance through federal programs.

Although the racial issue has greatly diminished, many of the political differences that characterized the debate in the '60s still persist over forty years later. Nonsouthern Democrats and liberals generally support compulsory insurance that is administered and funded by the federal government. Such insurance enables the federal government to prescribe uniform national eligibility requirements and enroll everyone who meets those requirements. It also provides a broad tax base of financial support from payroll taxes or general revenues. These sources of payment are "progressive" or "redistributive" because the amount paid varies with income. This differs from a program with fixed premium payments in which poorer people pay a larger proportion of their incomes than those who are wealthier.

Republicans and conservatives prefer to target benefits only to the needy as opposed to providing universal entitlements to everyone regardless of income. Their first preference is to provide direct medical services, often in clinics or community health centers. This allows them to specify the services offered and to limit government expenditures. Alternatively, they support tax credits or subsidies to encourage low-income individuals to purchase private insurance. Targeted tax credits and subsidies, however, require a means test. Liberals, who prefer universal social insurance, dislike means testing and oppose segregating services to the poor. They argue that health care should be a right of all citizens, regardless of income, and all citizens should be permitted to go to any provider, as in most other industrialized countries. If health care is means tested, they contend, it becomes a charity or welfare program and will become under-funded, stigmatized, and of lesser quality. Republicans, where they accept government involvement, prefer a state-administered program in which eligibility and benefits vary according to the dictates of each individual state. In addition, they oppose any government mandates and prefer voluntary participation by individuals and states.

Philosophical differences between liberals and conservatives existed throughout the history of health care reform and were the basis for passionate disagreements about the Obama health plan. Many of the issues that arose, both in the Medicare debate in 1965 and in the Obama plan in 2009, were a result of these philosophical divisions. They include the expanded role of the federal government, the amount of government spending, the federally created "public option," the intrusion into the private market, and the mandates for states, businesses, and individuals to participate in the plan. But 2009 was very different because government was already paying for nearly half of all health care expenditures, a radical departure from 1960.

## Kennedy Tries and Fails

Following his election in 1960, Kennedy followed up on his campaign promise by reintroducing Medicare legislation. Aware of the powerful opposition, the new King–Anderson bill was even more cautious than the Forand bill. No physician services were included, not even the doctor's bill for inpatient surgery. Eligibility was still limited to social security recipients, leaving out an estimated 3.75 million out of 17 million elderly citizens.[16]

For the bill to reach the House floor, it had to pass the Ways and Means Committee, the same body that had defeated the Forand bill 17–8. In 1961, the committee had fifteen Democrats and ten Republicans. Not unlike the Congress of 2010, all of the Republicans were expected to oppose the bill. This meant supporters would need thirteen of the fifteen Democrats. However, six of the Democrats, including Wilbur Mills, were from southern states and had opposed Forand. That left supporters four votes short, and the only possible chance to turn them was the persuasive power of Chairman Mills.

Mills, however, was not about to change his opposition, even for a Democratic president. And he had good reasons. The 1960 redistricting meant that Mills was going to have to run for office in Little Rock against an archconservative opponent. Supporting a federal social program that could integrate Little Rock hospitals was not something the politically savvy chairman was about to do. He was also not about to report out a controversial bill that might not have a majority in the full House. Furthermore, he did not want to see his own Kerr–Mills bill superseded in its first year.

In 1961, Kennedy needed Mills for his tax and trade legislation, both of which had to pass through the chairman's committee. Not wanting to alienate Mills, and understanding the lack of support in his committee, Kennedy eventually let the King–Anderson bill die quietly in Ways and Means without a vote.

In 1962, Kennedy still could not get King–Anderson through Ways and Means. Working with the liberal senator Jacob Javits (R-NY), he agreed on an alternative strategy. They planned to attach a version of King–Anderson on the Senate floor to a bill that had already passed the House and the Senate Finance Committee. However, that attempt was defeated 52–48 when all but four southern senators opposed the measure. Again, race was the underlying motive. The southerners did not want to set a precedent by circumventing the Finance Committee and going directly to the Senate floor. Such a precedent might encourage future attempts by civil rights advocates to bypass Judiciary, a committee the southern Democrats firmly controlled.[17]

## Lyndon Johnson and Wilbur Mills, the Seesaw Health Battles of 1964

If anyone knew how to work the Congress, it was Lyndon Baines Johnson. The biographer Robert Caro entitled his third volume on the life of LBJ, *Master of the Senate*, and indeed he was. As the Democratic majority leader, Johnson's ability to wield power was legendary. From the onset of his presidency he lobbied Wilbur Mills to change his opposition to Medicare. As early as January 27, shortly after Congress reconvened following the Kennedy assassination, Mills hinted to administration officials that he might consider a more comprehensive package of reforms as a way to support King–Anderson.[18]

For reasons cited earlier, Mills was reluctant to change. Nevertheless, he was aware that a consensus was building to do something about the uninsured elderly. His committee members were now evenly divided 12–12 on Medicare, and Johnson was pressing him to be the thirteenth vote; to champion the "Mills Bill," assuring him he would get the credit for a historic piece of legislation. Mills was cognizant of LBJ's power and knew it would only increase if the president was reelected.

Wilbur Mills was not going to be left out. If a bill was to pass, he wanted to make sure that he controlled the process. Hence, in 1964, under pressure from Johnson, he began to hedge his position. Then, in January, when John

Watts offered his support for King–Anderson (described in the beginning of this chapter), it appeared that Mills might be prepared to change sides. In a March publication, *Congressional Quarterly* claimed he would do so and Mills refused to issue a denial.[19] On June 9 and 11, Johnson prodded Mills in private telephone conversations to report out a bill, even urging him to expand it as Mills had hinted in his January memo.[20] To political observers, it seemed evident that at least some compromise on King–Anderson would come out of the committee. But, although Mills appeared to be forthcoming, the politically savvy president did not trust him and was already considering a fallback strategy: attaching Medicare to a bill in the Senate.[21]

Wilbur Mills no longer had to worry about his congressional seat in Arkansas. However, he still had numerous concerns about King–Anderson. After opposing it for so many years, he needed a credible way to change his position. For years, opponents had argued that King–Anderson was too narrow, providing little more than hospital benefits. Kerr–Mills and other Republican initiatives had offered broader benefits, but participation was voluntary rather than compulsory, and eligibility was charity- or means-based rather than universal. Mills was worried that people would see their taxes rise and then be surprised when doctors' bills and other medical expenses were not covered. "The public must be under no illusion regarding the benefits," Mills stated later in 1964. "Medicare does not refer to doctors' services or general outpatient medical care."[22]

Hence, one solution for Mills was a broader bill, giving him reasons to change his position. He certainly was being pushed that way by the president, although he must have known that LBJ and the Democrats would settle for much less. A broader bill presented other issues, however. It was uncertain whether a broader, more expensive bill would garner enough support in the full House. In addition, Mills was genuinely concerned about the budget. He feared that spending for Medicare, which was inherently unpredictable, could endanger the Social Security Trust Fund. Eventually he was to insist on keeping the two trust funds separate.

And then there was race. Wilbur Mills was not an ideologue on racial matters. Nevertheless, he was a practical politician who was not going to endanger his congressional seat by straying from the attitudes that prevailed in Little Rock, Arkansas. Mills had established his segregationist credentials by signing the 1956 "Southern Manifesto" that opposed *Brown v. Board of Education.* He also opposed the Civil Rights Act of 1960 and consistently opposed federal involvement in social issues. Most observers think Mills was moderate on race, but the politics of Little Rock forced him to the segregationist right and may have destroyed his opportunity to become Speaker of the House when Sam Rayburn died in 1961.[23]

Mills knew that his southern constituency would not be happy to allow federal involvement in health care—involvement that could try to force integration of health care facilities. If he had to go out on a political limb and support social security financing of Medicare, he wanted to be in a position to limit federal interference as much as possible.

### Round 1: Mills Tries to Bury Medicare

No one knows what Wilbur Mills might have done if the tobacco industry, bolstered by the AMA, had not pressured John Watts to change his position and oppose Medicare in 1964. But after Watts withdrew his support, LBJ's mistrust of Mills proved prescient. A 5 percent increase in Social Security benefits had been before the Ways and Means Committee. Benefits had not been raised since 1958, and the idea was widely popular in the 1964 election year. The increase would have raised the combined employer–employee Social Security tax to just under 9.5 percent. At the time, everyone considered 10 percent to be the absolute ceiling. The new rate would leave just enough room for King–Anderson, estimated to increase the rate by .5 percent.

After Watts's defection, Mills still refused to be the deciding thirteenth vote, and Medicare supporters withdrew the bill. But then Mills and the committee went a step further. In a move by a Republican conservative that would otherwise have been inexplicable, John Byrnes, the ranking minority member, proposed raising the Social Security increase to 6 percent. Medicare supporters were dismayed, realizing that the real purpose of the additional raise was to leave no room in the future to fund King–Anderson. Medicare opponents needed thirteen votes to pass the measure. As the votes were tallied, three southern Democrats, including Wilbur Mills and John Watts, joined nine Republicans to support the increase. Medicare supporters were in despair because the remaining vote belonged to Bruce Alger, perhaps the most conservative member in the entire Congress. Alger was so opposed to federal power that he was the only congressman to vote against the school lunch program! It appeared that Mills and his committee had dealt Johnson a deathblow on Medicare, perhaps for several years. However, to everyone's astonishment, Alger voted "nay." He later explained that since he opposed the whole concept of Social Security, he could not vote for an increase. Hence, on June 24, the day after Watts succumbed to the AMA–Tobacco lobby, Ways and Means sent the Social Security bill to the Senate with the original 5 percent increase and without attaching King–Anderson.

### Round 2: LBJ Succeeds in the Senate

Not to be outdone so easily, LBJ considered attaching King–Anderson to the Social Security bill in the Senate. It was a risky proposition because it could kill the social security increase, and no one wanted to risk losing the support of the elderly in an election year. In addition, King–Anderson would first have to be debated in the Finance Committee, because otherwise southern Democrats would again oppose a process that bypassed the committee for a direct floor vote. This presented two problems: First, a majority of the Finance Committee was opposed to Medicare. Second, the debate would delay any action until after the August convention.

Even if supporters eventually succeeded in attaching King–Anderson on the Senate floor (after it was debated and rejected by the Finance Committee), it would have to go to a House–Senate conference committee where Mills and other opponents held the balance of power. At best, they could expect a narrow, watered-down proposal to come out of the conference— something LBJ was apparently willing to accept in advance of the election. At worst, however, the conference committee could deadlock, not only defeating King–Anderson but also killing the Social Security increase.

A determined Johnson went ahead anyway. When the Finance Committee, as expected, reported out the bill without attaching King–Anderson, Johnson's forces intended to attach it on the Senate floor. Before they could do that, however, Russell Long, the Democratic senator from Louisiana, replicated Byrnes's strategy by proposing a 7 percent increase in Social Security benefits. Medicare opponents again appeared to be outmaneuvered as the Long amendment would push the Social Security tax close to the 10 percent ceiling. Despite Long's amendment, Johnson's forces did not give up. Albert Gore, the Democratic senator from Tennessee (and father of future vice president Al Gore), attached an amendment to the Long amendment providing for a fixed, seven-dollar increase in Social Security and a Medicare program that was essentially King–Anderson. Gore's amendment would bring the Social Security tax to nearly 10.5 percent, but, as an amendment to an amendment, it would be considered first.

The vote on the Gore amendment occurred on September 2, just two months before the election. Barry Goldwater, the Republican nominee for president, rushed back from Arizona, thinking he might be the deciding vote to oppose the amendment. The roll call initially resulted in a 42–42 tie. Immediately, nine senators who had hoped their votes would not be needed entered the chamber. Unexpectedly, five Republicans supported the amendment and it passed 49–44. Jacob Javits had secured their votes by including an antitrust exemption for private insurance companies to pool their risks for insuring the elderly. The entire bill easily passed a few days later, and for the first time, the US Senate had approved Medicare. LBJ and the Medicare supporters were jubilant. Barry Goldwater told the *New York Times* that the legislation "reveals a contempt for the intelligence and judgment of our people."[24] Now, the ball was back in the court of Wilbur Mills.

### Round 3: Mills Tries to Kill Medicare Again

No one was optimistic about a strong Medicare bill emerging from the House–Senate conference.[25] Three of the five House conferees, including Wilbur Mills, were opposed. Of the seven Senate conferees, only Gore and Anderson were in favor. However, the Senate conferees represented the whole Senate, and by long-standing tradition they had an obligation to support, at least initially, the Medicare bill that was passed by the full chamber. Nevertheless, if negotiations became protracted, it was understood they could go their own way. Few observers expected them to hang tough, but they did, conducting month-long negotiations with Mills. Despite their efforts, Mills would not be pinned down. He had a strong advantage because he figured the Democrats would not vote against the Social Security increase even if it was stripped of Medicare.

The Senate conferees were in a weak position, and Johnson's forces had few options short of total capitulation. Eventually they offered to accept a bill with only forty-five days of hospital benefits and nothing else, but Mills, after initially accepting, backed off. The Senate conferees were so frustrated they threatened to reject any conference report that excluded Medicare benefits. Wanting to avoid a confrontation, Mills told them to draft the compromise.

The conference vote was to take place on October 2, and Mills was expected to support the compromise. Lyndon Johnson, however, must still have been wary of Mills's support. On September 24, he had private telephone conversations with both Russell Long and George Smathers (D-FL), asking both of them not to reveal he had called.[26]

When the committee convened on October 2, Mills called for a vote only on the Social Security increase—stripping it of any provision for Medicare. The chairman was confident he would win. With three out of five votes in the House and five out of seven in the Senate, he would pass the popular Social Security increase and kill the Medicare bill until at least after the election.

### Round 4: An LBJ Surprise

Medicare supporters were distressed by Mills's decision. If the Social Security increase passed without Medicare, it would make it difficult to raise the tax again in the next Congress. At the outset of the committee vote, the two republican conferees in the House immediately supported Mills, securing the House side 3–2. Then, two Republican senators abandoned the position of the full Senate and voted with Mills. Robert Byrd abstained, wishing to uphold Senate tradition, but everyone understood he would stand with Mills if needed. The two Medicare supporters, Gore and Anderson, then voted against Mills as expected. At that point, the vote was 2–2, and Mills only needed one of the last two votes, along with Byrd's, to carry the motion.

It appeared the powerful chairman would prevail as he had every year of the Medicare battle since 1959. Only Long and Smathers were left, and they both were steadfast opponents of Medicare. Long had already tried to kill the measure in the Finance Committee, and Smathers had never voted against the AMA in nearly twenty years as a congressman.[27] Long's turn came next, and he cast his vote against Mills, astounding the chairman. It was then Smathers's opportunity to once again repeat his long-held opposition to Medicare and finally put the matter to rest. But Smathers also voted against the chairman. Mills was flabbergasted! He decreed that the committee was deadlocked and adjourned the conference. Both Medicare and the Social Security increase would have to wait until after the election.

It was rare, indeed, for Wilbur Mills to call for a vote he would not win. Few people counted heads as accurately as the chairman. It so happened that if Johnson won the election, Hubert Humphrey's position as majority whip would be left open. It was a post Russell Long coveted, but he knew he could not get it without the support of the party leadership. Long cast his vote with the Democratic supporters of Medicare and was subsequently elected whip when the party reconvened in January. Apparently no one knew why George Smathers had abandoned his long-held position and voted against Mills; so they asked him why he did it.

"Lyndon told me to," he said.[28]

## The Daisy Girl

If there was one political advertisement that changed the course of American political campaigns, it was the "Daisy Girl."[29] A cute little blond girl stands in an open field counting petals as she pulls them off a daisy. Then, a deep male voice in the background counts backward from ten as the camera zooms in on the girl's frightened eyes. Viewers then hear and see a horrific nuclear explosion. As the terrifying mushroom cloud rises, the twangy, Texas drawl of Lyndon Johnson is heard. "These are the stakes—to make a world in which all of God's children can live or to go into the darkness. We must either love each other, or we must die."

The Johnson campaign had hired the well-known advertising firm of Doyle Dane Bernbach. Tony Schwarz, the ad's creator, believed that a negative image could be more powerful in influencing voters than one that was positive.[30] After Barry Goldwater advocated the use of tactical nuclear weapons in Vietnam, the campaign seized on the message that Goldwater was dangerous. The one-minute ad ran only once, and it never mentioned Goldwater's name. Yet it was so powerful and controversial that it was credited with making a significant impact on the election. The Daisy Girl is considered to be the first of its kind—the genesis of negative political television advertising. As such, it was the forerunner of the "Harry and Louise" ads twenty-eight years later that helped kill the Clinton health plan.

Lyndon Johnson was elected in 1964 by a landslide, winning by a 22.6 percent margin and carrying forty-four states. It was the largest electoral margin since 1820. Swept in on LBJ's coattails, the country elected the most Democratic Congress since Franklin Roosevelt in 1936. Their margin in both houses was greater than two to one. With help from the Daisy Girl, Lyndon Johnson had enough votes in Congress to enact Medicare.

## Mills Changes Sides

Before most of the politicians and pundits, Wilbur Mills recognized that the battle was over. Even while he was confidently defeating the Medicare proposal in 1964, he was positioning himself to change sides if the election made Medicare inevitable. He had told Medicare supporters on his committee that if they went along with his position in 1964 (passing the Social Security increase without Medicare), he would address Medicare first in the next Congress. With Johnson running ahead in the polls, Mills gave an address to the Kiwanis Club in Little Rock and denied that he had ever obstructed Medicare. He then supported the idea of workers paying into a federal fund to insure their elderly health care expenditures. He told the Kiwanis Club, "I am acutely aware of the fact there is a problem here which must be met."[31] Then, on December 7, as mentioned earlier, he warned about angering the elderly by not including coverage for doctors' bills. After the landslide election, Mills understood that LBJ could pass Medicare without him, and, if he remained opposed, he could lose control of the legislative process.

Although Johnson had been lobbying Mills for the past year to consider a broader bill, the Democrats seemed less aware of the election's implications than Mills.[32] LBJ asked, and Congress agreed, to label the Medicare bills HR1 and S1, and to make them the first order of business in the new session. Yet the Democrats introduced the same King–Anderson bill with its narrow limits covering little more than hospital care.

The chairman was way ahead of them. He had a number of objectives he wanted to accomplish. He wanted to broaden the bill, both to provide a reason to change his position and to counter Republican criticism of the bill's narrow benefit package. He wanted to protect the Social Security Trust Fund. Most importantly, he wanted "to build a fence around Medicare."[33] In other words, he wanted to prevent future attempts to broaden the federal reach of the program and to endanger the Social Security Trust Fund. Medicare supporters now had a majority of 17–8 on the Ways and Means Committee, and the chairman knew he could have his way. The archenemy of Medicare for so many years was about to emerge as its champion. And Republican opponents were about to provide the vehicles to help him.

## The Three-Layer Cake

The AMA realized it was its last chance to defeat Medicare. On January 27, 1965, when the Ways and Means Committee convened to address King–Anderson, two committee members introduced a new bill by the AMA called Eldercare. It was essentially an expanded Kerr–Mills, providing a wide range of benefits for the needy elderly but still requiring matching funds and allowing voluntary participation. Kerr–Mills had been such a failure that no one took the bill seriously. However, the AMA launched an expensive ($900,000) campaign, claiming benefits in the King–Anderson bill were so narrow—with no doctor benefits—that it would only pay a small part of elderly medical expenses.

The next day John Byrnes, the ranking Republican on the committee, introduced his own bill. It was a voluntary program that provided a sliding-scale subsidy for each individual based on his or her social security income. The premium would be deducted from the participant's monthly Social Security check. Unlike King–Anderson, it provided a wide range of benefits, including doctor's services and prescription drugs. It was the first time a leading Republican had offered a program that was financed by general revenues. The Byrnes bill echoed the Republican argument that the narrow benefit package offered by King–Anderson was inadequate.

The committee met in executive session through the month of February. It had numerous bills to consider: King–Anderson, Eldercare, the Byrnes bill, an expansion of Kerr–Mills, the Social Security increase leftover from the previous session, and various other health insurance measures submitted by House members. On March 2, Mills asked Wilbur Cohen, the assistant secretary for legislation in Johnson's HEW department, to summarize the bills for the committee.

Everyone had assumed that Johnson had the votes to pass King–Anderson. There might be some congressional amendments, but eventually King–Anderson would pass and the other bills would be rejected. Everyone was wrong. After Cohen reviewed the bills, Mills startled everyone on the committee. Rather than choosing among them, he asked Cohen if Byrnes and Eldercare could be added to King–Anderson. It would create, in effect, a King–Anderson–Byrnes–Eldercare bill. This is what became known as the three-layer cake: King–Anderson provided hospital benefits funded through a payroll tax; Byrnes provided physician services through government subsidies and individual premiums paid from Social Security checks; and Elder-care, a beefed-up Kerr–Mills, provided a state-administered program of health insurance for the needy. These eventually became Medicare Part A, Medicare Part B, and Medicaid. The common assumption that Congress would choose among these proposals was wildly incorrect. Wilbur Mills had combined them.

Wilbur Cohen was stunned. Cohen had been an unrelenting advocate for health insurance since the administration of Franklin Roosevelt. He was considered the leading expert on Medicare-type legislation. At first, he thought Mills might once again be trying to kill the bill by overloading it. Upon consideration, however, he realized how wise the chairman had been. The AMA and Medicare opponents had launched huge campaigns supporting Eldercare and the physician benefits contained in the Byrnes bill. Mills had taken the very proposals from Medicare's opponents and made them a central part of the bill. It would now be difficult for them to oppose.

Regardless, Republican members of the Ways and Means Committee held firm and voted as a bloc to oppose the bill. The committee passed the measure 18–7 on a strict party-line vote. Democratic members were surprised, but also pleased, because they would get sole credit for the legislation, already being called the Mills bill. On April 8, when Mills rose to present the bill to the full House, he received a standing ovation. The bill passed easily in the House and, after much debate over minor provisions, easily passed the Senate. On July 30, 1965, the president and leaders of Congress traveled to Independence, Missouri, to sign the historic bill in front of the eighty-one-year-old Harry Truman. Lyndon Johnson had enacted the Civil Rights Act of 1964, Medicare, and Medicaid in his first two years in office. Wilbur Mills, the most stubborn obstacle to Medicare since 1958, had become its hero. And virtually every elderly person in the United States of America had health insurance.

## Sausage and Legislation: The Legacy of Medicare

"There are two things you don't want to see being made—sausage and legislation." The well-known quote is attributed to Otto von Bismarck, the German chancellor who brought social health insurance to all German workers in 1883. Just 126 years later, Rahm Emanuel, Barack Obama's chief of staff, responded to criticism about the compromises in Obama's health plan. "The goal isn't to see whether I can pass this through the executive board of the Brookings Institution. I'm passing it through the United States Congress."[34]

Emanuel spoke of the challenge of instituting major political change in a pluralistic society. The Medicare program was a landmark political achievement, and one of the most popular programs instituted in the twentieth century. At the same time, the political constraints confronting Medicare supporters and Wilbur Mills resulted in compromises that continue to plague the Medicare and Medicaid programs more than forty years later.

Most importantly, the organization and financing of care was fragmented by political necessities. The nonsouthern Democrats had accepted the fact that universal coverage was not achievable and focused on the elderly as a sympathetic group through which they might be able to expand health coverage. This focus divided access to health insurance by age, something that does not exist in any other country. Advocates figured it was just a first step and would gradually be expanded to include other groups and broader benefits. Of course, they turned out to be largely incorrect.

Wilbur Mills did not want to see the gradual expansion of Medicare. He was fiscally conservative and concerned about the Social Security Trust Fund. Hence, he attempted to "put a fence around Medicare." By expanding the Kerr–Mills bill into the Medicaid program, he essentially undercut any future demand to expand social security financing to the poor.[35] The Medicaid program also maintained state control (within limits) over benefits and administration. However, this further balkanized the system, instituting separate structures for the elderly and the poor, one administered by the federal government and the other by individual states. And, of course, it left most nonelderly nonpoor to secure private coverage if they could. No other country divides its system of care in such a fashion.

Mills was under pressure from Byrnes and the conservatives to limit federal encroachment into the private sector. At the same time, however, he feared citizens would be angry if the program raised their taxes and did not cover their doctors' bills. He reached out to the Byrnes constituency, replicating Byrnes's voluntary, premium-based program for physician and outpatient care. As a result, a system already divided by age and income and by federal and state administration was further divided by Medicare Parts A and B: separate systems for hospitals and doctors.

Furthermore, health care insurance was stratified by income. The non-poor elderly had a social insurance system that offered reasonably good reimbursement to providers and yielded good access to care. The poor had a welfare-based system that offered expansive benefits but paid providers lower fees and thus reduced access to care. Ironically, the poor elderly (called dual eligibles) were the one exception. They got the best of both plans: extended benefits under Medicaid and higher provider payments under Medicare. Instead of a coordinated system of health care, the country had numerous separate systems. Hospital and physician services were often financed separately and were neither coordinated nor integrated, and both were separate from long-term care. One important benefit that was included in the Byrnes bill but left out of the Mills plan was outpatient prescription drugs. Unlike today, there were only a small number of outpatient drugs that were considered important, and most were quite inexpensive. It also would have been administratively difficult for the government or its fiscal intermediary to process large numbers of small claims for drugs.

Political pressures not only resulted in fragmented systems of care, they also prevented legislators from instituting effective cost controls. Physicians and the AMA, who were about to lose their epic battle to kill Medicare, threatened to boycott patients who participated in the program. Afraid they would pass the legislation but not be able to implement it, lawmakers went out of their way to accommodate the industry. Trying to avoid confrontation, they made decisions that had severe budgetary consequences. Chief among these accommodations were decisions to pay hospitals whatever they billed, provided their fees were "reasonable;" and to allow physicians to bill the government based on their "usual and customary fees." Both policies were prescriptions for inflation. Moreover, in the case of doctors, they could charge patients additional fees in excess of the amounts they billed Medicare. This practice, called balance billing, infuriated many Medicare beneficiaries, who resented paying additional charges for services they thought were covered by the program. The government has since placed tight restrictions on the amount of these extra fees, and few physicians bother to balance bill.

Shortly after the legislation passed, some physicians were still threatening to boycott. However, the AMA discouraged them, realizing it had succeeded in molding reform to its own financial advantage. Nevertheless, there was more on the AMA agenda. Doctors and hospitals did not want to deal directly with the federal government. They preferred to operate through private intermediaries, utilizing many of the billing and payment systems that were already in place. Government officials had reasons to accommodate them. In less than a year, they had to create a system to enroll and serve nineteen million senior citizens. It was a gargantuan task. How could they start from nothing and implement such a program?

Into this void stepped Walter J. McNerney. In 1971, McNerney became president of the Blue Cross Association after directing the hospital administration program at the University of Michigan. Blue Cross was still closely affiliated with the AHA, and it was a separate organization from Blue Shield, which insured physician and outpatient care.

At the time, the Blue Cross Association was a very loose amalgamation of over seventy different state plans. Medicare was being hotly debated on Capitol Hill but was anathema to plan executives. Imagine an outsider stepping into the association and telling the presidents of seventy-seven private plans that he supported a government takeover of all their customers who were senior citizens. Essentially, though not overtly, this was what McNerney did.

Visionary, considering his position, McNerney understood two things well before his colleagues. First was that private insurance companies could not profitably provide health insurance to all of America's elderly. The elderly population, on average, simply had too high health costs and too low income. McNerney realized the government would have to provide assistance, and some form of Medicare was inevitable. Second, he realized that Blue Cross, by far the largest insurer in the country with fifty-eight million beneficiaries, including five million enrolled seniors,[36] had the knowledge and the systems in place that the government desperately needed.

McNerney's real genius was positioning Blue Cross to be an essential partner and beneficiary of Medicare without alienating his industry colleagues who all opposed the program. He never actually endorsed the legislation. Rather, he steered the association to a neutral position. All the while, McNerney testified repeatedly before the House Ways and Means and the Senate Finance Committee. The Blues possessed the knowledge that the government needed to implement the program, and McNerney met constantly with government officials, providing data and know-how that made him invaluable. And all the time, his message was clear: The government should not re-invent the wheel. Blue Cross already had all the machinery in

place to administer insurance to the elderly. Rather than duplicate from
scratch what was already there, the government should use Blue Cross as an
intermediary. McNerney told the Senate Finance Committee:

> A major matter of public policy to be decided by the action on this bill is,
> "How should government spend money for services to private individuals
> rendered by private institutions and practitioners?" There are two major
> alternatives. The government can work through the privately financed
> health care system, of which Blue Cross is a part, or around it.[37]

Although there were many in the single-payer community who wanted
the government to operate the system directly, Congress agreed with McN-
erney's reasoning. Of course, this fit the AMA's desire to work through private fiscal intermediaries and averted the threat of a physician boycott.
Moreover, it provided the government the only realistic option to meet an
otherwise impossible deadline for implementation.

The Blue Cross Association became the prime contractor for Medicare
Part A. Acting as fiscal intermediaries, Blue Cross Plans processed claims for
90 percent of the nineteen million seniors who enrolled in Medicare. Blue
Shield Plans became the largest Part B contractor, processing claims for 60
percent of beneficiaries.[38]

Although the use of private intermediaries was the most expedient and
probably the wisest choice, it assured that weaknesses in the existing system
would be replicated. The bifurcation of hospital and physician care between
Blue Cross and Blue Shield would now be ensconced in the Medicare program. More importantly, reimbursement for hospitals and doctors would be
cost-based, with no apparent limits on future increases.

By all accounts, the Blues performed exceptionally well. By the end of
the first year they were successfully processing one thousand hospital claims
and three thousand doctors' claims every hour.[39] Although it was their
responsibility to ensure that all charges were within program constraints, it
was ultimately the Congress that established the rules for reimbursement.
But the Congress, having focused on avoiding a confrontation with the
industry, had not provided the tools to control costs.

In fact, health care costs were about to explode. The average daily service charge in hospitals increased 20 percent during the first year of the program and continued to grow at double-digit rates into the early '70s.[40] The

rate of growth in doctors' fees more than doubled in the first year (from 3.8 to 7.8 percent) and averaged more than twice the rate of inflation over the next five years.[41] The rate of Medicare spending growth over the initial five years averaged 14 percent per year.[42]

Then there was the Medicaid program for the poor. The cost of Medicaid also grew quickly became a burden to the states. Although the program is state-administered, the federal government provides matching funds for 50 to 76 percent of total costs, the percentage match varying by state income.[43] States with lower average income receive a higher matching rate. The requirement to provide matching funds has been problematic in times of recession, because state revenues are reduced just when demand for services are at their highest levels. Unlike the federal government, states must balance their budgets each year. Frequent attempts to require the federal government pay a higher matching rate during recessions have failed to pass the Congress.

The growth in health care spending, initially triggered by the first five years of the Medicare and Medicaid programs, brought about a historical change in national health policy. Since 1970 the policy emphasis has shifted from expanding access to controlling cost. Since 1971, government has made numerous attempts to reduce the growth rate of Medicare spending. However, despite major changes in both the hospital and physician payment systems, growth in Medicare spending has far exceeded that of general inflation and national income. We discuss the government's repeated attempts and failures to control Medicare spending in chapters 9 and 10.

Despite its shortcomings, Medicare remains one of the most popular social programs in the country's history. It has been eminently successful in delivering access to health care to elderly Americans. In 1960, fewer than half of the elderly had any health insurance.[44] By 1970, the figure was close to 100 percent. The Medicare program also contributed greatly to reducing poverty among the elderly. The elderly poverty rate fell from 28.5 percent in 1965 to 14.6 percent in 1975 and 8.9 percent in 2009.[45]

In 1965, the Medicaid program was enacted with much less notoriety. However, it now serves over fifty-five million Americans,[46] enrolling more people than Medicare. It is the nation's public health program for low-income Americans, most of whom would otherwise be unable to afford private insurance. Until the Obama health plan, Medicaid remained categorical. The program was primarily limited to children, pregnant women, parents of children, and certain aged, blind, and disabled people—all of whom had to meet low-income eligibility standards that varied by state. In 2006, the program served nearly thirty million children, fifteen million adults, and fourteen million disabled individuals.[47] Although three-quarters of its beneficiaries are children and adults, 70 percent of the spending is devoted to the elderly and disabled, primarily for long-term, institutional care.[48] The program pays for 43 percent of all nursing home care and 34 percent of all home health care.

Medicare and Medicaid brought about a radical change in the ability of the poor to access medical care. In 1964 the nonpoor visited a doctor 20 percent more than the poor (and the poor have, on average, lower health status). By 1975, the situation was nearly reversed as the poor visited doctors 18 percent more than the nonpoor.[49]

Because of Medicare and Medicaid, the US health system functions at a much higher level of care. The programs have provided unprecedented clinical data, supported graduate medical education, and funded groundbreaking research. It is difficult to imagine the state of our health care system had these programs not been established.

Theodore Marmor said, "The outcome of 1965 was, to be sure, a model of unintended consequences."[50] Yet, to millions of Americans who access their health care through Medicare and Medicaid, it has kept them out of poverty, sustained their health, and saved their lives.

## Technical Appendix to Chapter 5: Medicare Benefits and Costs

The chart on the next page provides a summary of Medicare benefits and costs. Medicare Part A is principally a program for acute care hospitalization. Every citizen over sixty-five is automatically enrolled provided he or she has paid the Medicare payroll tax for at least forty quarters. Citizens who have not met this requirement can voluntarily purchase Medicare benefits.

Under Part A, all medically necessary hospital services are fully covered for the first sixty days of each benefit period after paying a deductible equal to the average cost of one day of hospital care. The deductible has risen from forty dollars at the time Medicare was enacted to $1,024 in 2010. A benefit period is the time from the first day of hospitalization to the sixtieth day after discharge with no readmission. From the sixty-first to the ninetieth day of hospitalization, the patient must pay a per diem coinsurance of one-quarter of the average cost per diem (this has changed from one-eighth when Medicare was enacted and was $256 in 2010). In addition, each patient has a lifetime reserve of sixty days and must pay a per diem coinsurance of one-half of the average cost per diem (this has changed from one-quarter when Medicare was enacted and was $512 in 2010). No patient can receive more than 150 days of coverage for any benefit period (ninety days plus whatever is left of the sixty-day lifetime benefit). This limitation was the main reason for the effort to enact catastrophic coverage (chapter 6).

Part A provides a very limited nursing home benefit (one hundred days maximum for each benefit period in a skilled nursing facility) that is only available after a hospital stay of at least three days. It also provides benefits for home health care and outpatient diagnostic services following a hospital stay. The home health benefit has been expanded in recent years. Hospice care has also been added to the original benefit package.

Although the benefits under the original Medicare program were quite extensive, four significant gaps existed:

Table 5.1
Summary of Medicare Benefits Enacted in 1965

| Service | Benefit | Deductible | Co-Insurance |
| --- | --- | --- | --- |
| **Part A** | | | |
| Inpatient Hospital (per benefit period) | First 60 days—Full coverage of all services after deductible | National average cost for one day of hospital care ($40) | |
| | 61st–90th day—Full coverage after co-insurance | | Per Diem cost of 1/8 of national average cost for one day of hospital care |
| | Lifetimereserve of 60 additional days—Full coverage after co-insurance | | Per Diem cost of 1/4 of national average cost for one day of hospital care |
| Nursing Home (per benefit period) | After at least 3 days of hospitalization—20 days of full coverage | | |
| | 21st–100th day—Full coverage after co-insurance | | Per Diem cost of 1/8 of national average cost for one day of hospital care |
| Home Health (per benefit period) | After hospital discharge—Full coverage for 100 days | | |
| Outpatient Hospital Diagnostic | Within 30 days of discharge—Covers 80% of costs after deductible | National average cost for 1/2 day of hospital care | 20% of costs |
| **Part B** | | | |
| Physician and surgeon care, outpatient services and other services listed below | After monthly premium ($3)—Covers 80% of costs after annual deductible | Deductible ($50) | 20% of costs |
| Home Health (100 visits), x-ray, lab, other diagnostic, radiation therapy, ambulance, surgical supplies, durable medical equipment, prosthetics, psychiatric services limited to inpatient (60 days per benefit period, 180 days lifetime maximum) and outpatient (lesser of $250 per year or 50% of costs), and other services. | | | |

Note: In 2010, Hospital inpatient deductible (average day) is $1,024; 61st–90th day is $256/day; 91st–150th day is $512/day.
    In 2020, Part B deductible is $155 annually. Part B income-related monthly premiums range from $96.40–$353.60.
Source: Authors' summary of legislation.

1. Inpatient hospital benefit was limited to 150 days.
2. Very limited coverage for long-term care.
3. No outpatient prescription drug coverage.
4. Considerable out-of-pocket costs for copayments and deductibles.

Prescription drug benefits were added in 2003, but the other gaps still exist. To fill them, many Medicare beneficiaries buy private, supplemental coverage or "Medigap" insurance. Some beneficiaries receive such coverage from current or past employers. The Medicaid program fills these gaps in coverage for their recipients. However, Medicaid eligibility is generally limited to low-income parents and their children (Until the Obama plan is implemented). Medicaid pays for long-term care, but recipients must "spend down" their assets in order to be eligible.

Medicare Part B is essentially a program for physician services and non-institutionalized (including nonhospital) care. It is a voluntary program and requires premiums, deductibles, and coinsurance. Originally, the premium was three dollars per month. That amount was intended to cover 50 percent of the cost of the program. In 2007, premiums became income-related. Thus, in 2010, monthly premiums ranged from $96.40 to $353.60. However, 73 percent of beneficiaries (those earning up to $85,000) have a maximum monthly premium of $110.50. These amounts are now intended to cover 25 percent of program costs. The balance is paid from general revenues. Because so much of the program is subsidized, over 90 percent of Medicare beneficiaries enroll in Part B. In addition to the monthly premiums, beneficiaries pay an annual deductible. That amount has increased from $50 in 1986 to $155 in 2010. Most services under Part B require a coinsurance charge of 20 percent.

Part B covers a wide range of services, some of which are listed on the chart. In 1973, Medicare added kidney dialysis and related services for people with end-stage renal disease (ESRD). Benefits for psychiatric care have changed frequently over time. "Medigap" insurance covers the cost of coinsurance and deductibles for many beneficiaries. The Medicaid program provides those benefits to its low-income participants.

The full list of both Part A and Part B services fills a fifty-four-page booklet published by the Centers for Medicare and Medicaid Services (CMS). It can be accessed online at the following URL: http://www.medicare.gov/Publications/Pubs/pdf/10116.pdf

# CHAPTER 6

# OOOPS!
# THE BRIEF LIFE AND DEATH
# OF MEDICARE CATASTROPHIC

In 1961, Ronald Reagan recorded a spoken record album for the AMA opposing pending Medicare legislation. He urged every citizen to send letters to their congressmen.

> "If you don't, this program, I promise you, will pass just as surely as the sun will come up tomorrow, and behind it will come other federal programs that will invade every area of freedom as we have known it in this country —until one day, as Norman Thomas said, we will wake to find that we have socialism. And, if you don't do this, and I don't do this, one of these days we are going to spend our sunset years telling our children and our children's children, what it once was like in America when men were free."[1]

On July 1, 1988, President Reagan signed the Medicare Catastrophic Health bill—the largest expansion of Medicare since the program was enacted in 1965. Then, on November 23, 1989, just eight months after Reagan left office, Congress repealed the entire program. The birth and death of Medicare Catastrophic starkly illustrates America's ambivalence toward government health policy.

## Government Is the Problem

When President Reagan was reelected to his second term in 1984, efforts to expand the Medicare program were a thing of the past. Democrats and liberals during the Johnson administration had believed that the initial Medicare legislation was just a first step. Once established, many thought it would be gradually expanded to include children and then other segments of the population. Liberals hoped it would be the first step toward single-payer health care.

However, at the beginning of the '70s, attitudes began to change. The focus of health policy efforts shifted from expanding coverage to controlling cost. The Medicare and Medicaid programs had helped fuel a precipitous rise in health care spending. In addition, the Hill–Burton program had encouraged so much hospital construction that many believed the country had too many hospital beds, and supply was creating its own demand. Both Richard Nixon and Jimmy Carter developed a number of programs to control health care costs (see chapters 9 and 10). By the time Ronald Reagan was elected president, budget deficits were an overriding concern, and many thought government spending for health and other social programs was out of control. Indeed, Reagan is remembered for stating in his inaugural address, "Government is not the solution to our problems; government is the problem."

In addition, public attitudes toward older citizens had changed. The combination of Medicare, Medicaid, and Social Security had alleviated poverty for many of the elderly. Between 1970 and 1986, elderly poverty rates fell by almost half, from 24.6 to 12.4 percent.[2] In 1982, for the first time the elderly had lower rates of poverty than the nonelderly. In fact, people began to think that too many government programs were benefiting the elderly at the expense of others. Terms such as "greedy geezers" and "intergenerational equity" reflected a growing resentment, especially toward those seniors who were well off. In 1982, the Greenspan Commission recommended a tax on Social Security benefits for upper-income seniors. For the first time, the popular social insurance program would be income-related, and net benefits for some would be reduced. In Ronald Reagan's second term as president, no one was talking about expanding Medicare. No one, that is, except Otis Bowen.

## Doc Bowen: A Man on a Mission

In 1985, President Reagan nominated the former governor of Indiana Otis Bowen to become secretary of Health and Human Services (HHS). Bowen (a distant relative of George W. Bush) was confirmed by a vote of 93–2, becoming the first physician to lead the department.[3] He had previously chaired Reagan's 1982 Advisory Commission on Social Security. The commission had recommended protecting the elderly against the cost of lengthy hospital stays by offering an optional insurance premium under Medicare Part B.[4] For forty-two dollars per year, the elderly could insure against all costs for unlimited hospital stays.

Bowen had good reasons to be concerned about Medicare's limited coverage. His first wife, Beth, had died of bone cancer in 1981, and he was all too familiar with the cost of lengthy hospitalizations. Only a small proportion of the elderly exceeded the sixty-day annual hospital benefit that was free from copayments. Still fewer exhausted the full 150-day coverage, but they were subject to out-of-pocket costs that could be truly catastrophic. In addition, Medicare coverage, in general, was exposing beneficiaries to increasingly wide gaps. Between 1980 and 1985, out-of-pocket costs increased by 49 percent for hospital care and 31 percent for outpatient and physician services.[5] In fact, the elderly were paying as much for out-of-pocket health costs in 1984 as they had in 1965 when Medicare was enacted.[6] Although 70 percent of the elderly had some form of supplemental insurance (or Medicaid), many policies were inadequate and had high administrative fees. Bowen's proposal was modest in scope, but it would help protect those with the highest out-of-pocket costs.

Almost immediately after becoming secretary, Bowen tried to convince Reagan to propose catastrophic insurance for Medicare beneficiaries in his 1986 State of the Union address. Initially, Reagan was supportive, but he later declined under pressure from the insurance industry, which did not want to surrender its lucrative supplemental business to the government. However, he told Bowen to form an advisory council to study the issue.[7]

The mild-mannered Doc Bowen turned out to be a pit bull on the issue of catastrophic insurance. Although he chaired the advisory council, he insisted at the outset that he did not want his own views to influence its conclusions. He went so far as to avoid attending the council meetings. However, his low public profile later appeared to be a ruse. Near the end of the council's deliberations in the fall of 1986, he inserted his own plan—nearly identical to one he published before he became secretary. Apparently he had intended this all along. Whether the president also intended this outcome when he authorized the advisory council is not clear.

Conservatives within the administration attempted to keep the proposal private while they lobbied the president to oppose the initiative. Knowing he had formidable opposition, Bowen acted boldly. Before opponents could coalesce, and without any White House review, he scheduled a news conference and made the details of his proposal public. The *New York Times* reported, "the unauthorized action outwitted and outraged conservatives, including some of the president's closest advisers."[8] Congressional Democrats immediately hailed his proposal and offered their support. Several drafted their own proposals, eight of which were filed in the House over the next several months.

Only one person in the entire Reagan administration could have driven this initiative. Thanks to Doc Bowen, Medicare Catastrophic was suddenly part of the public debate.

## The Bowen Proposal

Bowen's proposal provided catastrophic protection to Medicare beneficiaries by insuring all out-of-pocket medical expenses for hospitals and doctors above a threshold annual spending amount of two thousand dollars per year. The program paid for itself by raising the premium on all Part B policies by $4.92 per month. Thus it was budget neutral, financed by its own participants, and voluntary (Medicare Part B is voluntary, although most beneficiaries participate).

On the surface, Bowen's proposal seemed modest and straightforward. Yet, it contained the seeds of an invasive plant that would eventually sprout ideological controversy from both liberals and conservatives. To understand why, it is necessary to examine the age-old argument between liberals and conservatives about the value of social insurance.

## The Pros and Cons of Social Insurance

Social insurance is an agreement among *all* members of a society to pool their funds to protect against an unpredictable occurrence that might happen to *some* of them. Such society-wide programs are government-sponsored and mandatory wherein the governmental authority collects taxes from everyone and promises a specified set of benefits to those who will need them. The two major social insurance programs in the United States are Social Security and Medicare. Liberals contend that social insurance programs engender a great deal of social solidarity because everyone contributes, and, thus, everyone is deserving of benefits. Social Security and Medicare are both "intergenerational" programs. At any time, the benefits for the elderly are paid mostly by the younger generation of workers. Hence, there is a social compact that says, in essence, "I agree to pay for my parents' benefits knowing that, when the time comes, my children will pay for mine."

Many social insurance programs, including Medicare and Social Security, require "income-related" contributions. In other words, those with higher incomes contribute more than their proportional share. Hence, these programs redistribute money from the wealthy to the less well off, providing a social safety net for those in need.

Republicans and conservatives contend that social insurance programs are expensive, inefficient, and unfair, and they crowd out private insurance. Their reasoning is as follows: Social insurance programs are expensive and inefficient because they provide benefits to everyone—including the wealthy who don't need them. In an environment of scarce government resources, it is unwise to give benefits to the affluent that could otherwise be used to expand programs for the truly needy. Moreover, it is unfair to tax a low-income worker like "Joe Six-Pack" to provide benefits to someone like Bill Gates.

It is also unfair from an intergenerational perspective, because it transfers money from workers who are starting their careers and families to retired people who often have homes and other substantial assets. In addition, since the programs often have unfunded liabilities, the older generation often saddles the younger generation with increased debt.

Although it is important to provide citizens with security, it is also important to encourage responsibility. Otherwise, the government reduces the incentive for people to work, save, and provide for their own security.

Finally, many economists believe that increasing taxes and providing government insurance to everyone reduces the growth rate of the economy and destroys the market for private insurance. It is more economically efficient to reduce taxes, encourage private insurance, and provide subsidies targeted to those in need.

Democrats and liberals oppose programs that target only the needy. They contrast the Medicare program, which is popular and well funded, with the Medicaid program, which is frequently disparaged, underfunded, and subject to severe budget constraints. An old adage sums up the position of liberals: "Show me a program for the poor and I will show you a poor program." Targeted welfare programs require means testing, which liberals perceive as stigmatizing and demeaning. They contend that means-tested programs lack social support because those that receive benefits are not among those who contribute revenues. Marmor describes the difference as an "us–us rather than a we–them political dynamic."[9]

> The question is not what "we" (the affluent) do for "them" (the impoverished). Rather it is how we should manage the risks of economic misfortune that will befall some of us at any one time and threaten all of us over the course of our lifetimes.[10]

However, conservatives contend that Americans live in a supportive society in which the vast majority of people want to provide security for the needy. In the words of Stuart Butler, they just want to do it more efficiently.

> There is no need for us to give generous benefits to those who don't need them in order to "buy" their political support for programs for those that do.[11]

## A Foot in the Door

Medicare Part A is a universal social insurance program for the elderly and is close to the hearts of Democrats and liberals. Medicare Part B is voluntary and premium-supported. Nevertheless, because the government subsidizes 75 percent of the cost,[12] it has many of the aspects of social insurance. Many on the left would like to extend Medicare to all citizens, resulting in single-payer health care for the entire country.

The Bowen proposal threatened to take government health programs in the opposite direction. Under his proposal, the program had to be budget neutral and self-financed. Requiring the elderly to finance their own care was a departure from the model of social insurance typified by Medicare. Although it was government insurance, it was neither universal nor mandatory. There were no intergenerational transfers, and, under Bowen's proposal, there was no income redistribution. It more closely resembled the purchase of private Medigap policies, except, in this case, the government provided the insurance. In addition, the Bowen proposal did not protect against expenses for long-term care and pharmaceuticals, the catastrophic costs that most worried the elderly. In 1969, long-term care accounted for 42 percent of the elderly's out-of-pocket medical spending.[13] By comparison, a catastrophic hospital benefit would only help .5 percent of Medicare beneficiaries.[14]

Nevertheless, in the political environment of 1987, it was a foot in the door for liberals. Prior to Bowen's initiative there were no possibilities for expanding government-supported health insurance. Advocates faced a budget environment that was likely to be tightly constrained for the foreseeable future. Some reasoned that this kind of self-financing could be a blueprint for future expansions of social programs, but not all liberals agreed.

Republicans and conservatives certainly did not agree. The president's Domestic Policy Council was appalled. Bowen's program represented everything the Reagan administration had run against. It would expand the role of the federal government while crowding out private insurance that was already providing similar coverage. It would lead to increased government spending and larger deficits because costs would likely increase faster than Congress's willingness to raise premiums for the elderly. Once advocates got a foot in the door, Republicans feared a "Christmas tree effect."[15] When Congress began debate on the bill, Democrats would propose amendment after amendment, adding benefits like hanging decorations on a Christmas tree.

## The Christmas Tree

It was not long before the Republicans' worst fears were realized. The Democrats were flush from victory, having regained control of the Senate in the 1986 midterm election. Liberals, who had earlier supported Bowen's proposal, began to complain it was too narrow. Claude Pepper, the octogenarian Democratic senator from Florida, was leading an effort to enact long-term care legislation. Pepper threatened to attach his bill to the catastrophic bill unless Congress expanded the benefit package. That would have resulted in a certain veto from the president. In February 1987, Representatives Pete Stark (D-CA) and Bill Gradison (R-OH) appeased Pepper by reducing the out-of-pocket threshold to $1,700 from $2,000, adding benefits for skilled nursing facilities, and reducing copayments and deductibles.

The Ways and Means health subcommittee debated the bill in April. Committee members Stark and Gradison, urged on by the liberals, added further expansions to the bill. They doubled the Medicare home health benefit and required the states to pay all Medicare deductibles and copayments for Medicaid eligibles.

In May and June, it was the turn of the House Energy and Commerce Committee's subcommittee on health and the environment. Committee Chair Henry Waxman (D-CA) added benefits for respite care, mammograms, and prevention of spousal impoverishment. Meanwhile, the Senate Finance Committee, under Lloyd Bentsen (D-TX), adopted similar measures.

Still, liberal advocates were pushing for more. The AARP, a crucial constituency, had opposed self-financing from the beginning and had never given its support to the proposal. However, over the summer of 1987, it offered its support if prescription drug coverage could be added to the bill. No one was able to predict how much drug coverage would cost, but everyone knew it would be enormously expensive. Even many supporters in the Democratic leadership were opposed. Rostenkowski (chair of the House Ways and Means Committee), and Bentsen (chair of Senate Finance), as well as the moderate Republican Gradison, were all supporters of catastrophic legislation, and all opposed adding drug coverage.[16] Even Pete Stark, the liberal advocate from California, thought the elderly would not want to pay the cost of prescription drug insurance.[17]

Nevertheless, the AARP took its case directly to Jim Wright, the Speaker of the House. Wright thought his party "needed to put a Democratic stamp on what had been a Republican initiative,"[18] and he endorsed the proposal. After negotiating with the AARP and noting Wright's endorsement, Lloyd Bentsen also agreed. The Christmas tree was lit up and decorated to the hilt!

## The Paradox of Non-Social Social Insurance

Doc Bowen's modest proposal was originally going to cost beneficiaries $4.92 per month and have a five-year estimated cost of thirteen billion dollars. The estimated five-year cost of the final proposal was thirty billion dollars. Now there was no way that the low-income elderly would be able to afford their share of the premium. Still, the proposal had to be self-financed and budget neutral or it would be vetoed by the president. Since the drafters were unwilling to ask the nonelderly to support the expanded plan, they decided to finance the program by "income relating" the premiums. They would require upper-income seniors to pay a higher Part B premium so that lower income seniors could afford the coverage.

Conservatives have wanted to make Medicare income-related since its inception. Liberals have opposed those efforts, strongly supporting the social insurance nature of the program in which everyone shares equally in the costs and benefits. Liberals fear that if Medicare premiums become too expensive for the affluent, they will drop out, leaving only the poor, and Medicare will become a welfare program similar to Medicaid.

In the case of catastrophic insurance, however, both sides found reason to support income-related premiums. John Rother explained that AARP always opposed income-related premiums, but the opportunity to gain major new benefits softened its position.[19] "Liberals see it as a way to protect the poor, while conservatives see it as a way to avoid squandering federal money on the affluent."[20]

Since the Reagan administration, liberals and conservatives have flipped-flopped on the issue. Against conservative opposition, Bill Clinton eliminated the income limit subject to the Medicare withholding tax, thus raising the proportion paid by the affluent. Liberals supported this because the withholding tax was mandatory. Unlike optional premiums that might encourage the wealthy to drop out, the tax increase had the opposite effect—encouraging them to stay in and get what they had to pay for.

Then, in 2003, conservative George W. Bush "did a Ronald Reagan," puzzling many of his supporters. He enacted an expensive Medicare prescription drug benefit and financed it, in part, by income-relating Part B premiums. While most liberals opposed the plan for other reasons, they went along with the income-related feature to secure the benefit. Conservatives made the Medicare program more progressive.

Perhaps this history of waffling might explain how Congress badly underestimated public opposition to the catastrophic proposal. It was truly a departure from the popular Medicare program. The fact that it was budget neutral and self-financing was significant. But two other factors were even more important: It was the first time that income redistribution was so transparent to those who had to pay higher amounts. It was also the first time that social legislation would have clear losers. For higher-income participants, the costs would exceed the benefits. In 1989, the maximum supplementary premium would be $800 for individuals and $1,600 for couples, plus a fixed payment of $4.00 per month for everyone.[21] By 1993, that would increase to

$1,050 for individuals earning over $45,000 and $2,100 for couples earning over $75,000, plus a fixed payment of $10.50 per month for everyone. As a result, approximately 30 percent of beneficiaries would pay more than their benefits were worth.[22] Furthermore, premiums would be collected immediately, but benefits would be phased in gradually. For example, prescription drug coverage would not be fully phased in until 1993. Finally, the program further disadvantaged approximately 20 percent of Medicare recipients— those who already had catastrophic coverage from current or past employers.[23] Their employer benefits would be phased out, and those individuals would have to pay for what they formerly were receiving for free.

Stuart Butler of the Heritage Foundation explained that of the twenty-eight million Medicare enrollees, only about twelve thousand exceeded the annual hospital coverage limits—and most of those already had supplemental insurance.[24] "It is using a sledgehammer to crack a walnut," Butler exclaimed.[25]

Despite all of these factors, there was a real benefit to a substantial majority of enrollees, particularly those with the lowest incomes. Benefits would considerably outweigh costs for 70 percent of Medicare beneficiaries (all except the 30 percent with highest incomes). The lowest-income beneficiaries, Medicaid eligibles, would pay nothing at all. Only 36 percent of beneficiaries initially would be subject to the premium surtax, and only 5 percent would pay the maximum amount. Furthermore, benefits were not limited to the few who had long hospital stays. Beneficiaries would receive additional support for prescription drugs, home health care, skilled nursing facilities, respite care, and a number of other benefits. Hence, if every elderly person could have voted in their own economic self-interest, they would have supported the measure by a wide margin.

Instead, they erupted in protest!

## The Elderly Rebel

The crowd of elderly people surrounded Dan Rostenkowski as he entered his limousine. Screaming and jeering, they yelled, "Liar! Coward! Impeach!" Many of the aging protesters held wooden signs, and they started hammering them against the hood of the car. Rosty watched in alarm from the back seat as the anger swelled and the crowd became more aggressive. Realizing the car could not get through the crowd, he ducked out the rear door and drew the crowd backwards. When the limousine finally broke free, he ran back to the car, bent over for safety, and jumped in as the driver rode quickly away.[26] On August 18, 1989, the incident was seen throughout the country on the nightly news.

Ronald Reagan had signed the Medicare Catastrophic bill in the Rose Garden on July 1, 1988—the largest expansion of Medicare since its inception.

It hardly resembled the modest bill Doc Bowen had recommended. In fact, after the drug benefit was added, Bowen, and then the president himself, threatened a veto. But, as summer came to a close in 1987, another scandal was about to affect health care policy. The Iran–Contra affair revealed a secret agreement by the Reagan administration to supply arms to the revolutionary contras in Nicaragua. The deal clearly violated an earlier law passed by Congress. Either the president did not know about the deal, or he did know and faced possible impeachment.

Reagan needed to do something positive to deflect attention from the scandal and to show his administration could still govern. Rather than fighting with Congress over the details of catastrophic legislation, he used it as a vehicle to regain support. During August and September, the White House negotiated a deal with Lloyd Bentsen. The president agreed to include the drug benefit in return for some modest reductions in benefits and a promise that the bill would remain budget neutral and self-financed.

The protests began almost immediately after the bill was signed. The National Committee to Preserve Social Security and Medicare led a movement to repeal the bill. They were joined by the pharmaceutical industry, which was afraid the drug benefit would eventually lead to government control of drug prices. The "National Committee" was particularly vicious, distributing millions of pamphlets by direct mail. Much of their literature contained claims that ranged from over-exaggerations to complete falsehoods. The mass mailings scared many of the elderly into believing they were subject to the maximum $1,600 premium.

Stuart Altman recalled a discussion with his mother, Florence, who was then a widow in her eighties. "Back then," Altman recalled,

> I was chair of the Prospective Payment Assessment Commission. We recommended to Congress how they should pay hospitals under Medicare. I'm sitting at my desk, and I get this angry call from my mother. She's incensed

because her Medicare Part B is going to go up by $800. I told her not to worry, because unless she had a trust fund I didn't know about, she would not have to pay any of the extra premium. Moreover, she was going to receive lots of new benefits. Of course, my mother didn't believe me. She had just received a letter from James Roosevelt, the chair of the "National Committee" and the son of the beloved late president FDR. His letter warned that she would be forced to pay all this extra money for a few little benefits she didn't need. Who was she going to believe? Her fifty-one-year-old kid who worked for the government, or the son of Franklin Roosevelt? "You better make Congress repeal that law," she demanded, "I'm not giving away all my money to the government!"[27]

Perhaps the ugliest incident in the long catastrophic insurance debate involved AIDS patients. People with AIDS qualified for Medicare benefits (after a twenty-nine-month waiting period) because they were disabled. Under the catastrophic bill, Medicare would pay for AZT and other extremely expensive drugs (after a six-hundred-dollar deductible). Republican congressional opponents made public statements telling the elderly the bill would force them to subsidize the exploding cost of treating AIDS patients. Henry Waxman, trying to counter the argument, responded that it wouldn't matter because most AIDS patients died well before they were eligible for benefits. Philip Crane (R-IL) proposed sending the bill back to committee to ascertain the amount of money seniors would have to pay to support AIDS patients. His amendment was defeated, but the claims about supporting AIDS patients continued.[28]

Despite repeated efforts from the federal government and the AARP to explain the benefits contained in the bill, the opposition persisted. It was not terribly surprising that the wealthy protested because of the size of the premiums. However, polls indicated that the poor were almost equally opposed. Similar to Florence Altman, they feared being subject to the high premiums.

Nobody seemed to like the shift from universal to self-financing. The poor resented it as much as the wealthy. Projections by actuaries clearly indicated that most enrollees would be better off. Furthermore, Medicare Part B, as a whole, would still confer a net benefit to the wealthy, although the amount of the benefit would be smaller than it was before catastrophic was included. The message simply did not get through.

Support for Medicare Catastrophic had once been as high as 91 percent. By December 1988, just five months after passage, support had fallen to 65 percent. Between December and March, it plummeted to 46 percent. By the time Dan Rostenkowski spoke to the Illinois senior citizens in August, the elderly were fighting mad.

## Congress Changes Its Mind

Members of both houses of Congress were shocked by the turnaround in public opinion. The House had passed the measure 328–72, and the Senate 86–11. In the wake of determined protests, Congress considered a number of proposals to scale back the premiums and benefits and save the bill. They all failed to garner enough support. A last ditch effort by John McCain (R-AZ) proposed to charge beneficiaries only the flat premium and to cover little more than hospital, home health, and respite care. The proposal resembled Doc Bowen's original effort four years before. By that time, however, opponents had dug in and sensed victory. Even McCain's modest proposal failed.

The new president, George H. W. Bush, did not want to become entangled in the controversy and offered no support. Medicare Catastrophic, the largest social program enacted during the eight-year presidency of Ronald Reagan, was going down. On November 21 and 22, just before the Thanksgiving recess, both houses of Congress voted overwhelmingly to repeal the bill.

# CHAPTER 7

# TED KENNEDY AND THE REPUBLICAN CONGRESS
## HIPAA AND SCHIP ADD TWO MORE PIECES TO THE PUZZLE

### "Get Out In Front Of It Again"

Edward Moore Kennedy strode in to the Treaty Room on the second floor of the White House and greeted the president.[1] The room was named to commemorate President McKinley's signing of the 1898 peace treaty ending the Spanish–American War. It was where John F. Kennedy signed the partial nuclear test ban treaty the month before his death in 1963, and it now served as Bill Clinton's private office. The beleaguered president and his party had just suffered an ignominious defeat in the 1994 midterm elections, losing control of the House of Representatives for the first time in forty years. Kennedy, concerned about the direction the president might take following the election, was carrying a three-page strategic memo.

The pundits concluded that Bill Clinton was a one-term president. Some accounts predicted the president was so weak he was no longer relevant. With the ascendant Newt Gingrich about to push his "Contract with America" through the Republican-controlled Congress, the conventional wisdom was that the president should shift to the right to avoid being marginalized. Certainly the president's political advisor, Dick Morris, was pushing him in that direction.

Ted Kennedy was about to tell him otherwise. Kennedy had achieved a reputation in the Senate that was unique in American history. He had become the acknowledged leader of the liberal wing of the Democratic Party while, at the same time, becoming the one person in his party who could compromise best with conservative Republicans. It is a tribute to the character of the man that he could command respect from both ends of the political spectrum. Yet, time and again, he was able to reach practical compromises with his opponents without sacrificing his political ideals.

Above all else, the ideal he treasured most and pursued throughout his lifetime was universal health care. He had failed to achieve it under Richard Nixon and still regretted that he didn't compromise further with Nixon's plan. When Jimmy Carter pursued cost control rather than universal coverage, Kennedy became a bitter opponent and challenged him for the presidential nomination. He had urged Clinton to propose a simple employer mandate, as Stuart Altman and the transition team had recommended, and had watched the complex managed competition plan go down to defeat. But Kennedy never wavered in pursuit of his goals. If he could not win the entire battle for national health reform, he would continue to fight for it piece by piece.

Instead of counseling Clinton to move to the right, he advised him to energize his supporters and stand against steep cuts in education, Medicare, Medicaid, and Social Security. He also advised Clinton to resume the battle to expand health insurance. "You need to get out in front of it again," he told him "after lies about your plan."[2]

Although Clinton did drift to the right, particularly on welfare reform, he held the line on the steepest cuts to Medicare and Medicaid, allowing the government to be shut down rather than giving in to Newt Gingrich. Moreover, with Kennedy leading the congressional battle, two major health insurance expansions were enacted during Clinton's presidency: the Health Insurance Portability and Accessibility Act and the State Children's Health Insurance Program.

## The Health Insurance Portability and Accessibility Act (HIPAA): Job Lock and Senate Lock

America's private health insurance system was very expensive, but it worked fairly well for the majority of people who were insured. Americans' feelings about insurance companies resembled their feelings about Congress. They liked their congressional representatives but disliked congress in general; in the case of health insurance, most were happy with their own health insurances, but they disliked insurance companies. However, the way the insurance market was structured left some painful gaps in coverage for a significant minority of people.

One of these gaps occurred when people had preexisting conditions. If an individual applied for insurance and had experienced previous health problems, insurance companies might refuse to cover that particular health condition or refuse to cover the applicant entirely. Such a problem often occurred when workers with employment-based insurances changed jobs. An unfortunate consequence was "job lock," in which people stayed in jobs they no longer wanted because they would not be able to get health insurance if they left.

Preexisting conditions were also problematic for companies in the small group insurance market. Small companies who had one, or a few, very sick employees might get dropped by their insurance companies, receive large rate increases, or lose the ability to buy group insurance entirely.

Vilifying insurance companies for such practices is easy and often politically expedient. However, in a market where everyone is not required to purchase insurance, these companies confront "adverse selection," a problem we previously discussed. If individuals are allowed to wait until they are sick to buy health insurance, many will do so, and the market will fail. Insurance markets require a pooling of the healthy and sick so the pool is large enough to cover those who do get sick without anyone paying an extraordinary amount. Harry Truman explained the need to cover everyone in 1945, but it wasn't until 2010 that Barack Obama enacted an individual mandate, against much political opposition.

In 1995, it was politically impossible to enact an individual mandate, but Kennedy had another strategy. After the health reform debacle in 1994, he knew there was no chance for comprehensive reform. He was still determined to make headway, however, and, for the first time, he decided to pursue incremental goals. Having chaired the long markup sessions in 1994 in the Labor and Human Resources Committee, he knew there were pieces of the failed reform effort that Republicans had favored. If he could focus on those, he thought, there might be a chance to get bipartisan support for some specific reforms.[3] Fortuitously, he had been seated next to Nancy Kassebaum (R-KS) during the markup sessions for over four weeks, and he knew that she supported insurance reforms pertaining to insurance portability and preexisting conditions.[4] That was where he would start.

Kennedy had chosen wisely. By the spring of 1995, he and Kassebaum had introduced a bill in the Senate. The Kennedy–Kassebaum bill would limit underwriting restrictions on applicants with preexisting conditions. The AFL-CIO, AARP, and Blue Cross/Blue Shield, among others, recognized the problem and expressed support.[5] Not even the two large insurance trade organizations strongly opposed the bill even though it would limit their underwriting practices.[6] By the late fall of 1995, Nancy Kassebaum claimed to have eighty supporters in the Senate.[7]

Given the rules of the US Senate, however, eighty votes out of one hundred are not always enough. Senate Majority Leader Bob Dole refused to bring the legislation to the floor. Dole was seeking support to run for president in 1996 and needed to boost his conservative credentials with the right wing of the Republican Party. As described in chapter 2, he had earlier turned against his own health reform proposal (Dole–Packwood) to please the Party's conservative wing. At the very least, Dole and the Republicans wanted to include provisions in the bill to encourage the use of medical savings accounts (MSAs).

## What Are Medical Savings Accounts?

Medical savings accounts (MSAs) are tax-deferred savings accounts that can be used to pay for medical expenses. They are paired with high deductible health plans so that individuals can use the tax-free money in their medical savings accounts to pay their initial medical expenses each year until they reach their deductible limit, whereupon the health insurance plan kicks in. For example, you might purchase a health insurance policy with a three-thousand-dollar-deductible. Each year, you are allowed to put up to a certain amount—say two thousand dollars—of before-tax money in your MSA. Employers sometimes share in these contributions. For the first three thousand dollars of expenses in any year, you can use the tax-free money in your MSA. If you do not need all of it in any year, the funds in the account carry over to future years and can earn tax-free income from qualified investments.

Proponents of MSAs, most of whom are conservative, cite several advantages. First, high deductible plans are less expensive than standard insurance plans. Hence, they are accessible to more people, save money, and increase consumer choice. Second, because individuals are spending money out of their own accounts—until they reach the deductible—they will be more cost conscious. Proponents contend that the combination of lower premiums and increased cost awareness will reduce health care spending.

Opponents, most of whom are liberal, cite the following drawbacks: The wealthy will benefit most from the tax-free provisions of MSAs because of their higher tax rate and because they can afford the risk of high deductibles. The healthy will benefit because they will pay lower premiums and are unlikely to deplete all the funds in their MSAs. Conversely, the poor, who benefit least from tax savings, are less able to risk the expense of high deductibles. And the unhealthy are more likely to deplete their MSAs and have to pay out-of-pocket. Furthermore, the poor and unhealthy have an incentive to avoid needed care because of the out-of-pocket expense. The combination of the above will supposedly encourage the healthy and wealthy to use MSAs and the poor and unhealthy to stay in traditional insurance. As a result, this will take the healthiest people out of the traditional insurance pool, leaving a higher proportion of unhealthy people and driving up their premiums. Furthermore, opponents point out, the preponderance of health spending is for expensive procedures and chronic care. Those cost far more than the deductible and will not be affected by an MSA.

In practice, MSAs (which later evolved in to health savings accounts or HSAs), neither met the expectations of conservatives nor justified the fears of liberals. On the one hand, they never became very popular. On the other hand, those that utilized them were fairly diverse in terms of income and health and did not skew the insurance pool. Nevertheless, these insurance vehicles were the focus of heated political controversy when they were added to HIPAA and later to the Medicare Prescription Drug bill.

## The "Golden Rule" of Health Insurance

The Golden Rule Insurance Company, headquartered in Indianapolis, was one of many small- to mid-size insurers that were threatened by managed care in the early '90s. The company's revenues had grown from $330 million in 1987 to $820 million in 1993, but they declined in 1994 as the largest insurers with fast-growing managed care plans began to dominate the market.[8] However, the company's CEO J. Patrick Rooney had a plan. Starting around 1990, Rooney began proselytizing MSAs and contributing heavily to the Republican Party.

The Clinton health plan, based on competitive managed care, was a dire threat to Golden Rule and other small insurers. During the '93–'94 election cycle, Golden Rule was one of the country's largest contributors to Republicans, giving over one million dollars to oppose the Clinton health plan and to encourage legislation to support MSAs.[9] In 1996, Cynthia McKinney (D-GA) testified to Congress that Golden Rule had donated over $1.4 million to the Republican Party (Rooney claimed it was only $1.1 million since 1993).[10] Rooney thoughtfully targeted his contributions. He and Golden Rule's president, John Whelan, gave at least $152,000 to GOPAC, Newt Gingrich's political action committee.[11] Rooney also donated $30,000 to Bob Dole's Campaign America.[12]

MSAs were consistent with Republican philosophy. If people had "skin in the game," they would shop for providers and prices and the market would be more efficient. Furthermore, MSAs would expand consumer choice. By the time Kennedy and Kassebaum introduced their bill, Rooney was a darling of the Republican Right, MSAs were high on their health policy agenda, and Golden Rule Insurance Company was positioned to be the chief beneficiary.

In the spring of 1995, Kennedy began a campaign to pressure Dole, first on a minimum wage increase and then on Kennedy–Kassebaum. Dole's repeated refusal to call up the minimum wage bill played badly in the press and made him look mean. Kennedy had threatened to attach the two bills to every piece of legislation. In April, when the bill finally came before the Senate, Dole tried to add an amendment to include MSAs. Kennedy was able to get four Republicans and all forty-seven Democrats to defeat the amendment and embarrass the majority leader. The bill passed the Senate a few days later.

Still getting bad press on the minimum wage, Dole finally decided he could not run for president and be majority leader at the same time, and on May 15 he announced his resignation from the Senate. Meanwhile, the House had included MSAs in its version of Kennedy–Kassebaum, and the bill was in danger of being mired in conference. Clinton wanted the legislation passed before the Democratic convention, and Kennedy reluctantly agreed to a compromise. The final bill included a four-year MSA pilot program for up to 750,000 enrollees. Policies would be limited to the self-employed and firms with less than fifty employees. On August 21, 1996, the Health Insurance Portability and Accessibility Act, also known as Kennedy–Kassebaum, became the law of the land.

## What Does HIPAA Do?

The primary objective of HIPAA is to protect people who have preexisting conditions or a change in health status, particularly those who are already insured. The legislation mandates the following regulations:

1. Individuals who have been insured for at least eighteen consecutive months, and do not have a period of uninsurance greater than sixty-three days, cannot be denied insurance or be subject to new restrictions when they change jobs and/or insurance carriers.
2. Insurers cannot limit or deny coverage for preexisting conditions for longer than twelve months (the condition must be diagnosed within six months before the twelve-month waiting period). Waiting periods for pregnant women, newborns, or newly adopted children are prohibited.
3. Insurance companies must guarantee issue to small groups (two to fifty employees) and must renew for all employers except in cases of nonpayment or fraud.

Within an insured group, employers cannot discriminate against individual employees or their dependents on account of health status. Such discrimination includes excluding or dropping coverage or increasing rates.

The legislation was certainly not a cure-all. Most importantly, it did not restrict insurance companies from raising rates according to their risk assessment of insured individuals or entire groups. Hence, it did not ensure affordability. However, it was a workable and practical means of alleviating some of the worst shortcomings of the private market.

The legislation had a number of other significant provisions. It extended tax-deductibility of insurance to the self-employed. It provided tax incentives to purchase long-term care insurance and granted tax-free life insurance benefits for the terminally and chronically ill. It also had one set of provisions that actually became the most significant part of the bill: it initiated complex federal regulations regarding the electronic transmission and privacy of medical records. This is an important area that we do not attempt to address in this book. Finally, it made an important change in the way federal and state governments regulate insurance.

## The Employee Retirement Income
## Security Act of 1974 (ERISA)

Unlike commerce in most other industries, jurisdiction over the regulation of health insurance in the United States is divided between the federal government and the states. The states take precedence over the federal government in regulating all policies issued by health insurance companies within their boundaries. However, most medium and large businesses self-insure. They use commercial insurance companies only to administer their self-insured plans. About 40 percent of US workers are in such self-insured plans. These plans are considered to be employee benefit plans and can only be regulated by the federal government. It is a strange situation. Within each state, the federal government cannot regulate health policies written by insurance companies, and the states cannot regulate policies by firms that self-insure. How did this come about?

In 1944, the Supreme Court ruled that health insurance was interstate commerce. The states wanted to maintain their power to tax and regulate insurance companies within their jurisdiction, and insurance companies thought that states would be weaker regulators than the federal government.[13] Hence, both groups lobbied Congress, which responded by enacting the McCarren–Ferguson Act of 1945. The act not only gave states precedence in regulating insurance, but also immunized insurance companies from federal antitrust restrictions.

Congress enacted ERISA in 1974 to provide protection and standards for private employee pension plans.[14] The act preempted all state laws pertaining to employee benefit plans, leaving all such regulation to the federal government; however, the act "saved" state regulation of insurance companies under McCarren–Ferguson. The act also contained what became known as the *deemer clause*. The deemer clause banned states from declaring that companies' self-funded benefit plans were insurance for purposes of state regulation. ERISA was primarily concerned with federal protection of pensions, and it is not clear that members of Congress intended to bar states from regulating self-insured health plans.

In 1974, Stuart Altman was a senior official in HEW responsible for coordinating interdepartment legislation that affected health care. Like many, he was not aware of this provision. When he learned about it after the legislation passed, he was convinced the restrictions on state regulations of self-insured health plans would not be enforced. Not many self-insured plans existed at the time, and, regardless, many members of Congress assumed that a national health care bill was in the offing.[15] Apparently, however, House–Senate conferees who drafted the bill were aware of the clause's implications.[16]

ERISA has had far-reaching effects. The federal government has been virtually absent from regulating self-insured plans. Realizing they would be free from state regulation, many companies switched from commercial to self-insured plans. As a result, they did not have to comply with state insurance regulations or mandates. For example, if state laws required insurance companies to cover in vitro fertilization or bone marrow transplants as part of their minimum benefit packages, self-insured plans did not have to comply. Employees suffered, not only because some policies failed to meet minimally expected standards, but also because injured parties had no right to redress in the courts. Despite the fact that thousands of individuals had their rights abused, there had never been political support to change ERISA Large employers in particulr did not want ERISA eliminated. They insured employees in many states and wanted consistent national standards. Many national unions also opposed changing ERISA.

HIPAA is a significant departure from the regulatory status quo. It sets federal minimum requirements for all health insurance, whether commercial or self-insured. Although it leaves regulation to the states, it provides for the federal government to step in if the states do not comply or enforce the law. In her analysis of the bill, senior researcher Kala Ladenheim concludes, "The passage of HIPAA ends almost a century of federal deference to states in the matter of insurance regulation."[17]

It is particularly surprising that this expansion of federal powers occurred under the Gingrich-led Republican Congress of 1996 that at least professed to favor federalism and devolution of power to the states. Whether the federal government will build on this legislation to exert more regulatory power over health insurance remains to be seen. At the time of this writing, a number of states are suing the federal government over the individual mandate in the Obama health plan. One area of contention is the extent of federal regulation of health insurance that is allowed under the laws governing interstate commerce.

## Kennedy Strikes Again:
## The State Children's Health Insurance Program (SCHIP)

The same day that Congress enacted HIPAA, Ted Kennedy told reporters that covering uninsured children was his next goal.[18] Recently, Kennedy had met with John McDonough, who had conceived the idea of raising tobacco taxes to fund expansions in children's health insurance. McDonough, a member of the Massachusetts House and co-chair of the Joint Committee on Health Care, led a successful campaign in 1996 to enact such a children's health insurance expansion in Massachusetts. Kennedy knew McDonough from home-state politics and wanted to use his idea as a national model.

McDonough's idea has since been copied by many others, but at the time it was ingenious and simple. Nearly everyone supported the idea of insuring children, and nearly everyone disliked tobacco companies. Moreover, raising the cigarette tax would reduce health care costs and save lives— particularly those of young smokers. It would not have worked in a tobacco-growing state, but in Massachusetts it was the right idea at the right time. After meeting with McDonough, Kennedy teamed with John Kerry, the junior senator from Massachusetts, and introduced a bill in the fall of 1996 to expand children's health insurance. The proposal was funded by a seventy-five-cent tax increase on a pack of cigarettes.

Children's health insurance had been on the liberal agenda for a long time. When Medicare was enacted in 1965, liberals thought it would be expanded piecemeal until it became a single-payer and covered everyone. As the next most sympathy-deserving group after the elderly, many believed that children would be covered next. However, cost control took precedence over insurance expansions, and the number of uninsured steadily increased. In 1996, 41.7 million Americans lacked health insurance, and 10.6 million of them were children.[19] One out of every seven children in America (14.8 percent) was uninsured.[20]

The Clintons indicated concern about children's health insurance early in their reform effort. The Health Care Task Force, directed by Hillary Clinton, had developed a "Kids First" proposal in 1993. However, that was subsumed in the battle over comprehensive health reform. Bill Clinton gave public recognition to the issue in his State of the Union address in January 1997, proposing to expand insurance for five million children. The president then proceeded to set aside funds for a much less ambitious program in his budget proposal that included $3.75 billion in block grants to the states. Meanwhile, Tom Daschle, the Senate minority leader, had stated in a January press conference that children's health insurance was a top priority. Aiming to replicate the success of HIPAA, Daschle tried to appeal to Republicans and moderates. He suggested a program funded by tax credits that gave autonomy and flexibility to the states.

A number of proposals were filed in the first half of 1997. Trent Lott (R-MS) the Senate majority leader called the bills "Salami Slicing."[21] He claimed they were big-government bills that sought to expand public insurance slice-by-slice, just like many liberals wanted. Republicans, with strong support from the governors, did not want another federal entitlement program. Hence, they favored a budgeted program with block grants to the states. In fact, Clinton had vetoed a budget bill in December 1995 that contained a Republican initiative to change Medicaid to a block grant program. The Republicans and the governors wanted the states to have maximum flexibility to administer the program and to decide on such policies as eligibility, cost-sharing, and benefits. They were particularly wary of the Medicaid benefit package that included the Early Periodic Screening, Diagnosis, and Treatment program (EPSDT), which obligated them to provide services they otherwise might not have covered.[22] Given the political climate, Democrats were willing to support a federalist approach in which much of the decision making would devolve to the states. However, they wanted the states to comply with minimum national standards and wanted to ensure that all federal money was actually being spent for children's health.[23]

## The Odd Couple

Orrin Hatch (R-UT), the longest serving senator in Utah history, was first elected to the Senate in 1976. He has an 89 percent lifetime rating from the American Conservative Union.[24] A devout Mormon, he once served as a Bishop in the Mormon Church. He had six children and seventeen grandchildren, neither smoked nor drank, and, surprisingly, was a close friend to Ted Kennedy. Possibly the oddest couple in the Senate, Kennedy and Hatch were far apart ideologically, but they frequently worked together and cosponsored important legislation. When Kennedy needed a cosponsor for his children's health insurance bill, he sought out his nonsmoking friend, Orrin Hatch.

The Hatch–Kennedy bill was typical of Kennedy's political wisdom. It expanded health insurance coverage for children, it paid for itself from cigarette taxes, it provided block grants to states, and it applied ten billion dollars of the cigarette revenues to reduce the budget deficit. The bill gave states flexibility in administration and determination of eligibility, but it required them to provide the Medicaid benefit package. It truly had something for everyone.

The Gingrich-led Republican Congress did not want to allow a vote on the bill. It was an issue that would benefit Democrats, and it was not part of the Republican agenda. Covering children up to 200 percent of poverty, they claimed, would induce "crowd out"; meaning some parents of children who already had private coverage would switch to subsidized, government-backed insurance, costing taxpayers money and crowding out the private market. Republicans also wanted to curry support with governors as well as their political allies in tobacco-growing states. Conservatives expressed anger at Orrin Hatch for collaborating with Kennedy. Some called him a "latter-day-liberal," a play on words referring to his Mormon religion that Hatch did not appreciate.

Kennedy, however, knew he had a popular issue with which he could brow-beat the Republicans. He threatened to attach it to legislation until the Republican leadership allowed a vote. On May 21, Congress was debating the federal budget, and Senator Hatch proposed the Hatch–Kennedy bill as an amendment.[25] Kennedy, displaying the fiery and passionate language for which he was famous, stated, "Why can't we vote on whether the Senate stands with children or with Joe Camel and the Marlboro man?"[26]

The bill was popular, and Hatch and Kennedy expected to prevail. Hatch had testified that 72 percent of Americans favored the legislation. However, one crucial person sided with Trent Lott to oppose the amendment: the president of the United States. Although Clinton was in favor of the bill, he had spent months negotiating the budget with Republicans. The budget agreement contained sixteen billion dollars for children's health. Republicans threatened to unravel the whole negotiation if the thirty-billion-dollar Hatch–Kennedy bill was added. Together, Lott and Clinton managed to gather enough support to table the amendment by a vote of 55–45. Hatch thought that the president "caved," and Kennedy felt betrayed.

The liberal lion of the Senate, however, was not about to give up so easily. He immediately sought support from Hillary Clinton and Marian Wright Edelman, the president of the Children's Defense Fund. Hillary turned out to be instrumental in convincing the president to support a new version of the bill. Meanwhile, the Senate Finance Committee began work on a modified Hatch–Kennedy bill, adding eight billion dollars to the original budget amount and including a twenty-cent increase in the cigarette tax. The Senate bill did not require the Medicaid benefit package, although it contained minimum federal standards. Moderate Republicans, led by Orrin Hatch, convinced Trent Lott that it was politically harmful to oppose the popular bill. The president remained uncommitted.

On July 22, "an agitated Ted Kennedy" met personally with Clinton at the White House, urging him to publicly support the bill.[27] The president offered his public endorsement the following day. With Hatch, Lott, and Clinton on board, Gingrich agreed to a budget deal that included twenty-four billion dollars for children's health and an increase in the cigarette tax of fifteen cents per pack. SCHIP was signed in to law as part of the Balanced Budget Act of 1997.

## What Does SCHIP Do?

The purpose of the SCHIP is to expand insurance coverage for children of low-income families. The program is implemented through grants to the states that allow considerable state flexibility within broad federal guidelines.

### Three Choices for State Implementation

The states can expand their current Medicaid program, create a new program for SCHIP, or combine the two. If they expand their current Medicaid program, they have to meet or exceed all Medicaid requirements. If they create a new program, they can vary eligibility, copayments, and benefits, but must maintain minimum standards.

### Eligibility

Children under nineteen years of age are eligible if family income exceeds Medicaid eligibility but is less than 200 percent of poverty. States in which Medicaid eligibility is already above 150 percent of poverty can increase income eligibility by 50 percent. States can vary eligibility within federal limits, but they must insure lower income people before those with higher incomes.

## Minimum National Standards

The minimum standard for the benefit package is the actuarial equivalent of either the Blue Cross FEHBP option or the largest HMO in the state. Cost sharing is not permitted for families under 100 percent of the poverty level and is nominal for those below 150 percent.

## Federal Matching Assistance Program (FMAP)

Financing for SCHIP is shared between the federal government and the states similar to Medicaid, but the federal match for SCHIP is higher. The federal government pays 65 to 83 percent of SCHIP expenses (compared to 50 to 76 percent under Medicaid). Each state's FMAP percentage is determined by a formula. States are not allowed to lower their Medicaid-eligible guidelines to take advantage of the higher SCHIP match.

## Grants versus Entitlements

Federal SCHIP grants are limited by the budget allocation as opposed to Medicare and Medicaid that are open entitlements. If the funds are exhausted, the states can terminate their obligations. However, SCHIP is not a block grant. States must have an approved plan and must account for all expenditures before receiving federal payments.

## Waivers

States can apply for federal waivers for plans that do not conform to all of the federal requirements. For example, a number of states cover parents of SCHIP-eligible children under certain conditions.

## A Successful Program and the Kennedy Legacy

By all accounts, SCHIP has been enormously successful. The percentage of uninsured children under eighteen years old has fallen from 13.6 percent in 1996 to 10.0 percent in 2009.[28] During the same period, the percentage of uninsured adults under age sixty-five increased from 16.4 percent to 18.9

percent.[29] A more instructive measure is the change in the number of uninsured children whose families earn between 100 and 200 percent of poverty, the target income area of the program. Between 1996 and 2005, that figure declined from 22.5 percent to 16.9 percent, an impressive 25 percent decline.[30] Later figures (from a different statistical source) indicate a further decline to 14.4 percent through 2009.[31] In fiscal year 2009, 7.8 million children from all fifty states were enrolled in the program.[32]

Congress twice voted to expand the program during George W. Bush's administration, but the president vetoed both attempts. The first proposal would have increased SCHIP eligibility to 400 percent of poverty and the second to 300 percent. Bush maintained that he did not want to increase government coverage at the expense of the private insurance market. Research indicates a valid basis for his concern based on a substantial "crowd out" effect. The CBO estimated that at the current eligibility level (200 percent of poverty), between one quarter and one half of SCHIP enrollees are taken from the private insurance market.[33] Bush finally signed a two-year reauthorization of SCHIP in 2007 on terms similar to the original legislation.

The two-year extension was due to expire during the Obama administration in 2009. President Obama reauthorized the program through 2013. He increased spending by $31.4 billion over 4.5 years, an amount that will enable states to cover an additional four million children by 2013.[34] The increased spending was financed by raising the tax on cigarettes from thirty-nine cents to $1.01 per pack and by increasing taxes on other tobacco products.[35] The legislation will reduce the deficit by one billion dollars over CBO's ten-year estimating horizon.[36] CBO estimated that in 2010, the annual cost of each child enrolled in the program would be $813.[37]

It is a tribute to Ted Kennedy's skills and perseverance that the largest expansion of government health insurance since Medicare and Medicaid in 1965 was enacted under the conservative-dominated, Newt Gingrich-led Congress. Paradoxically, SCHIP was part of the Balanced Budget Act of 1997, the budget agreement that implemented the largest cuts to Medicare and Medicaid in the history of the two programs. Bill Clinton once said of Kennedy, "He's as good at what he does as Michael Jordan is at playing basketball. I mean, he can always see the opening. He's got lateral vision, and it's uncanny what he can do."[38]

## CHAPTER 8

# THE UNLIKELY SAGA OF THE MEDICARE PRESCRIPTION DRUG BENEFIT

### Policy and Politics

In 1999, the industry newsletter *Medicine and Health Perspectives* named Stuart Altman "Health Person of the Year."[1] He received the award for what he *didn't* do. He didn't provide the swing vote on the National Bipartisan Commission on the Future of Medicare to restructure the Medicare program. If the editor had a crystal ball, he might also have cited Altman for what he did do. He helped drag the issue of Medicare prescription drug coverage into the political arena where, against all expectations, it would become law just four years later.

On November 18, 2003, John Rother's mail was nothing less than abusive. The policy director and chief lobbyist for the AARP was about to see his organization lose sixty thousand members.[2] The day before, AARP endorsed the Republican proposal for a Medicare prescription drug benefit. A poll, taken by Peter Hart, found that only 18 percent of AARP's members supported the bill.[3] For the first time in the nation's history, senior citizens would receive a drug benefit, and they were fighting mad!

In the spring of 2003, Ted Kennedy joined with Max Baucus (D-MT) and John Breaux (D-LA) to support the Bush administration's effort to enact a Medicare drug benefit. Kennedy had spent years fighting for such a benefit expansion. However, on November 27, he led a filibuster to stop the bill. It passed anyway, and on December 8, 2003, George W. Bush, the conservative president, signed into law the Medicare Prescription Drug, Improvement, and Modernization Act (MMA), the largest expansion of the government health program since its inception in 1965. It is a peculiar story that reveals the entanglement of policy and politics that Barack Obama would have to confront six years later.

## The Voice of Reason

George W. Bush was not the first president or politician to recommend prescription drug coverage for seniors. As previously discussed, Congress considered including drugs in the original Medicare legislation in 1965 but demurred. An HEW task force recommended a Medicare prescription drug program to the Nixon administration in 1969, and the president included it in his proposal for national health care, but the effort failed. Prescription drugs were included in the Medicare Catastrophic bill that was enacted under Ronald Regan, but the legislation was repealed in 1989. President Clinton included Medicare prescription drugs in his Health Security Act, but the effort was defeated in 1994.

The National Bipartisan Commission on the Future of Medicare was created by the Republican Congress and the Clinton administration in the Balanced Budget Act of 1997. Its mission was to strengthen and improve the Medicare program to adequately serve the pending retirement of the baby boomers. The two co-chairs, Senator John Breaux (D-LA) and Representative Bill Thomas (R-CA), had a broader agenda. They believed the program had to be restructured. Their goal was to inject market forces so that private insurance, theoretically more efficient, would compete with, and eventually replace, the government-run program. Their proposal, called "premium support," would change the nature of Medicare, a thirty-four-year-old program that many conservatives had long opposed.

The concept of premium support was introduced in a paper by two well-known health policy experts, Henry Aaron and Robert Reischauer.[4] Simply stated, beneficiaries would receive a fixed sum of money from the government (or a voucher), which they could use to purchase a private insurance plan or the traditional Medicare fee-for-service plan. If they chose a plan that cost more than the voucher, they would have to pay the difference. If their choice cost less, they would receive money back. Proponents argued that competition among plans would reduce costs and give consumers additional choices. Opponents worried that competition would be unfair because seniors in traditional Medicare were older and sicker and, hence, would have higher health care costs. They were also concerned that the government-funded voucher might become less adequate over time. They favored the security of the guaranteed defined benefit over an untried program based on a defined contribution.

The seventeen-member Medicare commission was required to have an eleven-vote super majority to issue a report. All eight Republicans and two Democrats, Breaux and Bob Kerrey (D-NE), were in favor of restructuring the program. They needed to win one more Democratic vote.

The remaining seven Democrats had a number of concerns. They wanted to improve the Medicare benefit package because it only provided about half of enrollees' health expenses. Although a drug benefit would help achieve this goal, they wanted drugs to be provided within the Medicare program but strongly opposed the creation of a private system that would compete with traditional Medicare. In addition, they believed that future financial support should be derived from general revenues, or the Medicare withholding tax, and not from reducing benefits or shifting responsibility to the private sector.

Stuart Altman and D'Andrea Tyson were economists and were attracted to the goal of market forces and increased competition. Tyson, however, had served in the Clinton administration until 1996 and was somewhat constrained by party loyalty to support the Democratic position. It appeared likely that Altman could be the swing vote.

In an effort to entice Altman or other Democrats, the Republicans floated a bare-bones prescription drug benefit aimed at seniors earning below 135 percent of poverty. Altman, however, wanted a comprehensive drug benefit, not only because it was badly needed, but also because it would allow the traditional Medicare program to compete with private plans. He also wanted assurances that if there was a voucher, it would always be sufficient to purchase a reasonable benefit package. The Brandeis professor was the eleventh and deciding vote, and as the deadline approached for the commission to issue its report, he had to make a decision. In the end, the Republicans would not offer a full Medicare drug benefit or sufficient guarantees of adequate funding. Altman was sympathetic to premium support, and he received no pressure from the Clinton administration to support the Democratic position. However, he was not willing to put the traditional Medicare program at risk. He refused to budge, for which the editor of Medicine and Health called him "the voice of reason."

The commission never got eleven votes for any proposal and failed to issue a report. The momentum for restructuring withered, and Medicare remained unchanged. However, the newly discussed Medicare prescription drug benefit rose to the top of the political agenda. President Clinton

proposed a drug plan with a Medicare Part D, and a number of other proposals were filed in Congress. None of them were adopted, but Medicare
prescription drugs became an important issue in the 2000 presidential
campaign.

## Health Policy in a Democracy—
## Bridging the Philosophical Divide

George W. Bush pursued a Medicare drug benefit throughout the first three
years of his term. Why would a conservative Republican president want to
add an expensive new entitlement to a federal program that many in his own
party thought was bureaucratic and out of control? It was counterintuitive.
It seemed reminiscent of Nixon going to China, Clinton ending welfare, or
Reagan supporting Medicare Catastrophic. Yet, a confluence of events may
explain his decision.

Many people were upset about the price of drugs. Between 1998 and
2002, prescription drug spending per person in the United States had
increased more than 13 percent every year.[5] Employers had been cutting back
health benefits, especially to retirees, and many private Medicare plans (then
called Medicare + Choice) had reduced coverage or exited the market completely after cutbacks from the Balanced Budget Act of 1997. Nearly one
quarter of Medicare beneficiaries had no drug coverage.[6] More importantly,
the budget situation was unique. In 2001, the CBO projected a $5.6 trillion
surplus over the next decade.[7] The Bush administration had money to spend!

Economic factors were not the only reasons that may have influenced
Bush's agenda. Controlling the presidency and both houses of Congress, the
Republicans had their first unified government in over forty years. The
opportunity existed to enact substantive change, and the Medicare program
had long been in the crosshairs of Republican conservatives. Bush saw an
opportunity to use prescription drugs as an enticement to change the nature
of the program and shift it back toward the private sector. At the same time,
by providing a prescription drug benefit to seniors, he could usurp the
Democrats' long-held advantage with the Medicare population. It was a win-
win situation—seemingly too good to pass up.

In the first two years of the new administration, Bush and congressional
Republicans proposed several limited drug programs. Bush initially proposed a

program that targeted low-income seniors and would be administered as block grants to the states to help the needy purchase private insurance. The Republican House also advanced proposals that provided funds for low-income Medicare beneficiaries to purchase insurance from private plans. Democrats, however, did not want a means-tested benefit and wanted drugs to be part of traditional Medicare. The Republican plan passed the House, but the Senate was more liberal, and the Democrats had regained the majority in 2001 when Jim Jeffords from Vermont left the Republican Party to become an independent. The Senate easily defeated the proposal, and no action was taken.

The midterm elections in 2002 altered the political landscape. The Republicans again held the presidency and both houses of Congress. George Bush was near the height of his popularity, having rallied the country after the terrorist attacks on September 11, 2001. The president, known to be bold in his initiatives, seized the opportunity to reorient Medicare toward the private sector. He proposed spending $400 billion over ten years, and he outlined a program that permitted Medicare beneficiaries to purchase drug coverage, but only by joining private health plans. Those in traditional Medicare would be limited to purchasing catastrophic drug coverage that would only cover annual drug expenses over $5,500.[8] Bush reasoned that many seniors would switch from traditional Medicare to private (Medicare + Choice) plans in order to get the more comprehensive prescription drug benefit.

Many Senators, however, worried about offending senior citizens. Rural states had few Medicare + Choice plans, and many rural residents would not have access to a drug benefit under Bush's plan. In addition, 89 percent of Medicare beneficiaries were still in the traditional Medicare program and might not be pleased if Congress pressured them to move. It appeared that the four-year deadlock on the Medicare drug benefit might continue.

Then, on June 6, 2003, Chuck Grassley, the Republican chair of the Senate Finance Committee, announced an agreement he had reached with Democrats Max Baucus and Ted Kennedy. The compromise was an artful blend of policy options that was another example of Kennedy's ability to forge agreements with his political opponents. In this case, Kennedy knew he would have to accept a program that would keep within the president's budget limits and provide support for private sector initiatives. He was willing to privatize the purchase of all prescription drugs, a significant compromise, if he was assured that the private plans and traditional Medicare would have substantially equivalent benefits.

The proposal allowed Medicare beneficiaries to join private, single, or multistate health plans that would provide prescription drug coverage as well as other extra benefits. It also allowed people who were enrolled in traditional Medicare to purchase private drug-only plans. If no plans were available in an area, the government would provide a fallback plan.

The most difficult issue was how to structure the benefit and keep within the president's ten-year, $400 billion budget. The two standard choices for insurance were catastrophic or first-dollar coverage. Under catastrophic coverage, enrollees would pay all of their annual prescription drug expenses up to a threshold limit. The program would then provide coverage for all annual expenses beyond the limit. The reasoning behind the catastrophic option was that most seniors who were not Medicaid-eligible could afford an average amount of drug spending. It was only those with extraordinary drug expenses that needed protection. Many economists favor a catastrophic program because it is consistent with the way insurance works—it protects against an unlikely but unaffordable occurrence. In addition, it makes people more cost-conscious because they have to pay for their own drugs until they reach the catastrophic threshold.

Under the first-dollar option, the program would pay for all of an enrollee's prescription drug expenses with the exception of small deductibles and/or copayments. Many economists do not like first-dollar coverage because it is expensive and prone to overuse. Furthermore, the program could not possibly provide first-dollar and catastrophic coverage and remain anywhere close to the president's budget limit. However, first-dollar coverage is much more politically popular than catastrophic because nearly everyone receives benefits. Under catastrophic, everyone pays a premium, but only a small proportion who have high drug expenses receive a tangible benefit. A similar structure angered seniors and led to the repeal of Medicare Catastrophic. Politicians were wary of making the same mistake again.

In this case, necessity was the mother of the donut hole. The senators figured out a way to combine the two types of coverage and remain within the budget. In order to provide some front-end coverage, the Senate plan paid 50 percent of prescription drug expenses up to $4,500 after an initial annual deductible of $275. Then, there was no coverage between $4,500 and $5,800—the infamous donut hole. The program would then provide catastrophic coverage by paying for 90 percent of all expenses above $5,800. The size of the gap in coverage was totally dictated by the need for the plan to stay within the ten-year budget of $400 billion. A similar structure was also included in the drug benefit plan proposed in 1999 by Bill Clinton but received little attention. The compromise bill was a convoluted but creative way to satisfy both the policy and political imperatives. Everyone appeared to get some of what they wanted, and no one's principles were violated. The legislation immediately drew bipartisan support, and, in lightening speed (for Congress), easily passed the full Senate on June 27 by a vote of 76–21.

In the more conservative House, however, ideology trumped compromise. Reviving a strain of premium support, the House bill tied future increases in Medicare premiums to cost increases in the type of plan (private or traditional Medicare) in which an individual was enrolled. Hence, over time, Medicare prices would have to compete with prices of private plans. This pleased conservatives, who trumpeted the ideal of greater competition. However, Democrats and liberals contended that enrollees in private health plans were younger and healthier than those in the traditional Medicare program. With an older and sicker population, costs in traditional Medicare—and thus premiums—would have to rise faster, pushing more and more people into lower-cost private plans and leaving the sickest population in traditional Medicare where prices would rise even further. Democrats foresaw a "death spiral" in traditional Medicare, a goal some believed was the underlying intent of the Republican proposal.

The House plan had other controversial measures. It required low-income seniors to prove their incomes and assets were below a threshold level in order to qualify for the program. It also related benefits to income, raising the catastrophic threshold for beneficiaries earning over sixty thousand dollars. This was reminiscent of measures that angered seniors and caused the repeal of Medicare Catastrophic. It also violated the social insurance philosophy of Medicare in which all citizens, rich or poor, received the same benefits. Despite the provisions in the House bill, many conservatives were still unhappy. They objected to $400 billion of spending for a new entitlement program, particularly since it was funded almost exclusively by general tax revenues with practically no offsets from other sources of funds. They also believed the legislation should have had stronger measures to push people into private Medicare health plans. When the bill reached the House floor on June 27, the Republican leadership did not have enough votes. Even an unorthodox visit to the chamber by Vice President Cheney was unable to turn the tide. The leadership finally offered an increase in tax reductions for those who established health savings accounts, a favorite policy of conservative Republicans. That plum, estimated to cost an additional $174 billion over ten years, apparently outweighed the concerns about spending, and the bill squeaked by the house on a 216–215 vote.

The House and Senate had passed very different versions of a Medicare Prescription Drug benefit, and the two bills had to be reconciled in conference. Controlling both houses of Congress, the Republican leadership stacked the conference committee in favor of the conservatives. Bill Thomas, the chair of Ways and Means and an ardent supporter of premium support, chaired the conference. Thomas, a brilliant legislator, was a big-picture kind of guy. He foresaw an opportunity to change the stodgy, thirty-eight-year-old program to a more dynamic and competitive model. He conceptualized much of the bill and was truly the force behind much of the political maneuvering. Thomas, however, angered the Democratic leadership. He allowed only two Democratic senators—John Breaux and Max Baucus, both of whom were sympathetic to restructuring—to attend the deliberations. He then excluded all Democratic House members including the minority leader Tom Daschle. The conference began in August, and four months later, in November, there was still no agreement. The hot-tempered chairman, who favored premium support and wanted to shift Medicare beneficiaries into private plans, was not inclined to compromise. He had heated confrontations with Iowa senator Chuck Grassley, who worried about the lack of private plans in his rural districts. A congressional staffer remarked, "Premium support had a constituency of one—Bill Thomas."[9]

Finally, in November, Dennis Hastert (the Speaker of the House) and Bill Frist (the Senate majority leader) took control of the conference. Both realized that Thomas was not going to make the compromises needed to pass the legislation. They had to stay within the president's $400 billion budget limit. They had to satisfy liberals and representatives of rural states by granting a near-equivalent drug benefit to seniors in traditional Medicare while still satisfying conservatives with incentives to switch people to private plans. In addition, they had to negotiate with the AARP and the pharmaceutical industry to win their support while avoiding opposition from insurers, employers, doctors, hospitals, and other powerful lobbies, any one of which could torpedo the narrow support for the plan. It was a prescription for politics to overwhelm the policy.

## Details of the Plan: A Cauldron of Policy and Politics

The 2003 MMA was a lengthy and complex bill. Those wondering why the Obama health plan (or the Clinton plan) was so complicated and abstruse might have more appreciation for the complexity of health care reform by reading the 148-page CMS summary of the plan, or a shorter summary from the Kaiser Family Foundation.[10]

MMA was the largest expansion of Medicare since it was enacted in 1965. It was estimated to cost $395 billion dollars and increase Medicare spending by 30 percent over the next ten years.[11] Yet it would only cover one-fifth of the amount Medicare beneficiaries would spend on drugs. The following is a summary and explanation of the major aspects of the plan:

### Voluntary Enrollment in Private Plans or Traditional Medicare

The program was entirely voluntary. Medicare beneficiaries had three options: they could keep their existing coverage, whether or not it included prescription drug coverage; they could remain in traditional Medicare and purchase private, drug-only insurance policies; or they could join private Medicare insurance plans that included drug coverage (renamed Medicare Advantage, superseding Medicare + Choice). Medicare Advantage plans were authorized in Part C of the Medicare program and the drug-only private plans became Part D.

### Benefit Design with the Donut Hole

The benefit design for traditional Medicare was the oddest part of MMA, and many beneficiaries found it baffling. However, as we explained previously, the cost of the legislation had to be less than the arbitrary figure of $400 billion that was specified in the 2003 budget resolution. If it exceeded that amount, the president had threatened a veto. In addition, any senator could raise a "point of order" and it would require a sixty-vote majority to override the budget rule. Because the bill's supporters did not have sixty votes (and certainly not sixty-seven to override a veto), supporters on both sides of the aisle endeavored to keep within the budget.

Hence, the bill was designed with premiums, a deductible, and a "donut hole;" but the combination was less generous than the original Senate bill.

Part D premiums began at $35 per month with a $250 deductible. Medicare paid 75 percent of annual expenses between $250 and $2,250. Medicare did not pay anything for annual expenses between $2,250 and $5,100 (the donut hole). Medicare then paid 95 percent of annual expenses exceeding $5,100. In addition, beneficiaries had to make small copayments. Premiums could be paid directly or deducted from Social Security checks.

### Stand-alone Drug Plans and the Medicare Advantage Advantage:

The political compromise required private, stand-alone drug providers for the great majority of seniors who would elect to remain in traditional Medicare. Some worried that if the design benefited mostly sick people, (i.e., those with high drug costs), then mostly sick people would sign up. If that was to occur, it could be a classic case of adverse selection. What private insurance company would provide insurance to people who knew they were going to need it? And if they did provide it, wouldn't it have to be so expensive that no one would buy it? That conundrum prompted Tom Scully, the administrator of CMS, to tell Congress that, "stand-alone drug coverage does not exist in nature."[12] Many worried that there would not be enough private drug-only providers to serve the traditional Medicare population.

On the other hand, the bill was very advantageous for Private Medicare Advantage Plans (MAs). They would now be paid for drugs that they previously offered essentially for free to attract enrollees. In addition, they could create cost-saving efficiencies by substituting drugs for more expensive treatment regimens. These benefits allowed them to offer drug coverage with a zero premium and low deductibles—a strong incentive to attract seniors who were enrolled in traditional Medicare to switch to their private plans.

However, few MA plans existed in rural areas or in cities with relatively low Medicare expenses. In rural areas, the sparse population made it difficult to support networks of providers. In low-cost areas (as elsewhere) the benchmark reimbursement rates were pegged to the regional fee-for-service rates in the traditional Medicare program. In regions where those rates were low, it was difficult to offer the added benefits that would attract enrollees from traditional Medicare. Politicians from those areas argued that in order to attract private MA plans, the government would have to pay rates that were significantly higher than those paid for traditional Medicare. With strong support from rural members of Congress, particularly Senators Baucus and Grassley on the Senate Finance Committee, benchmarks were raised in rural and low-cost areas. In addition to the regional adjustments, a fourteen-billion-dollar stabilization fund was established nationwide to encourage private plan entry and retention. Furthermore, the government implemented a program to share financial risk with private plans initiated under the new program.

The regional adjustments were substantial. In some areas, government reimbursement exceeded the cost of traditional Medicare by as much as 20 to 30 percent. In addition, both stand-alone and MA plans were allowed to structure their own drug benefits as long it was actuarially equivalent to the government standard. Over time, all of these advantages enabled MA plans to attract many seniors from traditional Medicare. By 2007, 19 percent, or 8.3 million, Medicare beneficiaries were enrolled in private plans, and the CBO projected an increase to 26 percent by 2017.[13] Because of these advantages, the program created political controversy and cost the government substantial amounts of extra money. Conservatives argued that the existence of private, competitive plans would lower the government's cost over the long run. However, liberal members of Congress, who were opposed to private Medicare plans in the first place, believed that such plans should only exist if they were more efficient and cost less than traditional Medicare. In 2007, the CBO projected that if the benchmark reimbursements for MA plans were reduced to the same as traditional Medicare, the government would save $149 billion over the 2009–2017 period.[14] Reducing these subsidies became a major source of funds to support the Obama health reform bill.

## Protecting the Private Sector

In addition to the subsidies and the requirement that private insurers provide drug coverage, the bill had controversial provisions that protected the pharmaceutical industry. Medicare, which had enormous market power, was expressly prohibited from negotiating drug prices with private pharmaceutical companies. Conservatives generally believe that markets function better without government interference. In this case, they were particularly concerned that the monopsony power of Medicare could unfairly drive down prices and endanger the pharmaceutical industry's ability to develop new drugs. Of course, it also would have serious negative consequences for the profitability of the industry.

This infuriated Democrats, who never supported incentives for private

Medicare plans and wanted to keep the drug benefit within traditional Medicare. They maintained that prohibiting Medicare from negotiating lower prices was a wasteful giveaway of taxpayer money to the pharmaceutical industry.

How much of a giveaway this was is subject to dispute. The Veterans Administration (VA) negotiates prices directly with drug companies. A Families USA study in 2005 found that the Medicare prescription drug plan paid 48 percent more than the VA for the top twenty drugs used by seniors.[15] However, the CBO did not think the savings would be substantial. They maintained that the VA obtains most of its negotiating success by limiting its formulary so that they can steer all their business to one drug in each class— something that Medicare would be politically unable to do. Liberals contend that Medicare could still save a considerable amount of money, and they cite the success of foreign countries that often pay less than US citizens for American-manufactured drugs. Liberals would like to save money by reimporting those drugs, but an additional provision in the bill expressly prohibited reimportation. Both prohibitions caused many liberals to oppose the bill.

## Poor and Low-Income Seniors Receive the Greatest Benefit

The largest beneficiaries of the plan were poor and low-income seniors. Medicare assumed financial responsibility from the states for all low-income Medicare recipients, called dual eligibles (seniors enrolled in both Medicaid and Medicare). Dual eligibles received a 100 percent federal subsidy regardless of income or assets. Other Medicare enrollees with incomes below 135 percent of poverty received a full premium subsidy if they had assets below six thousand dollars for an individual or nine thousand dollars for a couple. The subsidy was set at the weighted average premium for a basic plan in the region, but at no less than the least expensive plan available. Enrollees with incomes up to 150 percent of poverty received a sliding scale subsidy and also had to pass an asset test (ten thousand dollars/individual; twenty thousand dollars/couple).

Because Medicare took over payment responsibility from the states for former Medicaid recipients, states were required to remit maintenance of effort payments to the federal government. These requirements were called "claw back" provisions and caused much opposition from the states. Under these provisions, the federal government would claw back eighty-eight billion dollars of an estimated $115 billion state savings over ten years.

## The Rich Pay More with Income-Related Part B Cost Sharing

The elderly poor would receive the greatest benefits from the program, but wealthier Medicare recipients would have to pay part of the bill. Cost sharing for Medicare Part B would be income-related beginning in 2007. Medicare beneficiaries had been paying 25 percent of their Part B expenses, and the government had been paying the balance. Under the income-related provisions, beneficiaries would have to pay more as their incomes increased. The following schedule was phased in over five years:

The difference in cost for high earners was substantial. For example, those earning over $200,000 would see their costs more than triple. Charging higher payments for wealthier beneficiaries was a significant departure from traditional Medicare. Democrats and liberals had always supported the social insurance nature of Medicare wherein every working citizen contributed and everyone received the same benefit. As we discussed previously, if the cost for wealthy seniors were too high, they might drop out of the program, rendering it a welfare program like Medicaid instead of universal social insurance. Indeed, seniors were so angry about similar provisions in the Medicare Catastrophic Act that they had the entire legislation repealed.

Table 8.1

| Annual Income | % of Part B Costs That Beneficiaries Would Pay |
|---|---|
| Less than $80,000 | 25% |
| $80,000 – $100,000 | 35% |
| $100,000 – $150,000 | 50% |
| $150,000 – $200,000 | 65% |
| Above $200,000 | 80% |

Source: Henry J. Kaiser family Foundation (prepared by Health Policy Alternatives, Inc.), "Prescription Drug Coverage for Medicare Beneficiaries: A Summary of the Medicare Prescription Drug, Improvement, and Modernization Act of 2003," December 10, 2003, http://www.kff.org/medicare/upload/Prescription-Drug-Coverage-for-Medicare-Beneficiaries-A-Summary-of-the-Medicare-Prescription-Drug-Improvement-and-Modernization-Act-of-2003.pdf (accessed December 28, 2010).

The income-related provisions were estimated to yield thirteen billion dollars over ten years and would initially affect 3 percent of beneficiaries (increasing to 6 percent in 2013).

### Encouraging Employers to Maintain Retiree Drug Coverage

If Medicare provided a prescription drug program, employers might stop providing drug coverage for their retirees, saving the expense and letting their former employees obtain coverage from the government. If that happened, the government would incur the added expense of subsidizing seniors who were previously receiving private benefits. Hence, policy makers decided to provide a subsidy to employers to encourage them to maintain coverage.

The size of the subsidy was difficult to determine. If it was too small, many employers still might drop coverage, shifting the cost to the government. However, if it was too large, the government would be needlessly providing taxpayer's money to large corporations. Policy makers decided to provide a 28 percent subsidy that was estimated to cost eighty-six billion dollars over ten years.

### A Compromise on Premium Support

The bill specified that premium support would be "field tested" by funding demonstrations in six localities beginning in 2010. Generally based on the Aaron–Reischauer design, it would establish competition between traditional Medicare and private Medicare Advantage plans. It was a compromise that worried liberals but only gave conservatives a small piece of what they wanted.

### An Attempt to Cap Medicare Spending

The bill included a provision to limit the amount of general tax revenues expended for Medicare. The Medicare Trustees were required to issue seven-year projections of expenditures for the Medicare Trust Funds and for general revenues required to support Medicare Parts A, B, and D. During the seven-year window, if projected general revenue payments exceeded 45 percent of total Medicare spending, a Medicare warning had to be issued. The warning required the president to submit legislation within that year to bring general revenue funding below 45 percent.

Conservatives were worried that the cost of the drug benefit would increase much faster than predicted and, as a result, would drain general tax revenues and increase the deficit. The provision was first suggested by Bob Kerrey, but Thomas knew it would encounter opposition, so he waited until the conference to insert it into the bill.[16] Liberals opposed the measure, fearing that, over time, the budget cap could weaken the guaranteed Medicare entitlement.

## Dealing with Stakeholders and Special Interests

The provisions of the MMA revealed the deep philosophical differences between Republicans and Democrats that have always haunted efforts at health care reform. The Republicans wanted to limit cost, reduce the role of government, and shift transactions to the private market. The Democrats wanted to utilize the power of government to provide universal social insurance for citizens' basic needs and to protect citizens from market failures and/or abuses of corporate power.

Interest groups had scuttled many previous attempts at health care reform, always insisting on the particular policy prescription most beneficial to their own needs. The MMA was no exception. Special interests had played a major role in defeating the Clinton health plan, and the Bush administration, acutely aware of the politics, had no intention of suffering a similar fate. Bush's strategy was not as aggressive as Obama's, which actively pursued negotiations with every important stakeholder. Nevertheless, the Bush team successfully bargained with the most important industries and was more than receptive to the lobbying efforts of others. The provisions of the final bill were not only shaped by different philosophies but bore the imprint of private interests who had much to gain or lose. Perhaps Barack Obama fashioned his more aggressive stakeholder strategy in light of Bush's success with the MMA.

Among the most important interest groups was the AARP. Although it is generally known as an advocacy group for seniors, the organization derives most of its revenue from the sale of various products and services. The sale of health insurance policies alone exceeds its revenues from membership. With over forty million members, it is a powerful interest group, and it is likely that MMA would never have passed without its endorsement. The

Republican leadership worked with the AARP throughout the long process, and in return for its support, they largely yielded on the organization's three most important demands: an adequate Part D subsidy for low-income beneficiaries, a subsidy for employers to encourage them to maintain retiree drug coverage, and a pared-down premium support effort limited to the six demonstrations in 2010.

Many AARP members were furious with the organization's decision to support the bill. However, the AARP leadership felt that the Republicans had alleviated its most important concerns. Furthermore, with a looming budget deficit and a Republican administration, they thought this might be their only chance for many years to secure the long-sought drug benefit.

The pharmaceutical industry was the next most important stakeholder. They had previously opposed every attempt to enact a government drug benefit. Spending over one hundred million dollars each year on campaign contributions, the industry had been one of the most powerful lobbies in the country, and it is doubtful that the administration could have passed the drug bill without its support. In the case of MMA, their support was well-rewarded when the legislation acceded to their three most important demands: all prescription drugs had to be supplied through the private sector, government would be barred from direct price negotiation, and reimportation would not be allowed. The pharmaceutical companies stood to gain from the purchases of an estimated forty-one million seniors who would enroll in the program, thirteen million of whom had no previous coverage for prescription drugs.

Any important piece of legislation on Capitol Hill attracts the close attention of industry lobbyists, but a bill of this magnitude was particularly important to all stakeholders in health-related industries, and they lobbied the administration intensively. With opponents from the liberal and conservative wings of both parties, the Republican leadership could hardly afford further opposition from other stakeholders. As a result, the lobbyists were able to extract a boatload of generous provisions. Judy Feder, a seasoned health policy expert said, "There's a tremendous amount of money floating in this bill. While we think it's about prescription drugs, the promoters of this bill put money into every interest group—physicians, hospitals, rural providers, cancer doctors, (and) on the drug side, the pharmaceutical and insurance industries, and it's tough to fight all those bucks."[17]

The insurance industry was well-compensated. They would be the beneficiaries of a huge new subsidized market for drug insurance. Their Medicare Advantage plans would receive substantial sums to develop new plans and expand enrollment in rural and low-cost areas. In addition, the government would initially share financial risk with some private plans to protect them against unforeseen losses.

For some time, the Business Roundtable and other large industry groups had been seeking relief from the government from the cost of their retiree health benefits. Indeed, a number of companies had rescinded health benefits they had promised retirees—a highly controversial policy, but one that was legally permitted under their labor contracts. Lobbyists for business wanted subsidies from the government in return for maintaining their drug coverages. As we previously explained, there was mutual interest because the Medicare program would have to assume the entire cost of enrolling any senior whose coverage was dropped. Hence, employers received the aforementioned 28 percent subsidy to maintain coverage they were previously providing at their own expenses.

The AMA also got a piece of the pie. Doctors had been scheduled to receive a 4.5 percent reduction in Medicare reimbursement in accordance with existing regulations. Instead, under the MMA, they received a 1.5 percent increase. Hospital reimbursements were also increased, and a temporary moratorium was established to halt the increasing competition from specialty hospitals. Additionally, to shore up support among rural senators, Medicare reimbursement to rural providers was increased by twenty-one billion dollars over ten years.

The fingerprints of special interest groups were all over the final thousand-page bill.

## Political Shenanigans

On November 21, 2003, Nick Smith (R-MI) and about twenty other conservative Republican congressmen met for dinner in the back room of the Hunan Dynasty.[18] Later that evening, they would have to cast their votes for or against MMA. They discussed the pressures they were getting from the Republican House leadership that included the loss of a subcommittee chair and the threat of future opposition from Republican opponents. Possibly, none of the members had been lobbied as hard as Smith, who had been promised money and political support for his son's upcoming congressional campaign.

Despite all the enticements that had been inserted into the bill by the conference committee, many conservatives were still opposed to what they considered an expensive, unfunded government entitlement. Smith and twenty-four of his Republican colleagues would later vote their conscience and oppose the bill. In fact, on the floor of the House at 3:15 a.m. on the early morning of November 22, it appeared MMA would be defeated. Although the roll call was supposed to be completed in fifteen minutes, Republicans held the vote open, attempting to pressure a few congressmen to convert. For more than an hour, they were two votes short. Tommy Thompson, the secretary of HHS, broke with tradition and lobbied on the House floor. President Bush, who had just returned from London, made personal calls from the White House in a last-ditch attempt to get a few members to change positions. After two hours and fifty-one minutes, the longest roll call in the history of the House, the leadership succeeded, and the bill passed the House 220–215 with the support of sixteen Democrats.

A few days later, on November 25, the bill came before the Senate. Ted Kennedy, who was instrumental in forging the compromise that produced the Senate version of the bill, was now bitterly opposed. It is an "attack on Medicare as we know it," Kennedy said, and he organized a filibuster. Despite liberal sympathy for his position, the Senate easily ended the filibuster with a 71–29 vote for cloture. Then, Kennedy and Minority Leader Tom Daschle raised a point of order, claiming that the bill exceeded the $400 billion spending limit in the budget resolution. Republicans needed sixty votes to suspend the budget rules, and for some time the vote stood at 58–39. It appeared that the unusual combination of Republican conservatives and Democratic liberals would prevail. However, Trent Lott and Lindsey Graham (R-SC), both loyal Republicans who opposed the bill, changed their position and supported the motion. That allowed a floor vote and the bill eventually passed 61–39, with most Republicans supporting the expansive new Medicare entitlement and most Democrats opposing their long-held goal of providing a Medicare drug benefit. After voting for the motion that allowed the floor vote, Lott returned to his original position and voted against the bill.

It stood as the most divisive and bitter congressional battle in several decades, surpassed only by the vote on the Obama health plan in 2010. The Republicans invited only two Democrats to the signing session. Ironically one was Max Baucus, the man who would shepherd the Obama plan through the Senate (the other was John Breaux). During the signing, opponents held a rally on Capitol Hill, where a bitter Ted Kennedy famously shouted to the crowd, "Who do you trust? The HMO-coddling, drug-company-loving, Medicare-destroying, Social-Security-hating Bush administration? Or do you trust Democrats, who created Medicare and will fight with you to defend it every day and every week of every year?"

## Epilogue

Back on June 20, 2003, in the midst of debate over the Medicare drug bill, Rick Foster, the Chief Actuary for Medicare, peered into his computer monitor and clicked on an e-mail.[19] The message was from Jeffrey Flick, the top aide to Medicare's administrator, Tom Scully. Flick warned Foster not to release his cost estimates of the Medicare drug bill to Congress until he spoke with Scully. The ominously worded e-mail read, "The consequences for insubordination are extremely severe."[20]

In January 2004, the month after Congress enacted MMA, Cybele Bjorkland heard the familiar sound of an incoming message on her office fax machine. Ms. Bjorkland worked for the Ways and Means Committee chaired by Bill Thomas. Since June, she and Thomas had been requesting Foster's cost estimates for MMA. On June 11, she had asked Scully directly for the estimates. Bjorkland claims that Scully replied, "If Rick Foster gives that to you, I'll fire him so fast his head will spin."[21] Scully denies he said this and contends he never threatened to fire Foster. However, an internal HHS investigation concluded that Scully did indeed threaten to fire Foster.[22] Since 1912, the law has protected the right of federal employees to communicate with Congress.[23] Nevertheless, the HHS investigative report agreed with the Bush justice department opinion that Scully had "the final authority to determine the flow of information to Congress."[24]

By the time Bjorkland received the fax, she probably was not surprised. Foster had estimated that the cost of MMA from 2004 through 2013 would be between $500 and $600 billion, 25 percent to 50 percent more than the White House was telling Congress.[25] Had members of Congress known about the chief actuary's estimate, it is highly unlikely they would have voted to enact the MMA.

On January 29, less than two months after MMA was enacted, the Bush administration publicly revised their estimates. Instead of the original $395 billion, they projected the MMA would cost $530 to $540 billion over the next ten years.[26] Douglas Holtz-Eaton, the director of the CBO, estimated the bill would cost between one and two trillion dollars in its second decade.[27] At the time of passage, the projected cost of the bill was a real problem. But it was not the only problem the administration had to confront. The initial implementation of the law in 2006 was a disaster. Because of "bureaucratic and computer problems," tens of thousands of elderly and disabled people had difficulty getting needed medications.[28] Instead of too few stand-alone private drug plans, there were so many that the elderly did not understand how to choose. The Medicare telephone help lines were severely inadequate, and Medicare beneficiaries could not get any information. In an effort to prevent unnecessary deaths, the Bush administration tried to require insurers to provide ninety days of additional coverage for all ongoing courses of medications, but pharmacists and beneficiaries reported widespread noncompliance.[29] And six million dual eligibles who lost their Medicaid coverage on January 1 were having difficulty getting their medication from Medicare. It appeared the most dire predictions about the legislation were coming to pass.

But that was not the case.

By the summer of 2006, after a difficult transition, most of the problems had been ironed out. And then the program began to work better than anyone expected. Many experts had believed that private drug-only plans would never materialize because of fears of adverse selection. However, the plan was wisely devised to avoid such an occurrence. In order to prevent seniors from waiting until they were ill to enroll in the program, the legislation instituted a 1 percent penalty for each month seniors delayed enrolling after becoming initially eligible. Hence, if a healthy sixty-five-year-old waited to enroll until he or she was sixty-seven, the monthly premium would be 24 percent higher. In addition, to help encourage the formation of stand-alone drug plans, the legislation established risk corridors, guaranteeing the government would pay private plans for any substantial losses.

The response was the opposite of what many had predicted. In nearly every state, more than forty plans were available.[30] Competition among the drug-only plans reduced premiums beyond expectations. Every state but Alaska had at least one plan with premiums priced at under twenty dollars per month.[31] By the end of the first month of the program, the administration reduced its cost estimates by 20 percent. Medicare actuaries reduced their estimated monthly costs of a drug-only plan from thirty-seven dollars to twenty-five dollars, a decrease of nearly one-third.[32] And enrollment in the program was strong.

At the time this chapter was written, the latest projections by CMS for the years 2004 through 2013 predicted $516 billion of federal expenditures offset by $119 billion of revenues from premiums and state maintenance of effort payments.[33] That translated into net spending for the first ten years of $398 billion, almost exactly equal to the predictions made by the CBO.[34] In the year 2008, the program distributed forty-nine billion dollars in benefits and had an administrative cost of just .6 percent. It is exceptionally difficult to predict the cost of a complex new program like MMA, and nearly everyone had great respect for Rick Foster. This time, however, he was wrong.

Many of the worst fears of liberals and Democrats never came to pass. The demonstrations for premium support simply never occurred. Democrats were worried about the stabilization provision requiring a "Medicare Funding Warning" if general revenue contributions exceeded 45 percent of Medicare spending. However, they had nothing to worry about because there was no enforcement mechanism. In fact, a warning was issued, the president responded, but his proposed actions were largely ignored by the Congress.

Two of the Democrats' chief concerns were the competition from private Medicare Advantage plans and the impact of the donut hole. The Obama health plan has apparently nullified both. The Medicare Advantage plans cost the government more than traditional Medicare, and the Obama plan derived some of its projected revenues by reducing or eliminating some of the Bush-era subsidies. And, in a political deal reminiscent of MMA, the pharmaceutical companies agreed to close the donut hole and support the Obama health plan in return for a government promise not to directly negotiate the price of prescription drugs.

Many of the players maligned in the MMA battle appear wiser in hindsight. Although he was the target of much liberal criticism, John Rother, the policy director of AARP, is happy about his organization's endorsement. Most seniors, particularly those with low incomes, are better off under the plan. In addition, the concessions given to the AARP were sufficient to satisfy its primary concerns. Rother told us in 2010, "The program is successful, I think, by almost any measure."[35]

Bill Thomas endured much criticism for his heavy-handed leadership of the congressional conference committee. Nevertheless, with a budget of only 20 percent of projected elderly drug spending, he helped formulate a plan that worked for most seniors. He was the force behind the plan, keeping it within the budget and successfully structuring private sector options for the Medicare population. Thomas failed to get a full-blown premium support program, but he did get the provision that would allow a series of premium support demonstrations beginning in 2010. Although he was not completely satisfied, he told us he got nearly everything he wanted.[36]

Tom Scully also endured much criticism. The HHS investigation showed that Scully was caught between a rock and a hard place, clearly acting on orders from the White House. Scully always maintained that the executive branch was not required to share its research with Congress. Whether he believed that to be true, whether he was being a loyal soldier, or whether he should have resigned in protest is for the reader to decide. Had he released the inaccurate projections, however, the bill probably never would have become law.

George W. Bush will never be considered a hero for enacting the Medicare drug benefit. Unfortunately for Bush, he never received the popular political support from the elderly that he had hoped to gain. Yet he employed three key strategies that Bill Clinton failed to utilize but that might have been instrumental to Barack Obama's success. He negotiated with all of the important interest groups to blunt opposition. He did not attempt to enact a large entitlement and cut costs at the same time. And he presented a broad framework of his program to Congress and left it to them to hammer out the details.

For several years, Ted Kennedy was bitter. He had shepherded the bill through Congress, but he had no control over what happened in the Republican-dominated House–Senate conference. He could only watch as the deal he constructed changed so drastically that he led a filibuster to oppose the bill. Despite his misgivings about the altered provisions, however, Kennedy eventually saw that the drug benefit was working better than he ever expected.

The MMA is still a convoluted piece of legislation. It is certainly not the most cost-efficient way for Medicare to administer a drug benefit. Furthermore, it is one more separate piece in our uncoordinated piece-by-piece health care system. Nevertheless, it is working. It is less expensive than most people thought. And, for thirty-two million senior citizens who have signed up in the first two years of the program, it has provided affordable access to prescription drugs.[37]

The MMA is our last example of access expansions before we discuss the Obama health plan. It helps set the scene for the final chapters because the major themes that have shaped health reform efforts for the past one hundred years played important roles in the story: the long-standing philosophical differences between liberals and conservatives; the power of major interest groups; and the piece-by-piece attempt to build an insurance-based private health care system. But the final piece of the puzzle cannot be appreciated without understanding one more overwhelming force that has shaped the nature of health care policy: the irrepressible rise in the cost of health care has been at the very heart of policy and political decision-making and continues to challenge every phase of the American health care system. It is to that challenge we turn next.

# PART 3

# WHY CAN'T AMERICANS AFFORD THEIR HEALTH CARE?
## THE BATTLE TO CONTROL HEALTH CARE COSTS

# CHAPTER 9

# CONTROLLING HEALTH COSTS
## MANY ATTEMPTS BUT FEW SUCCESSES

## Unsustainable Health Care Costs

Have you ever wondered just how much a trillion dollars really is? To dramatize the magnitude of a trillion dollars, Governor of Oregon John Kitzhaber, MD, often tells his audience that a million seconds ago was just last week, a billion seconds ago Nixon resigned the presidency in 1974, and a trillion seconds ago was 30,000 BCE. In 2009, the United States will spend $2.5 trillion for health care. This amounts to over eight thousand dollars for every person in the country.[1] In contrast, countries like Canada, Germany or France spend less than half that per person.[2]

For the average worker, wages grew by about 20 percent between 2000 and 2008, but health insurance premiums grew by almost 100 percent during the same period—five times higher than wage growth! Granted, the United States is a rich country, but is it rich enough to spend almost one-fifth of its annual income to support this one sector of the economy? That is the question that bedeviled President Obama as he and much of the Democratic Party attempted to cover the forty-seven million Americans who lacked any health insurance coverage. Many argued that the United States should cut costs before expanding coverage. The country was already spending about 17.5 percent of its annual income on health care, and costs were increasing three to four times faster than national income. Obama rejected that argument. Covering the uninsured was his primary focus. Although the health reform plan he signed included some cost-saving provisions, they were limited in scope. Obama knew that controlling health costs would be far more difficult than adding coverage. The technical and political difficulties of controlling costs have been learned the hard way by government and private insurers over the past forty years.

Those lessons will be crucial for future efforts, because the current rate of cost growth is not sustainable over the long term. As Herb Stein, the former chairman of the Council of Economic Advisors under President Nixon said, "If something cannot go on forever, it will stop." It is to understand past efforts and their failure to control health costs that we now turn.

## Nixon Imposes Nationwide Wage and Price Controls

It was a warm August morning in Washington, DC, when Stuart Altman entered his spacious fifth floor office. Just a month earlier he had been appointed deputy assistant secretary for Health Planning and Evaluation at HEW. He was met by his assistant with a concerned look. Secretary Richardson wanted to see Altman right away. The previous evening, Sunday, August 15, 1971, President Nixon had signed an executive order freezing all wages and prices in the country. This was no ordinary event. Other than in war time, the United States had never imposed such tough measures on the national economy. Overall, inflation was becoming a serious economic problem. The Nixon team was especially concerned about the rapid growth in government spending for health care that had followed the enactment of Medicare and Medicaid six years earlier. The White House asked HEW Secretary Elliot Richardson to send over those at the department who were knowledgeable about health costs. Richardson wanted Altman to lead the team. Although Altman's HEW position was technically political, Richardson had received a commitment from President Nixon that he could select individuals for his policy office that had appropriate expertise, even if they were nonpartisan. Altman, who was on leave from the economics department at Brown University and had just completed a book on the shortage of nurses, fit that bill.[3]

The president's wage and price freeze, although unprecedented, was permitted under the Economic Stabilization Act that Congress had passed the previous year to control inflation. To implement the freeze, Nixon created a Cost of Living Council under the chairmanship of the secretary of the treasury John Connally. After the initial ninety-day freeze, a more permanent organizational structure was formed with Donald Rumsfeld as its director and Richard Cheney as his deputy.[4] Both Rumsfeld and Cheney would later become secretaries of defense, and Cheney would serve two terms as vice president under George W. Bush. A separate committee on the Health Services Industry was formed to advise the council on the workings of the health industry and to recommend how to combat health cost inflation. Altman was appointed deputy director of the committee and he assembled a team to undertake the task. The team included Dorothy Rice from the Social Security Administration, which was the home of the Medicare program at that time, as well as Richard Berman and Joseph Eichenholz from Altman's staff at HEW.

## What Constitutes a Unit of Care?
## The Precursor to Modern Hospital Payment Systems

After the initial freeze, The Cost of Living Council ruled that physician fees could only grow by 2.5 percent per year. Hospitals could not increase prices by more than 6 percent per year unless they received prior approval. These were much smaller increases than had been occurring during the previous five years. Measuring price increases in health care, however, turned out to be a difficult problem. First, the unit of care was vague. For example, if a patient visited a doctor for a broken arm, was the unit of care on which the price was based a fully fixed broken arm or each separate component of care? As the control program progressed, physicians found ways to separate care into more and more units. Although the price for each unit increased less than the approved limit, total spending for physician services grew much faster.

Similar problems existed for hospital prices. Was the unit of care the price of the total treatment, the price of each individual service, or the price per day spent in the hospital? At the time, hospitals were paid by private insurance and the government on a per diem cost basis. They received a certain amount for each day a patient was in the hospital, regardless of what services were provided. The government determined the per diem amount by calculating the average cost per patient per day over the entire year (i.e., total costs/number of patient days).[5] This was a crude measurement for each patient, since some patients would cost much more than others, but it was accurate for all patients over the entire year. Blue Cross also paid hospitals on a per diem basis, although its payment included an additional amount for profit.

The regulatory system was problematic because hospitals were paid according to their unregulated per diem costs rather than their regulated prices. Hence, they posted prices that conformed to regulations, but they were paid according to their costs, which were actually increasing by 11 to 12 percent annually.[6] Clearly something different had to be done.

By 1973, Nixon's council had removed controls over most wages and prices in the economy. However, two sectors, construction and health care, continued to exhibit strong inflationary pricing and were kept under controls. George Shultz had replaced Connally as chair of the council and John Dunlop became the executive director.[7] Both Schultz and Dunlop were university economics professors—Schultz from the University of Chicago and Dunlop from Harvard. Schultz in particular was a strong proponent of the antigovernment "Chicago School" of economics in which wage and price controls were an anathema. Altman was also trained as a "Chicago School" economist. He often joked that he went to a "farm school" of the University of Chicago called UCLA. But like Dunlop, he was more eclectic in his views about government controls. In Nixon's second term, Casper Weinberger replaced Richardson as secretary of HEW and joined Dunlop and Schultz on the council. Weinberger, as readers may remember, had previously been head of the OMB and was known as "Cap the Knife" because he was so tough on government spending. Surprisingly, when he joined HEW, Weinberger became a strong supporter of Nixon's universal health plan.

The three cabinet secretaries were ultimately responsible for deciding how to control inflation in the health sector, but they left many of the technical issues to Altman and his team. Altman and the council staff realized that if they were to have any impact on controlling true medical inflation they would need to change the way the council regulated pricing. At the heart of the issue was the need to change the unit of control. They reasoned that since patients enter hospitals for specific medical conditions—and have little input about the individual services provided—the unit of care should be the whole hospital stay to treat each condition. They also realized that basing hospital payments on the average cost of a day of care, as did the Blues and Medicare, encouraged hospitals to keep patients in the hospital for more days than were necessary. It was well known that the final days in a hospital were much less costly than the initial days, when most of the procedures were performed. If patients stayed in hospitals a day or two longer, hospitals would continue to receive per diem payments based on average costs; an amount that was considerably higher than the actual cost of the extra days. Thus, the council proposed that cost per admission should be the new unit of control. Hospital costs would be based on the average cost per admission each hospital incurred during the previous year (i.e., total costs/number of admissions). Under such a system, a hospital would no longer have the incentive to keep patients beyond the minimum time recommended for their illnesses.

This revolutionary way of looking at hospital pricing was not well received by the industry. As Altman recalls, he was asked to discuss the new regulatory proposal at a special meeting of the AHA on Mother's Day night 1973. From Altman's perspective, he considered it the "Mother's Day Massacre." He and his sidekick, Joe Eichenholtz, were attacked from all sides.

Many hospitals complained that it was unfair to limit their price or cost increases to an average cost for the previous year's admissions because they might treat much sicker patients the following year. Hospitals also objected to the idea that the unit of care should be the cost of all the services provided during a patient's total stay in the hospital. They argued that sicker patients need more services during their hospital stays, and the council's methodology had no mechanism to pay higher rates for sicker patients. The council, on the other hand, worried that if it permitted higher payments for sicker patients, too many hospitals would claim they had sicker-than-average patients. Unfortunately, there was no acceptable method to measure the variation in sickness among hospital patients.

As it turned out, the new "per admission" regulations were never implemented. Before the technical issues could be resolved, Congress repealed Nixon's authority to regulate wages and prices. Never again would the federal government attempt to control the prices or costs of all health care services throughout the country.

Although the per diem payment system continued, the concept of paying for a total hospital admission set in motion a number of research projects to see if it was possible to measure a patient's degree of sickness. John Thompson from the Yale School of Medicine received a grant from HEW to study the question. Thompson, a nurse trained in the military during World War II, was convinced it was possible to develop a system to categorize differences in treatment costs based on the medical diagnosis of the patient. He wanted to use such a system to find out why the cost of care for similar patients seemed to vary by as much as 100 percent among Connecticut's thirty-five hospitals.[8] Thompson was a clinical diagnostician and he needed the help of a "systems engineer." Hence, he teamed up with Robert Fetter who was a professor in the Yale School of Organization and Management.

Together they created the Diagnosis Related Grouping system (DRG), a hospital pricing system that is currently used throughout much of the world.

The DRG system was adopted by Medicare in 1984. It is based on the average cost of treating an individual patient with a particular diagnosis during his or her total stay in a hospital. This was the same pricing unit proposed by Altman and his team at the "Mother's Day Massacre" in 1973, eleven years before it emerged as an international standard.

## The '70s: Rate Regulation and Health Planning

During the early '70s America experimented with several other approaches to control health costs. Whereas Nixon's wage and price controls were designed to lower spending for all health care services, both public and private, other efforts were specifically aimed at slowing the growth in Medicare spending, a major concern to federal policy makers. When Medicare was passed in 1965 it was estimated that in 1967, the first full year of operation, it would spend $2.2 billion.[9] Instead, actual spending was $4.2 billion.[10] It continued to grow much faster than estimates. Hospital spending for 1970 was projected to be $7.1 billion and was actually $15.1 billion—more than double the original estimate.[11] The degree of concern was reflected in a statement by the chairman of the Senate Finance Committee Russell Long when he called Medicare a "runaway program."[12]

Thus in 1972, Congress modified its "hands off" approach toward Medicare and required limits on payments to some doctors and hospitals.[13] In future years, analysts would look back on these 1972 amendments as a major break from the "politics of accommodation" that formed the basis of the original law.[14] Robert Ball, who had been the head of the Social Security Administration when Medicare was enacted, told Altman to remember this period, because the relationship between government and the medical community would never be the same. "Perhaps we were a bit naive," Ball said. "We thought that if we paid medical providers appropriately they would increase spending in a reasonable way. Well, their definition of reasonable and ours were not the same."[15]

The original law modeled Medicare's payment system after the approach used by Blue Cross and Blue Shield. Physicians were paid in accordance with their "customary" charge for a particular service, provided it was within the bounds of the "prevailing" fees in the community. To keep Medicare spending in check, the law limited the prevailing fee to the seventy-fifth percentile of physician fees in the community.[16] In concept, the customary and prevailing payment system was designed to pay physicians no more than they charged private patients. However, a dynamic set in whereby physicians increased their rates beyond what they usually charged private patients in expectation that in future years the higher rates would become the new accepted Medicare fees.

Hospitals were paid on a per diem basis according to the costs they incurred in treating Medicare patients. Medicare regulations, as opposed to Blue Cross, required that the costs incurred needed to be "reasonable." Initially, Medicare's payment system generated few restraints on spending. Hospital spending for new equipment and facilities grew rapidly, as did the wages paid to hospital personnel.[17] Some analysts predicted this would happen, but even their projections were much less than what actually occurred.[18]

Attempting to curtail spending, the 1972 Medicare amendments limited the increase in physician fees to growth in medical inflation. An index was developed to measure inflation in the services used by physicians, such as rent and wages. The amendments also established limits on per diem payments to hospitals. The restrictions on hospital costs were written to minimize any negative impact on the quality of care provided to Medicare beneficiaries. Hospital costs were divided into two categories: routine (room and board) expenses and ancillary costs. No restrictions were placed on ancillary costs because they were believed to be related to the medical condition of patients. However, room and board costs were regulated. Dr. Jim Morgan, a senior staff member of the Senate Finance committee, summarized the thinking of Congress in an interview when he stated, "We understood that people (patients) might be sicker and have different (higher) ancillary costs, but by God the routine or 'hotel' costs ought to bear some similiarity to all other hospitals."[19]

Initially, the new regulations were quite timid. Hospitals were placed in separate groups based on their bed size as a measure of the complexity of their patients. Hospitals with more beds were assumed to treat more complex patients. Within each group, the per diem routine costs of each hospital were ranked, and only those that fell beyond the ninety-fifth percentile were considered excessive or "unreasonable." Hospitals that charged beyond the limit were given one year to lower their costs. Each year the federal government estimated how much Medicare would save under this provision, and each year the savings disappeared. Frustrated by its inability to lower hospital spending, Medicare kept lowering the unreasonable level, but the savings continued to vanish. Altman and his staff determined that hospital administrators learned how to redefine what had been a routine expense into an ancillary cost, thereby avoiding any reductions in payments.[20]

The 1972 amendments did more than constrain Medicare spending. They authorized the federal government to experiment with alternative forms of hospital reimbursement. They also expanded coverage for certain categories of patients, including those under sixty-five suffering from end-stage renal disease and those with severe disabilities. In the end, the increased spending generated by the new coverage provisions far exceeded the meager savings that resulted from cost containment. As a result, Medicare spending for hospital care doubled between 1970 and 1975.[21]

## State Regulation in the '70s

Often overlooked in many studies of the '70s were the cost control efforts of the states. During that period eight states established mandatory rate regulation, mostly for hospital costs. Another four required officials of state government to issue advisory opinions on any cost increases, and fifteen required some form of voluntary regulation. The first mandatory program was instituted in New York in 1970, actually predating the cost control efforts of the federal government. Although the state programs varied in design, all focused on limiting hospital spending, and all received waivers from the federal government to include Medicare and Medicaid patients in addition to those who were privately insured. Of the eight mandatory control programs, only the Maryland system was in operation in 2010. In every other state, pressures from the regulated hospitals to end controls were strong enough to push state legislators to eliminate the programs. Most states also found that they could receive more federal funds if they dropped their regulatory systems and accepted Medicare payments instead.

Were there any positive outcomes from rate regulation in the '70s? This question is currently being raised as states grapple with the rapid growth in health care costs. We support the conclusions of Professor Frank Sloan, who conducted the definitive study of the impact of the rate regulation activities.[22] He concluded that of the state-level activities of the '70s, only mandatory controls had any positive impact on controlling costs.[23] In a more recent meeting in Massachusetts, he refined his earlier conclusion and said that many of the initial successes in cost regulation did not last as the control programs matured, and providers developed political alliances to minimize their impact.[24]

In addition to rate regulation, the federal government experimented with various techniques to slow the growth of health spending by limiting the availability of expensive medical services. The most ambitious was the creation of a national system of local planning agencies that would help determine what services and institutions were needed in each geographical area.

### Creating a National Health Planning System

Did you know there is a mountain range that splits the state of Washington and separates two distinct health care delivery systems? This was news to a boy who grew up in the Bronx and had only been west of the Hudson River by airplane. This geographic lesson was taught to Altman and his staff at HEW as they attempted to create planning agencies throughout the country that could rationalize the health care system at the local level. It was believed that a major reason for inflation in health spending was the uncontrolled growth in the supply of health care facilities and expensive equipment. Once a facility was built or equipment was purchased there were few constraints on its use, whether it was needed or not. A well-known professor of public health at UCLA, Milt Roemer, coined the phrase, "A built [hospital] bed is a filled bed."[25]

In an effort to control this growth, President Ford signed the National Health Planning and Resource Development Act in January 1975. The law required each state to establish local planning agencies to prepare detailed plans on what facilities and services were needed in their areas. Before any new facility could be built or expensive equipment could be purchased, the planning agency had to recommend a Certificate of Need (CON) for the project. The governor of each state had the ultimate authority to grant a CON. If a project was not granted a CON, Medicare and Medicaid would not pay for any of its costs. Since the federal government would be paying all the costs of running the local area and state agencies, the secretary of HEW had to determine how many agencies were needed in each state. That assignment was given to Altman and the HEW group. Altman's group initially awarded one agency to the state of Washington based on its population. However, when the governor informed HEW that it was not easy for residents in the eastern part of the state to receive medical care in the western part because of the mountain range, two planning agencies were permitted. After several other geography lessons, the HEW group approved more than two hundred local agencies. Each was governed by an independent board of consumer and provider representatives and staffed by professional health planners. Although the local health system agencies (HSAs) had a number of responsibilities, by far the most important was the review and approval of CON applications in their area.

The proponents of the health planning law did not believe that markets or peer pressure alone could restrain cost growth. Extensive insurance and government subsidies shielded patients and providers from the true cost of care and, as a result, induced both provider and consumer demand for health care goods and services. Regulation was inevitable, and the most effective form of regulation was to limit the availability of unnecessary and expensive facilities and equipment.[26] Nevertheless, when the law was passed there was much skepticism that local area agencies would be willing or able to use the CON process to regulate the health care system. Several state officials tried to stop the legislation, fearing that they would lose control to local independent organizations. Provider groups were concerned that planners would dominate the agencies and would demonstrate more concern about the cost of care than its availability. Some of their concerns were validated. Many area agencies became tough regulators, particularly when asked to approve the construction of new beds. State officials, concerned about the rapid growth in Medicaid spending, often supported restrictions on new construction. The American Health Planning Association studied the actions of 139 HSAs over a two-year period and reported in 1978 that the local agencies denied 25 percent of requests for new bed construction, amounting to 5,717 short-term beds.[27] Nevertheless, as time passed, those seeking to expand services became more successful in gaining approval for their projects. They hired sophisticated consultants and lawyers and sought political help from state legislators who wished to develop new jobs in their areas. Although support for the program did not end until the early '80s under President Ronald Reagan, independent analysts were questioning the value of the planning effort as early as 1976.[28]

## Carter and Kennedy: Controlling Costs versus Expanding Coverage

With the limited success of both the health planning program and the hospital spending restrictions, Medicare spending for hospital care grew at double-digit rates after Nixon's controls ended in 1974.[29] When Jimmy Carter became president in 1976, liberals hoped he would move aggressively to propose national health care reform and universal coverage. Instead he focused on cost control, which he believed was the chief health care concern of most Americans. Hospital spending was the largest component of health care costs, and the president could direct his efforts there and not antagonize the politically powerful physician community.

Carter proposed the Hospital Cost Containment Act of 1977, which limited the payments hospitals could receive from all payers, including government programs, private insurance companies, and individuals. The CBO undertook an analysis of the legislation under the supervision of Stanley Wallack and Robert Reischauer. It estimated that under the legislation, increases in any hospital's total revenues would be limited to 10.6 percent in 1978 and 8.9 percent by 1981.[30] Applying today's standards, Carter's limits would seem quite generous, but not in 1977 when spending for hospital care had increased by 31 percent over the previous two years.[31] The proposed legislation also established a national global budget on hospitals' capital expenditures. Budgeted funds would be allocated to planning agencies according to population.

As in previous legislative battles on health reform, most urban, northern Democrats supported the Carter plan, but opposition from southern and Sunbelt Democrats and most Republicans led to a series of political defeats for the president. Opponents argued that limits on hospital spending would favor those areas that already had high costs and adequate services. The restrictions, they believed, would unduly restrain revenue for hospitals in regions experiencing population growth. The hospital industry strongly opposed the Carter plan, and it was defeated twice during his presidency. In the end, Congress supported an alternative approach developed by the AHA. It called for a voluntary commitment by hospitals to limit future price increases to overall inflation. Even the powerful chair of the House Ways and Means Committee, Dan Rostenkowski, supported the voluntary plan.

For a while, the voluntary plan seemed to work.[32] Hospital spending grew by less than inflation in 1977 and 1978. But pressure within the industry could not be contained. By 1980, spending growth skyrocketed to 17 percent and grew even faster in 1981.[33] A similar failure had followed a voluntary program advanced by President Ford in 1976. History strongly suggests that voluntary regulation of the health care industry is not likely to be effective.

While Carter focused on cost control, liberals were unhappy that the administration had not advanced any proposal for expanding health coverage for the uninsured. Kennedy met with Carter in June of 1978 and elicited promises from the president that he would propose such legislation. However, Carter was reluctant, focusing on hospital cost control and welfare reform and wanting to balance the budget.[34] The two met again in July and Carter refused to support comprehensive reform. Instead, he wanted to propose an incremental bill with "triggers." If any phase became too expensive, the next phase would be postponed.[35]

Kennedy knew that a long-range, incremental bill would be picked apart by industry opponents, and the triggers would present continuous opportunities to kill the legislation. Exasperated by Carter's repeated delays and incremental approach, he finally broke with the president. It was a turning point in national politics as Kennedy eventually decided to challenge Carter in the 1980 elections, splitting the Democratic Party in an election they might have lost anyway to Ronald Reagan.

Within the Carter administration there were differences on how to proceed with health reform. The secretary of HEW, Joseph Califano, asked well-known economist Alain Enthoven from Stanford University to develop a plan to provide universal coverage and control health care spending. As we discussed in chapter 2, Enthoven's "managed competition," plan required a substantial restructuring of the entire health care delivery system.[36] Carter, supported by Califano, rejected the Enthoven model and instead recommended a more conservative approach.

In June of 1979, Carter finally submitted a proposal for national health reform. Maintaining his incremental approach, he recommended a program that would be phased in over a long period of time. The proposal was for universal catastrophic insurance implemented by an employer mandate. Carter negotiated with Russell Long (D-LA) to push the first phase of the bill. This was the same Russell Long that had proposed catastrophic insurance in opposition to Nixon's universal health plan. By the time Carter submitted his proposal, however, the election was only a year and a half away and he was dismally unpopular. In addition, it was clear that health reform, particularly a costly expansion of health insurance, was never one of his priorities. The long-awaited proposal never got out of committee.

In 2010, Carter published a book in which he blamed Kennedy for the failure of his health reform proposal. "The fact is that we would have had comprehensive health care now, had it not been for Ted Kennedy's deliberately blocking the legislation that I proposed," Carter stated. "It was his fault. Ted Kennedy killed the bill."[37]

In the opinion of these authors, history suggests otherwise. It was clear that Carter opposed any large expansion in health insurance that would add to the budget deficit. He much preferred to focus his efforts on cost control. When he finally proposed a program, it was far too late for such legislation to be considered, even if he had been popular. In addition, Kennedy was most likely correct in his assessment. Long-term, phased-in reform with cost control triggers could never survive the opposition of powerful special interests and political opponents. It is difficult to imagine Ronald Reagan phasing in the next part of Carter's program. It was certainly true that Kennedy opposed the legislation. Furthermore, the country had become more conservative, and Kennedy's bill had no chance of success in the Congress. Nevertheless, Carter's program was a half-hearted effort that never had a chance of being enacted, and, even if it had, it almost certainly would have failed.

## Ronald Reagan and the '80s: DRGs and a Procompetitive Approach to Government Regulation

Ronald Reagan's victory over Jimmy Carter ushered in the decade of the '80s. A strong champion of free markets and limited government, Reagan was faced with serious challenges. The US economy was entering one of the worst downturns since the Great Depression of the '30s, and unemployment was approaching 11 percent.[38] Total health care spending, particularly for hospital care, was growing far faster than the economy. This created financial problems for Medicare because expenses were rising at the same time that fewer Americans were contributing to the program. The solvency of the federally financed program was in jeopardy, and Reagan had no interest in solving the problem with a tax increase, but he needed to slow the growth in Medicare spending.

The Reagan team was not about to strengthen the failing health planning system or ask Congress to reconsider its rejection of Carter's rate regulation proposal. Both efforts allowed the government to control *all* health care spending, both public and private. This was too much government interference for the new Reagan team. They also could not count on the hospital industry to voluntarily hold down spending. Two failures had convinced even friends of the industry that outside forces were needed to control spending. The government needed to come up with something new. With the Senate now under Republican control, there was an opportunity for a more market-oriented approach, or an approach that minimized the role of government in controlling the way hospitals operated.

Reagan asked his newly appointed secretary of HEW, Richard Schweiker, to come up with a plan. Before being appointed secretary, Schweiker had been a senator from Pennsylvania and the ranking minority member of the Senate Finance Committee. He understood the uncontrolled nature of the way Medicare paid hospitals for inpatient care. Fifteen years of watching hospitals bill the government for whatever costs they incurred was enough to convince Schweiker that a totally new payment approach needed to be found.

Schweiker appointed a committee of HEW and Medicare staff to develop new approaches to pay hospitals under Medicare. While Schweiker and his team were working on these new approaches, Congress passed legislation that substantially toughened the hospital payment limits established in the 1972 legislation. Although the Reagan administration preferred to end cost-based reimbursement and government controls, it supported the congressional plan because it limited spending only for government programs. The new restrictions on Medicare payments to hospitals were contained in a law that changed many Internal Revenue tax codes, the Tax Equity and Fiscal Responsibility Act (TEFRA). Although the section that focused on hospital costs was only six pages long, many health analysts consider it a major piece of health policy legislation.[39] The 1982 law restricted Medicare payments for all inpatient hospital expenses, including ancillary costs. This was in marked contrast to the 1972 law that only disallowed excess routine (hotel type) costs. What was more significant is that TEFRA changed the unit of control from average costs per diem to average costs per case. This was the same unit of control suggested by the Nixon Cost of Living Council in 1973. Once again, the hospital industry was not happy. It was concerned that TEFRA restricted payment growth to a substantially lower rate than was occurring in the early

'80s.[40] Furthermore, a technique still needed to be found to differentiate hospitals based on the complexity of the patients treated. Although Congress knew this was a problem, it did not have a clear solution. Thus, it directed the secretary of HEW to develop patient "case-mix" indexes for each hospital and then assign hospitals to appropriate peer groups based on these indexes. The peer groupings were a crude technique for differentiating hospitals in relation to the complexity of the patients treated.

Many who worked for the Congress in 1981 knew the TEFRA rules were far from perfect. It was widely believed that they were only a temporary stopgap to slow Medicare spending until a more permanent solution could be found.[41] In fact, the legislation specifically directed the secretary of HEW to develop a proposal for a "prospective payment" system and to submit such a plan by the end of 1982. What was most unusual was that the legislation called for the secretary to work in consultation with the Senate Finance and House Ways and Means Committees and to have the work completed in just five months. Clearly, a plan had already been developed between Schweiker and his former colleagues on the Senate Finance Committee. This was also a bipartisan approach since staff of the Ways and Means Committee were controlled by Democrats.[42] David Durenberger, a key member of the Senate Finance Committee, later told Altman that he and Schweiker had already worked on a plan that could replace TEFRA by 1983. When the hospital industry saw how easily Congress adopted such tough regulations, it realized that changes in the Medicare payment system were inevitable. If it wanted a "better" system from HEW, the hospital industry would have to work with Congress on its design and support it through the legislative process.[43]

## The Birth of DRGs

The HEW team had three goals in designing the new Medicare hospital payment system. It wanted to end cost-based payments, create an annual budget for hospital spending, and provide a financial incentive for hospitals to lower the cost of care. Similar to TEFRA and Nixon's wage and price controls, the plan incorporated per-case expenses as the unit of payment. Rather than the imprecise case mix adjustment used in TEFRA, the HEW plan used the DRG system developed by Thompson and Fetter at Yale University.

As the name implies, patients would be assigned to a DRG based on their diagnosis when they entered the hospital.[44] Each DRG was assigned an index number based on the expected cost of the resources needed to treat that diagnosis. The expected resources needed per DRG were determined by analyzing actual patient usage throughout the country in the years prior to implementing the program. The more resources needed, the higher the index. An important component was the average number of days required for treatment. A different DRG for the same diagnosis was assigned if the patient required surgery. In order to make the system manageable, the thousands of potential diagnoses were combined into 467 DRGs. Each DRG included diagnoses that were similar in terms of medical characteristics and patterns of resource use.

The index was structured such that a base rate of 1.0 was assigned to a normal hernia repair. Diagnostic groups would receive more or less than the base, according to estimated resource use. For example, kidney transplants had one of the highest DRG indexes.[45] The final step in the process was for the government to determine what it would pay for the base DRG with a weight of 1.0. This was called the "standardized amount" and was derived such that total Medicare spending for inpatient hospital care would be consistent with the budget set by Congress each year.[46] However, Medicare was an entitlement, and if total spending for Medicare exceeded the budget, the government would still pay the difference.

For each hospital, an average DRG weight was established based on the types of patients it treated. Thus, hospitals that treated more complex patients received a higher average weight and, therefore, more revenue.

Fortunately for the planners of this new system, a version of the DRG system had been used in New Jersey since 1976. It was developed with the cooperation of the New Jersey Hospital Association and Blue Cross and covered all payers. To gain the acceptance of the hospitals and private insurers, the state agreed to build in payments to hospitals for charity care and bad debt.[47] The president of the New Jersey Hospital Association, Jack Owen, became a strong supporter of the DRG system and later advised the HEW team.[48] The original DRG system was intended to be a management tool and needed to be modified to be used as a payment system. Although many of the changes were made during the New Jersey experiment, the HEW group created modifications so that the system could be used for the entire nation.

## Prospective Payment

The system proposed by Schweiker was prospective in that both hospitals and government would have a reasonable estimate of what Medicare would pay the following year. Under the previous system, the amount of Medicare spending was determined by whatever costs the hospitals incurred. Hospitals were ultimately in the dark about their payments since government did not generate a final check until years later; after they had done a careful audit to ensure that the cost figures were accurate. The Schweiker/Reagan plan was supported by the hospital industry and encountered little opposition. Few legislators took the time to learn the intricacies of what is generally considered the most complex system in the world for paying hospitals. Dan Rostenkowski, the chair of the House Ways and Means Committee, included the provisions in a bill that strengthened Social Security. With millions of seniors dependent on their monthly Social Security checks, holding up such legislation to debate technical issues about paying hospitals was not a high priority, and the legislation passed quickly and easily.

Some critics of the new Medicare Prospective Payment System (PPS) labeled it a "Rube Goldberg"–administered pricing system that would ultimately lead to rationed care.[49] The Reagan administration dismissed such criticisms and viewed PPS as a promarket system that created incentives for hospital efficiency and helped reduce the federal deficit.[50] Hospitals had a strong incentive to treat patients efficiently because if they spent less than the prospective DRG payment, they could keep the difference. Patient advocacy groups were concerned that the financial incentives were too strong and patients would be forced to leave the hospital too soon.[51] While some examples of premature discharges were uncovered, they were quite rare. Physicians provided an important safeguard against early discharges. They were responsible for discharging patients and they were not paid under the DRG system. If a patient claimed he or she had been discharged too early because the government would not pay for additional care, the hospital was subject to a significant penalty.

## Outliers

One issue subject to much debate was how to pay hospitals for "outliers." These were patients whose total cost of care far exceeded the DRG average.

Outliers were usually patients who entered a hospital for a particular diagnosis but developed other problems or complications while being treated. Hospitals wanted to be paid for the extra costs, but the government did not want to encourage hospitals to spend excess amounts on patients. Nor did they want them to be rewarded for not doing enough to prevent such complications. If Medicare decided to pay for outliers, there was the issue of funding. The Reagan budget group, headed by David Stockman, wanted the new system to reduce the budget deficit—or at least be budget neutral.[52] They decided to pay hospitals only a portion of the extra costs for treating outlier patients and to fund the extra payments by withholding 5 percent of Medicare payments to all hospitals.[53]

## Teaching Adjustments

The American Association of Medical Colleges (AAMC), the organization representing major teaching hospitals, had serious reservations concerning the legislation. They believed the proposed system failed to reflect the higher cost associated with training the next generation of physicians.[54] Originally, Medicare paid for the cost of education, recognizing it as a legitimate patient care expense. The proposed new plan set the same DRG payment for all hospitals. If the teaching hospitals were correct, an adjustment was needed for medical education expenses. Researchers determined that medical education expenses fell into two categories, "direct" and "indirect." Direct expenses were straightforward and included the salaries for professors and the stipends for medical residents. But the existence and amount of the indirect expenses were more controversial. The AAMC argued that teaching hospitals incur higher costs of providing care to Medicare patients because medical students participate in the delivery of care while they are learning.[55] This necessarily increases the time to treat a patient and often results in additional tests and procedures. Research at Brandeis University, under contract with Medicare, validated these additional costs. The Carter hospital cost containment plan had included an extra payment of 6 percent for indirect medical education expenses. The drafters of the PPS proposal wanted to include the same adjustment in the new system, but the AAMC argued that it was too low.[56] Not wanting to antagonize such a powerful group, Congress doubled the original estimate.[57] Analysts later recognized that this hasty decision overpaid teaching hospitals by hundreds of millions of dollars.[58] Since the introduction of PPS in 1984, the indirect teaching adjustment has been cut almost in half.[59] How much Medicare should pay hospitals for teaching students is still a very controversial topic.[60]

## What to Do About DRG Creep

The Prospective Payment legislation included a provision to establish an independent advisory group to provide Congress with an annual assessment of how the new system was working. This was considered particularly important since a payment system as complicated as PPS had never been tried anywhere in the world. Congress established the Prospective Payment Assessment Commission (ProPAC) and chose Stuart Altman as its first chair. The commission had seventeen members representing different constituents of the health care industry and included a number of independent health analysts. ProPAC was important not only because it advised Congress and Medicare on the operation of PPS, but also because it established a model for independent federal advisory groups. The commission had its own staff and did not report to any federal agency. Its budget was approved by Congress, and the chair reported directly to the two congressional committees with responsibility for overseeing the Medicare program.

ProPAC had been in existence for somewhat over two years when Altman received a call at his Brandeis office. It was a reporter from a Texas newspaper. She had been studying the financial condition of one of her local medical centers. She was surprised to find that it was earning very substantial profits from treating Medicare patients. Before she printed the story, she asked Altman if he would review her findings to see if she was correct. He agreed, but suggested that it was highly unlikely since PPS had been designed to limit spending and profits on Medicare patients. Altman asked the ProPAC staff to analyze her worksheets. They were shocked! The hospital under study was receiving so much more revenue than its costs, that its profits from Medicare patients alone exceeded 10 percent. It seemed impossible, but it was true. As the story unfolded, the ProPAC staff and those at Medicare discovered a serious problem. When PPS was designed, the Medicare actuaries were asked to determine the amount that should be paid for each DRG such that overall spending would be the same as if hospitals were paid under the previous system. The actuaries assumed that patients would be assigned to DRGs in a manner similar to the way they were during the test years. Instead, hospitals became acutely aware that the DRG codes determined their payments, and they became very aggressive in using the highest codes possible. This became known as "DRG creep" or "code creep." Many consulting firms were formed to help hospitals maximize their revenues by adjusting the coding. How much of this up-coding was legitimate and how much bent the rules for higher payments was never resolved, but up-coding did generate higher payments. A 1 percent average code increase for all Medicare hospital admissions in a year would cost the program $400 million dollars. The actuaries had recognized the possibility of some DRG creep and had built a 3 percent increase into their estimates. The real number turned out to be closer to 9 percent. This generated excess spending of close to $2.4 billion a year (six times $400 million).[61] Other reasons that PPS payments exceeded expectations existed, but by far the major reason was the coding problem.[62] When Congress learned about these overpayments, it cut the future growth rate in PPS payments below the level of medical inflation. Nevertheless, it took six years for Medicare to get back to the spending amounts it had anticipated when the program began.[63]

The reaction of Congress to the overpayments also highlighted the benefit of PPS. For the first time Congress had a tool to regulate what it wanted to pay for hospital care under Medicare. How it used that tool is another matter. There are many examples where Congress bowed to political pressure and added new spending to the program. The ongoing controversy of urban versus rural payments is a good example.

## Geographical Differences in the Cost of Health Services

In the original PPS plan, each DRG payment represented the average cost of care throughout the entire country. The higher-cost urban areas argued that this would necessarily underpay their hospitals. Research showed there were indeed major differences in the cost of treating the same type of patient based on where a hospital was located. Pacifying the urban hospitals, two separate expense groups were established for each DRG. Higher rates were established for urban hospitals and lower rates for those in rural areas.

Health planners believed it was perfectly appropriate for less intensive, smaller hospitals in more remote locations to send their more complex patients to big hospitals in more populated areas. Groups representing rural hospitals, however, strongly objected to being paid less for the same DRG.

They argued that smaller payments prevented them from purchasing new equipment and forced them to send too many patients to urban hospitals. As a result, many rural hospitals would be forced out of business. In the old cost-based system, a rural hospital with low occupancy would be paid its higher costs per admission (fewer admissions generated higher costs per admission) and be able to stay in operation. Under PPS, a hospital was only paid for the patients it treated and was not compensated for having vacancies. During the popular NBC *Today Show*, Jane Pauley grilled Altman about why the government was destroying rural hospitals. Altman explained that rural hospitals were not suffering because of low government payments, but because patients in rural areas often chose to go to bigger hospitals that were better equipped to deal with complex illnesses. His explanation did not convince either Pauley or the supporters of rural hospitals. With their strong lobby groups in Congress, rural hospitals gradually were able to reduce the differential in the two rates and eliminate it entirely by 1995.[64] Today, many rural hospitals are classified as "sole community hospitals" and are again paid on a modified "cost" basis instead of DRGs.[65] Advantages certainly exist in maintaining vibrant rural hospitals. They are often the largest employers in their communities and they keep patients closer to home. However, substantial extra government spending resulted from these payment adjustments, and some of our most financially secure hospitals are now located in rural areas.

Although the implementation problems were considerable, the successes of the PPS system far outweighed the negatives. Its design was built on a decade of careful research and its passage into law was a textbook example of bipartisan cooperation. The government worked with the hospital industry but did not let it dominate the process. The wasteful and inappropriate incentives of the cost-based system were replaced with a much fairer mechanism for differentiating hospitals in terms of the types of patients treated. For the first time, the federal government had a payment system it could use to establish how much it wanted to spend on inpatient hospital care. Although many adjustments added to the cost of the program, they have mitigated most of the geographic and other problems that could have destroyed the system.

PPS provided strong incentives to reduce patient length of stay. And, it was able to do so without reducing quality or discharging patients "sicker and quicker," as some had feared. From 1980 to 2006, the average length of stay in US hospitals decreased from 7.3 to 4.8 days.[66] Perhaps the ultimate compliment is that almost every industrialized country has included some form of a DRG mechanism in its hospital payment system.

## Outpatient PPS

Prospective payment, however, was only an "inpatient" hospital payment system. Changes in the practice of medicine and the introduction of new technologies have moved many patients and procedures to the outpatient department of the hospital—or out of the hospital altogether. PPS was partly responsible because it provided an incentive for hospitals to treat patients in the cost-based outpatient department rather than the PPS-regulated inpatient setting. Responding to those changes, Medicare established an outpatient PPS in the year 2000. What is still needed over ten years later is a payment system for all sites of care that creates better incentives to use only the medical care that provides appropriate value for money spent.

## Physician Payment Reform

After the federal government instituted DRGs and the PPS to pay hospitals, it turned its attention to doctors and created a new physician payment system. As discussed previously, Medicare initially agreed to pay physicians their usual and customary fee per procedure. Although this retrospective payment method was modified in 1972, it still permitted significant differences in the rates paid to physicians. Often younger, less experienced physicians were paid more than older physicians because they could establish a higher "usual" rate when beginning practice. Congress and the Reagan administration recognized that a system of national rates was needed, with adjustments for differences in regional costs.

Reagan instructed the HEW secretary to report to Congress by 1985 on the feasibility of inpatient physician DRGs. The AMA strongly opposed the concept because physicians could lose the independence that the AMA had fought so hard to preserve when Medicare was enacted. The Reagan administration did not want to antagonize organized medicine, whom they viewed as friendly to their antiregulation, procompetition philosophy.[67] Hence, the legislation allowed physicians a choice. They could accept the government-established rate as full payment (known as "assignment") or they could bill a higher rate and charge the patient the difference (known as "balance billing"). Patient advocates opposed the latter option, arguing that a Medicare beneficiary would never know what they would be required to pay if they became ill. Furthermore, patients could not ascertain whether a physician would accept assignment when they or their families required emergency care. Stuart Altman was soon to appreciate these problems firsthand.

### Stuart's Mother Gets Balance Billed

When Florence Altman was diagnosed with a detached retina, she immediately called her son in Boston. Stuart, of course, knew health care people all over the country, and he was able to find his mother a highly regarded surgeon near her home in New York. After the surgery was completed, his mother was surprised to receive a bill which was far more than what Medicare would pay. Florence, who had always gone to physicians that accepted Medicare fees, had no idea what to do, so she again called her son, the Medicare expert. Stuart told her either to discuss the issue with the surgeon or not pay the bill. Still having a large bandage over her eye, not paying the bill seemed like a bad idea. Florence smartly chose to discuss the issue with the surgeon, who cut the difference in half. She had less luck with the anesthesiologist who demanded a substantial balance that Florence reluctantly paid. After her eye had healed, Florence asked her son, "Who designed this crazy system?"

In later years, this reimbursement policy was modified to limit how much a physician could charge above the Medicare rate, and today only about one percent of physicians across the United States do not accept assignment. However, in 1983, when only 51 percent of physicians accepted assignment, it was a real issue.[68]

If Congress included physician payments in the new Medicare PPS, physicians would have to accept assignment, just as hospitals had done. The policy was not able to gain much traction, given the strong opposition of physicians, and soon lost favor by both the Reagan team and the Congress.[69] The Reagan administration never viewed physician payment reform as a top policy issue and finally delivered the mandated congressional report in September 1987, two years after its due date. Although the report summarized various payment options, it did not recommend any fundamental changes.[70]

## Resource-Based Relative Value Scales (RBRVS)

There still remained a need for physician payment reform, and Congress created its own advisory group, the Physician Payment Review Commission (PPRC). Included in the 1985 Consolidated Omnibus Budget and Reconciliation Act, and similar in structure to ProPAC, PPRC reported directly to Congress.[71] Unlike ProPAC, however, PPRC was asked to help Congress devise a new physician payment system. Congress and many members of the PPRC favored a national fee schedule but did not have the expertise to create one. Hence, they asked a group at the Harvard School of Public Health to work with the AMA to develop a schedule based on the relative value of resources used in the provision of each physician service. The director of the project, William Hsiao, a former Medicare actuary, worked with a series of expert physician panels to develop the relative value of different procedures within each specialty. They devised a technique to create a relative ranking of specialties based on years of training and the complexity of the services provided.[72] Although the designers of the RBRVS worked hard to cross-link specialties so that payment rates were fair, a strong bias emerged against non-procedure dominated specialties such as primary care.[73] Nevertheless, RBRVS gained credibility and support from most physician groups.

An important component of RBRVS was the value of "work." Researchers decided the value consisted of both the time it took to do a procedure and the intensity of effort. Time was easy to calculate, but intensity was highly subjective. Ultimately, intensity included three components: (1) mental effort and judgment, (2) technical skill and physical effort, and (3) stress due to patient risk.[74] Although these concepts made sense, they also reinforced the bias in physician payment. Routine and diagnostic tasks received much less value than procedures—particularly procedures that included substantial medical risk.

PPRC also had to address the problem of regional differences in physician fees. The same issue confronted PPS, but the outcomes were different. PPS initially paid hospitals based on prevailing differences in regional costs, but, ultimately, it paid rural hospitals considerably more than their relative costs, allowing many rural hospitals to survive. This was not so for physicians. RBRVS permitted regional differences in payment only for "practice costs." These were defined as direct operating costs such as rent and local wage differentials. Today, there are growing physician shortages in rural areas, partly as a result of these lower payments.

## A Regulatory Problem that Will Not Go Away

One policy issue nearly killed congressional approval of physician payment reform. Policy makers knew that a limit on fees would not, by itself, control Medicare spending. The volume and intensity of physician services would also drive spending.[75] Policy experts and others debated if the plan should include a mechanism to limit the growth in the volume of physician services and, if so, how it could be done. However, the AMA threatened to block passage of the plan if it included a mechanism that was too restrictive. In a surprise move, the American College of Surgeons (ACS) agreed to support the plan if it included a separate volume adjustment for surgery. The ACS understood that the number of surgeries in the future was likely to decline, and a negative volume adjustment would produce higher fees. Years later, they proved to be correct. Other physician specialty groups, particularly those representing primary care, also supported the plan, believing it would generate higher fees for them as well. This forced the AMA to pull back from its opposition.

The House passed the Medicare Physician Payment bill, including a limit on excess volume increases. Support for the plan in the Senate was not as strong. Several state physician associations lobbied their senators to oppose the legislation, fearing it would negatively affect their incomes and impose government standards on what was appropriate medical care.[76] Again, one of the main sticking points was whether the plan should include any restrictions on volume growth. After much debate, the Senate Finance Committee, chaired by Senator Rockefeller, passed a plan that included a "Volume Performance Standard." It was more like an advisory guideline rather than a specific target.[77] The plan eventually passed the Senate using budget reconciliation, the same technique Democrats employed to pass the 2010 Health Reform plan. Although both Houses had passed the legislation, the difference in the type of volume restrictions led to a protracted and controversial set of conference committee meetings. The odds makers of the day gave passage of any legislation a low probability.[78] But they were wrong. In the final hours before congressional adjournment on November 21, 1989, the Omnibus Reconciliation Act of 1989 finally passed. The legislation included restrictions on volume growth that were somewhat stronger than the Senate proposal but weaker than the House version. The regulations were scheduled to begin on January 1, 1992, and provided for a ten-year implementation period.

The argument over the volume adjustment mechanism in the 1989 leg-islation was just the beginning of what remains a major issue confronting Medicare. The Balanced Budget Act of 1997 (BBA) significantly strength-ened the volume adjustment formula for physician payments. In a little-debated provision, the government instituted the Sustainable Growth Rate (SGR). It specified that if the annual growth in total spending for Medicare physician services (fees × volume) exceeded a targeted amount, doctors' fees in future years would be reduced to bring spending within the budget. Two factors would primarily determine the SGR target: the percentage change in the fees paid for physician services and the ten-year average annual per-centage change in per capita real gross domestic product (GDP). Although these two factors look reasonable, they represent a major departure from previous experience. For the first time the federal government was going to limit the growth in a major component of Medicare spending to the growth in the national economy. It was akin to a global budget for physician services.

For the first two years after the BBA was signed, actual and target spending were aligned. Beginning in 2000, however, substantial growth in the volume of physician services pushed actual spending above the target, and the gap has grown every year. Congress repeatedly has been required to cut physician fees, but has been reluctant to do so because of opposition by doc-tors and the AMA. As a result, the gap became large and politically difficult to close. Although Congress did allow payments to decrease by 4.8 percent in 2002, it has since postponed every reduction and has actually authorized five small fee increases. As a result, the cumulative reduction in fees that would be necessary to close the gap reached 21 percent in 2010. Medicare fees are already only 78 percent of commercial rates, and such a reduction, aside from wreaking political havoc, could have serious implications for Medicare ben-eficiaries' ability to obtain physician services. Each year Congress has consid-ered eliminating the required cuts and revising the SGR formula, and each year it has put off the decision. The reason is quite simple. It would now cost nearly $250 billion over a ten-year budget horizon. The saga of the SGR again highlights just how difficult it is to reduce health care spending growth.

## Halfway Competitive Markets and Ineffective Regulation

The Reagan administration aggressively sought to control Medicare spend-ing but was strongly opposed to any government regulation of private health spending. The administration succeeded in dismantling the national health planning system and its CON controls. Thus, the states became responsible for limiting the availability of new health care facilities and equipment. Most states either ended or weakened their CON programs by the late '80s. The defeat of the Carter hospital cost containment plan ended any federal attempt to limit nongovernment health care costs.

Although the Medicare program adopted PPS in 1983, few private health plans followed, relying instead on paying providers on a fee-for-service basis. Insurers discussed the idea of market competition between alternative health delivery systems, but took no action. Private health plans were more interested in adding new members than in controlling premiums. Between 1980 and 1990, average health insurance premiums grew by 300 percent.[79] This acceleration in spending was aided by a rapid growth in the number of hospital beds and practicing physicians. American medical school capacity doubled in the early '70s. Combined with the inflow of foreign-born doctors, the growth in the number of practicing physicians far outstripped the growth in population. Between 1980 and 1990, physicians per one hundred thousand population increased from 202 to 238, a rise of nearly 20 percent.[80] In a 1988 journal article, Altman named the '80s the decade of "halfway competitive markets and ineffective regulation."[81]

# CHAPTER 10

# THE LAST TWENTY YEARS
## HEALTH CARE SPENDING
## KEEPS GROWING

### The 1990s: Big Business Worries about Health Care Costs

V isiting Little Rock, Arkansas, in December is not high on many people's list. But, for several hundred of the most prominent economic and business leaders in the United States in December 1992, it was the place to be. President-elect Bill Clinton had organized a two-day economic summit in Little Rock to discuss the nation's economic problems and the policies his new government should undertake. High on the president-elect's list was the rapidly rising cost of health care. The previous decade had seen the biggest increase in health care spending in recent times. On a per capita basis, health care spending grew from $1,100 in 1980 to $2,814 in 1990.[1] One can measure spending growth by comparing it to national income. In the '70s, annual growth in health spending exceeded that of national income by 2.2 percent. It reached 3.1 percent in the '80s. In contrast, the average for the same measure in European countries during the '80s was 0.8 percent.[2]

Many CEOs of large American companies were sounding the alarm that if something wasn't done to slow this cost growth, the international competitiveness of US products would be seriously compromised. Jobs would be sent overseas as American companies transferred production to less expensive countries. For this reason, Bill Clinton asked the CEO of Ford Motors, Harold "Red" Poling, to address the summit. Following Poling's remarks, the Clinton presidential transition team asked Stuart Altman to discuss what the United States could do to slow the growth in health care costs.

Poling discussed how much the Ford Motor Company was spending on health insurance and how rapidly it had grown in the last ten years. Of particular concern to large manufacturing companies like Ford that had been in business for many years was the substantial expenses it incurred each year to provide health coverage for retired workers. Such extra costs were not incurred by foreign auto companies, even those producing cars in the United States, because they employed younger workers and had few retirees.

Some economists questioned whether the health costs of current workers hurt the competitiveness of US firms because higher health costs eventually were offset by lower wages. However, the president-elect took Poling's concerns seriously, and so did Altman.

Altman outlined a number of reasons why large manufacturers, such as automakers, paid higher premiums than other employers. One reason was their workforces were older and used more services. In addition, they often paid for spouses who worked for smaller firms that offered no coverage. They also provided wraparound coverage to supplement their retirees' Medicare benefits. And they paid higher rates to help providers in their communities pay for the uninsured. Altman reiterated the argument that if all Americans had adequate coverage, some of these higher expenses would disappear. Nevertheless, he cautioned, until the United States changed its payment and delivery systems, much of the growth in health costs would continue.

## Managed Care Reduces Cost Growth in the Mid-1990s

When Bill Clinton's health reform effort failed in 1994, American businesses had to find other solutions for their health cost problems. Many firms arrived at the same solution that was at the heart of the Clinton health plan—managed care. After Nixon enacted the Health Maintenance Act of 1973, enrollment in managed care grew slowly. By 1988, only about 16 percent of American workers were covered under such plans.[3] But that changed dramatically in the '90s. Most of the large health insurance companies developed HMO-type managed care plans with the following attributes: the plans selected a limited panel of hospitals, doctors, and other providers who would accept lower payments because plans would send them more patients; plans reviewed the utilization of providers in their panels to ensure best practices—but also to save money by limiting overuse; and some providers agreed to capitation arrangements in which they would guarantee to provide services for all of a patient's needs for a fixed annual payment. Studies suggested that a well-run HMO plan could substantially reduce costs and unnecessary services by employing these strategies.

Many providers agreed to these arrangements, not only because they expected the plans to supply more patients but also because they feared losing patients if they were left out of the panels. In addition, managed care companies were able to negotiate lower prices because many communities had an excess number of hospital beds and a growing supply of physicians. It was estimated that the occupancy rate of hospital beds in 1995 was close to 65 percent, much below the ideal 85 percent level.[4] Having lower costs, managed care companies enticed businesses to enroll in their plans by offering multiyear commitments with very low premiums if the firm required all employees to join the plan. As a result, enrollment in managed care plans soared in the mid-1990s.

By 1996, the percentage of workers with some form of HMO coverage reached 31 percent.[5] After many years of large premium increases, managed care delivered on its promise to tame costs. Health insurance premiums, which had been rising at double-digit rates in the late '80s, declined dramatically beginning around 1992, and were held to low single-digit increases and even small decreases in the early to mid-1990s.[6] But many Americans were not happy. Physicians and hospitals bitterly complained that they were not receiving adequate compensation for their services, and their expected increases in volume never materialized. Stories spread that HMOs were denying care to patients in order to save money. The press soon picked up the cause, presenting vivid examples of patients who were denied services.[7] Movies such as *John Q, As Good As It Gets*, and *The Rainmaker* vilified managed care. Inevitably, many politicians joined the attack.[8]

Surely there were reasons to question some of the decisions of the managed care companies. Was it really necessary to limit payment for a normal delivery to one day? Was there always clear evidence when rejecting an unnecessary service? How many clinical decisions were being made for financial rather than clinical reasons? Were the payment limits to physicians and hospitals too restrictive?

Part of the backlash came from employees who were forced to enroll in HMOs. Sidney Garfield was the founder of Kaiser Permanente, the largest HMO in the country. He believed that only those individuals that wanted to be in a managed care option should be encouraged to join. Therefore, he required employers who wished to enroll their employees in Kaiser to give their workers a choice of the type of insurance coverage.[9] By requiring all employees in a firm to be in the HMO plan, the managed care plans of the '90s violated Garfield's rule.

In addition to all of these concerns, one could argue that the backlash against managed care was also an attack on reducing the growth in health spending. Everyone wants lower health care costs, but not if it affects their care or their freedom to choose any physician. Americans would like access to unlimited services, but they do not want to pay the price. That is a painful lesson that policymakers have learned many times in the last forty years.

## Medicare Policy 1995-2000:
## Government Shutdowns and the BBA

Although private health plans constrained their spending in the mid-1990s, providers still increased their revenues. The revenue loss from private plans was offset by accelerated Medicare spending. Medicare payments to hospitals grew at much higher rates than costs through the early '90s, and profits from treating Medicare patients approached 10 percent by 1995.[10] Similar increases in Medicare spending were recorded for other services, including home care and outpatient hospital care.[11] As a result, the federal trustees of the Medicare Program warned that the Medicare trust fund that financed hospital and home health services for seniors could be bankrupt by 2001.[12]

The 1994 congressional elections were a disaster for both the Democratic Party and President Clinton. Both houses of Congress switched from Democratic to Republican control. Key to the Republican victory was a strategy developed by Newt Gingrich called the "Contract with America." Among the ten provisions of the contract was a commitment to balance the federal budget. The Republican Congress attempted to achieve this goal by passing a series of bills in 1995 that would have substantially reduced spending in the Medicare and Medicaid programs.

Reductions in Medicare spending were supported by both political parties as a way to preserve the fiscal integrity of the program. The only major difference was how much spending should be cut. The severity of the reductions proposed by the Republicans, combined with their proposal to lower federal tax rates, angered both the Democrats in Congress and President Clinton. Clinton vetoed several budget bills sent to him by the Republican Congress. This led to two shutdowns of the federal government, including one that lasted from December 16, 1995, to January 6, 1996, the longest shutdown in the history of the country.[13] The Democrats used these budget battles to label the Republicans as "Medicare killers" and were able to win back some congressional seats in the 1996 election. Most importantly, President Clinton, despite facing widespread attacks on his personal activities, won reelection. Ultimately, both political parties agreed that something needed to be done to slow Medicare spending and balance the federal budget. After much negotiation, the Balanced Budget Act (BBA) was signed by President Clinton on August 5, 1997.[14]

The BBA was designed to generate the largest reductions in Medicare spending in the history of the program. It succeeded beyond what policy makers expected. In July 2000, Gail Wilensky, chair of the Medicare Payment Advisory Committee, testified before a congressional committee.[15] "Since the enactment of BBA in 1997," Wilensky reported, "Medicare outlays have increased at a rate well below what was projected at that time." The cuts were so severe that Medicare spending growth was flat in 1998 and declined in 1999. This prompted many providers to petition Congress and the president for help—and help was on the way. The Balanced Budget Reform Act of 1999 and the Budget Improvement and Protection Act of 2000 ameliorated some of the spending reductions. However, the net reductions were still substantial, and, combined with vigorous economic growth, the projected bankruptcy of the Medicare trust fund was pushed back from 2001 to 2026.[16] With the reductions in Medicare spending, total health expenditures increased more slowly between 1997 and 2000, and at much lower rates than in the '80s.[17] The excess of health care spending above income growth during the decade of the '90s fell to 1.07 percent per year from 3.11 the previous decade.[18] However, the trend toward lower growth was about to end.

**Turn of the Century: Americans Prefer Unmanaged Care**

Following the managed care backlash, Americans demanded, and insurance companies supplied, managed care options that had fewer constraints. PPOs grew rapidly and became the dominant form of health insurance in the United States. PPOs provide patients with a wider choice of physicians from a plan's "preferred provider" panel than the choices typically offered by an HMO. Patients can select a provider outside the preferred list, but they may be required to pay a higher copayment or pay more than the plan's usual charge. PPOs have weaker utilization controls on the kinds and amounts of health care services that can be used. Because these plans are less managed, they spend more, incurring higher patient costs than HMOs, and they charge enrollees higher premiums.

Private spending also increased because hospitals aggressively sought higher payments to make up for losses they incurred from treating Medicare and Medicaid patients and the uninsured.[19] The burden of providing care to the uninsured varied widely among hospitals. Some hospitals, particularly rural and public facilities, reported uncompensated care costs as much as 15 percent or more of their total costs.[20] Most hospitals made up for these shortfalls by charging privately insured patients considerably more than the cost of their care (cost shifting). In effect, the US health system imposes an indirect tax on privately insured patients and their employers. Institutions with a significant proportion of privately insured patients and strong market power within their communities were able to secure such higher payments and increase their profits. In 2008, the most profitable quartile of hospitals had profits of 6.9 percent or greater. However, many hospitals lost money, particularly those treating more uninsured and fewer private patients. The bottom quartile sustained losses of 1.8 percent or more.[21]

Hospitals were also able to price aggressively because there was much consolidation in the industry. The number of hospitals underwent a steady decline from 1980 to 2000 as many hospitals consolidated, merged, or joined integrated systems, and some simply closed. Gradually, hospitals gained market power relative to the insurance companies with which they negotiated prices. The above factors led to an increase in premiums of over 90 percent between 2000 and 2007. In comparison, salaries grew by only 20 percent over the same period.[22] When Barack Obama began his presidential campaign, the cost of health care was again a prominent issue.

## Controlling Health Costs: Should We Care, and What Can We Do about It?

In 2010, the United States spent over 17 percent of GDP on health care—far more than any other country. So what? Why should we be concerned? No one questions how much we spend on automobiles or televisions. What separates health care services from other services or products? The answer is threefold. The first reason lies in the nature of health insurance. Most of us try to protect ourselves from the catastrophic costs of serious illnesses by purchasing insurance. The elderly in Medicare and the poor who qualify for Medicaid receive insurance from the government. However, once we are insured, and thus protected from having to pay the true cost of providing care, there is a propensity for patients to want many services; some of which provide limited or no medical value. As we explained earlier, economists call this moral hazard. At the same time, there are temptations for providers to offer extra services. Most providers are paid per service, and they know the patient will not have to pay much of the cost—a situation that does not encourage tight restrictions on the provision of services. Second, as a compassionate society, we do not let people suffer for lack of health care. Hence, if anyone is uninsured and unable to pay, all of us pay for that person's care, either through taxes or higher private insurance premiums. Third, the amount we tax ourselves and spend to govern our society is limited. Hence, to a considerable extent, the tax dollars we spend on health care are dollars that cannot be spent on education, housing, defense, and other societal needs. Health care is therefore different than other goods and services, and it does matter how much we spend for them, which is why we have tried so hard to control costs.

Several years ago, a beer commercial pitted two rival groups arguing why their beer was better. One group believed it tasted great. The other group maintained it was less filling. In the end, the beer company did not care which group you supported as long as you bought their beer. In the health world, two groups are arguing over why health care spending is growing so rapidly, and why it is so much more expensive in the United States than in other countries. One group believes that patients in the United States use too much care. The other side maintains that prices are too high. Similar to the beer commercial, both arguments have merit, but a deeper understanding is important if we are ever going to solve the health care cost problem.

## Cost Drivers

What can or should be done to limit the use or restrain the price of medical care? We could limit the availability and types of insurance. One option would be to eliminate the tax deduction that subsidizes the purchase of insurance. A less drastic option would be to reduce the tax deduction for policies that offer excessive benefits. This option was included in the Obama health reform legislation—but only after a big political battle. High-deductible health plans that require patients to pay most of the cost of care below a catastrophic threshold are another approach.[23]

Economists believe all of these options would lower overall health spending. However, they have negative consequences. Eliminating or reducing the government subsidy to buy insurance would increase the number of uninsured. Imposing a high deductible discourages people (particularly those with low incomes) from using beneficial services, such as preventive care. It is doubtful, however, how much these strategies would save because most expenses are for high cost care and chronic illness, neither of which would be affected by these limits on coverage.

Alternatives to limiting insurance coverage include government regulation of prices and/or the supply of services. We reviewed numerous regulatory techniques that were tried in the '70s. Many were effective initially, but, without exception, all were ended. Opponents of regulation concluded they did not work. Although that is partly true, a more complete reason is that the US political system would not let them work.[24] Controlling costs means controlling prices or limiting use of certain medical services. It is easy to talk about controlling costs, but what we are really controlling is spending. Not surprisingly, those who stand to lose by these controls try to neutralize them by exercising political power or by finding ways to game the regulatory systems. In contrast to the United States, most other Western, industrialized countries have developed successful techniques to regulate health care spending and use. They have restricted the availability of expensive services and regulated the amounts paid to providers, technology manufacturers, and pharmaceutical companies while increasing access to preventive and low-cost care. The success of these cost control techniques has a downside. They restrict use and conjure up the dreaded *r* word: *rationing!* Americans thus far seem to prefer spending more for their health care than accepting such restrictions.

Another strategy to control service use is managed care. We reviewed efforts in the '90s when managed care plans implemented utilization restrictions that limited choice of doctors and required physicians to get second opinions before ordering expensive services. Health insurers took these actions because they believed there was overuse of many expensive medications and procedures, some of which had limited medical value. Studies indicated, for example, that Americans received far too many MRI and computerized tomography (CT) scans.[25] Unfortunately, we have little evidence-based knowledge whether one drug or procedure produces a better clinical outcome than another. Although the Food and Drug Administration is required to determine if a drug or device is safe and effective before it can be used, only limited studies are undertaken to show if a drug or service is medically superior to those already in use. The Obama administration funded a program for comparative effectiveness research (CER). The purpose of CER is to help doctors and patients compare different treatment regimens to determine which is the most clinically effective. Unfortunately, critics in the United States have disparaged CER, arguing that it will be used by the government to restrict treatment options with the intent of saving money. In fact, the CER legislation explicitly forbids any consideration of cost (we discuss this in chapter 14). However, Americans seem to have an abject fear of anything that might lead to health care rationing. Some of the opposition to CER came from people who confuse comparative effectiveness research with cost effectiveness analysis. The two sound similar, but they are very different.

Cost effectiveness analysis monetizes the benefit of a given drug or treatment regimen and compares it to the cost. It is used to answer a question such as the following: If a new drug costs ten times more than an existing drug, but only confers a marginal benefit, should doctors prescribe, or should insurers pay for, the more expensive drug? Such decisions become very controversial if life-extending treatment is involved. For example, if a new drug costs one hundred thousand dollars but, on average, extends life for one month, is the benefit worth the cost?

Cost effectiveness analysis is currently used in the United Kingdom as well as in some other countries. For a procedure, device, or drug to be added to the public treatment protocol in the United Kingdom's National Health Service (NHS), it must be shown to have an acceptable "Cost-Effectiveness Ratio." To make such a determination, the United Kingdom created the National Institute for Clinical Effectiveness (NICE), which analyzes the medical effectiveness of the procedure under review in comparison to existing standards of care or to no treatment. The benefit is calculated in terms of patients' additional "quality-adjusted life years" (QALYs). The measure includes not only how much longer patients will live, but also the quality of their additional time. If the cost per QALY exceeds their guideline, NICE will recommend that the intervention should not be covered by the National Health Service.[26]

NICE and the use of cost effectiveness by the NHS has received considerable criticism. From an individual patient perspective, as opposed to a societal one, denying a treatment because of its costs can seem unconscionable or even mercenary; all the more so because wealthy patients can pay for treatments with their own funds. Nevertheless, the use of cost effectiveness is supported by the UK population as an appropriate technique for balancing the needs of its sick population with the amount the country is prepared to spend for medical care. The NICE website states: "With the rapid advances in modern medicine, most people accept that no publicly funded health care system, including the NHS, can possibly pay for every new medical treatment which becomes available. The enormous costs involved mean that choices have to be made."[27]

Current US policy prohibits any form of rationing based on price. However, many policy analysts believe that the United States will never be able to control health care costs if every possible treatment is available regardless of cost or efficacy. The United States already spends almost double what other countries spend per person for health care, and much of that is spent in the last year of life.

Some libertarians and conservatives, who distrust the government, worry that CER will morph in to cost effectiveness analysis. That was one source of worry about "death panels." Although that concern should not be dismissed, the two are very different. CER simply focuses on the best medical practice while cost effectiveness analysis involves a host of difficult ethical and social policy decisions. If the cost of health care continues to grow at an unsustainable rate, however, cost effectiveness analysis is likely to emerge as an important policy issue.

## Too Much Use

Do Americans use too many health services? How do we compare with other industrialized countries? Here, the evidence is mixed. The Organisation for Economic Co-operation and Development frequently publishes data for its thirty-two member nations. They include extensive health data and statistics that can be used to place US data in context. For several services such as hospitalizations or visits to the doctor, the results are quite surprising. Recent data shows an average discharge rate of 157.8 per 1,000 people across OECD countries compared to 126.3 in the United States.[28] Residents of OECD countries had 6.8 physician visits per year compared to 3.8 in the United States.[29] The United States also had fewer hospital beds and doctors per capita than most European countries.[30] On the other side of the ledger, the United States used far more expensive medical procedures, such as cardiac cauterization, kidney dialysis, and transplantations.[31] Defenders of the US style of medicine argue that American doctors use expensive procedures more intensively to reduce the time patients stay in the hospital. It is true that the length of stay of patients in the United States is considerably shorter than in most industrialized countries. For example, the average length of stay for a hospitalized patient in the United States was 5.5 days, compared to 7.2 in the United Kingdom and 7.8 in Germany.[32] Nevertheless, the cost of the American style of care is high. As we stated previously, Americans spend about eight thousand dollars per capita, more than twice the average spent in Europe. If the comparative utilization of medical services does not provide a definitive explanation for this higher spending, what about a comparison of prices?

## Too High Prices

Here the evidence is clear: prices in the United States are much higher. The following table compares prices in the United States and OECD countries.

Table 10.1

All amounts in USD

| Fee Type | Procedure | Canada | France | Germany | Netherlands | Spain | UK | USA Average/ Low-end | USA High-end | USA Medicare |
|---|---|---|---|---|---|---|---|---|---|---|
| Scans and Imaging | CT Scan Abdomen | 83/530 | 248 | 319 | 258 | 161 | 179 | 750* | 1,600 | 400 |
| Physician Fees | Routine Office Visit | 30 | 31 | 22 | 32 | 15 | Primary care | 59 | 151 | 72 |
| | Normal Delivery | 498 | 1,023 | TBD | 622 | 1,041 | capitation specialty salaries No Fees | 2,384 | 4,847 | 1,601** |
| Hospital Charges | Ave.Cost of hosp. stay | 9,043 | 9,840 | TBD | 3,535 | 2,261 | | 12,549* | 40,680 | 12,000 |
| Total Hospital and Physician Costs | Bypass Surgery | 14,111 | 11,916 | TBD | TBD | 15,761 | 12,868 | 56,472* | 116,798 | 22,092** |
| | Hip Replace | 8,483 | 8,200 | 8,500 | 7,600 | 9,152 | 8,347 | 32,093* | 67,983 | 17,500 |
| Tests and Cultures | Pap Smear | 27 | 14 | 26 | 16 | 20 | See note above | 24 | 64 | 17 |
| Drug Prices | Lipitor | 33 | 53 | 48 | 63 | 32 | 40 | 125 | 334 | No Medicare Rx fees |
| | Nexium | 65 | 67 | 37 | 102 | 36 | 41 | 154 | 424 | |

Non-US fees shown above came from both government sources and data files of IFHP member plans. For countries with multiple health plans or multiple regions with different payment systems, the fees reflect a representative sample of estimated average prices.

Canadian scans include the government "reading" fees and the charges used by private scanning facilities for patients who pay their own expenses. There are no government fees associated with MRIs because this equipment is typically purchased by local health authorities and is included with fees for facility-level use.

*Represents USA average fees rather than USA low-end fees.

** Representative Medicare fees from Portland, Oregon market or CMS Medicare average for tests and cultures; all other Medicare fees are averages provided by a global consulting and actuarial firm.

Source: International Federation of Health Plans, "2009 Comparative Price Report: Medical and Hospital Fees by Country," http://voices.washingtonpost.com/ezra-klein/IFHP%20Comparative%20Price%20Report%20with%20AHA%20data%20addition.pdf (accessed December 28, 2010).

The differences are striking. A routine visit to the doctor was between two and ten times more expensive in the United States than in Canada and in several European countries. Procedures, diagnostic tests, and pharmaceuticals were also several times more expensive in the United States. Although the price of a one-night hospital stay varies considerably in the United States, the average rate was 25 percent higher than it was in the most expensive European countries.

Why are health care prices so much higher in the United States? Unfortunately there is no one answer. American physicians and health workers earn higher salaries than their counterparts in Europe.[33] This is true even when earnings are adjusted for our higher GDP. Hospitals and consumers in the United States pay considerably more for drugs and devices.[34] Higher malpractice costs and substantial regulatory requirements add additional costs in the United States.[35] Furthermore, there is the complexity of the US payment system. Every health provider employs large numbers of workers simply to process the bills it sends to private and public payers. Regardless of what one thinks about a single-payer system, it does reduce administrative costs.[36]

However, the factors leading to higher medical prices and overall medical spending in the United States go far beyond administrative costs and will not be solved by a single-payer system. Much more fundamental changes are needed in the way we organize and deliver care and the way we pay for personnel and services. Solutions will ultimately involve controlling both use and price. Until now, neither American consumers nor the health care industry have been willing to support such reforms. In the final chapter, we discuss several ways that are being contemplated to make such changes.

# PART 4

# SUCCESS AT LAST!

# CHAPTER 11

# OBAMA DEVELOPS HIS PLAN

## Early Pressure

"Let's be the generation that says right here, right now, that we will have universal health care in America by the end of the next president's first term."[1] Announcing his run for the presidency on a frigid February morning in Chicago, Barack Obama made it clear that health care reform would be a major focus of his upcoming campaign. Generalities, however, would not suffice, and Obama immediately faced pressure to outline his proposal. During the first televised candidate's forum on April 27, 2007, John Edwards chided Obama for not offering specifics about his health plan. "Highfalutin language is not enough,"[2] said Edwards, who had released his plan in February. Pressure also emanated from Obama's front-running opponent, Hillary Clinton. Having engineered her husband's health reform effort, she made it clear the issue would be a focal point in her presidential campaign.

After enduring repeated criticism from Edwards and other primary opponents, Obama released the details of his plan on May 29. The *New York Times* reported that the plan was based on the advice of several economists, including Austan Goolsbee, David Cutler, and Stuart Altman.[3] It was immediately apparent that the plan built on the current private, employer-based system. It required all but the smallest employers to provide coverage or pay a penalty. It sought to include lower income individuals and small business by a combination of tax credits, subsidies, and an insurance exchange with a public option. It promised to reduce costs by providing government-sponsored catastrophic reinsurance. The plan required insurance companies to cease unpopular underwriting practices such as exclusions for preexisting conditions and lifetime limits on coverage. And it included a limited, individual mandate requiring children to have insurance. Obama also promised that the plan would be paid for—it would not add to the federal budget deficit.

Almost immediately, his plan was derided by both Democratic and Republican opponents. Republicans called his proposal government-run health care. Democrats criticized his plan for not requiring an individual mandate for everyone. Without such a mandate, his liberal opponents claimed, he could not achieve universal coverage. Throughout the primary campaign, Obama was forced to defend the lack of a mandate. Both Clinton and Edwards insisted that Obama's plan fell short of the Democrats' long-sought goal. Only their plans, they claimed, would cover America's forty-five million uninsured. Obama countered that a combination of subsidies and incentives would entice nearly everyone to purchase insurance. It was a weak argument, and one that Obama would have to reverse shortly after becoming president.

In most other respects, however, his original proposal provided the framework for the eventual legislation. Despite a bitter year-long battle, and differing bills by five congressional committees, the general outline of his plan remained mostly unchanged. Certainly, he had to concede a few of his original recommendations. In addition to the individual mandate, he would give up the public option and the ability of Medicare to negotiate prices with drug companies. Nevertheless, the framework of his proposal would remain intact, and the reason is quite simple: Barack Obama had learned the lessons of history from his predecessors.

He was not going to propose a wholesale restructuring of the health system like Bill Clinton. Neither was he going to embrace a government-run single-payer system favored by liberals. He would build on the current private system, retaining Medicare and Medicaid and not requiring those who already had insurance to change their coverages. His plan resembled universal proposals by Democrats and Republicans who had come before him. In fact, every serious plan for universal coverage had embraced these basic principles.

Contrary to what most people believe, the general characteristics of the plan Obama developed during the campaign and the one adopted by the Congress and signed into law are not difficult to understand. In the following section, we outline the framework of Obama's original plan, and we note the significant changes between the original proposal and the actual legislation.

## Substance Built on History: The Substantive Framework of the Obama Health Plan

### Universal Coverage

Barack Obama was committed to universal or near-universal coverage. It was a core issue throughout the presidential primaries, and all three Democratic candidates had set forth comprehensive proposals. Democrats and liberals had sought this final piece of social protection since FDR enacted Social Security in 1935, and their failures have been detailed in earlier chapters. Obama put the matter succinctly before a joint session of Congress in 2009. "I am not the first president to take up this cause," he stated, "but I am determined to be the last."[4]

### Employer-Sponsored Insurance System

Richard Nixon understood that an employer-sponsored insurance system was the only practical way to attain universal coverage. A single-payer system, regardless of its advantages and disadvantages, was not politically possible. Tax credits were hard to target, making them prohibitively expensive, and they still required public insurance programs. As recently as 2000, presidential candidate Bill Bradley proposed a system based on tax credits. In order to provide generous enough subsidies to approach universality, however, large amounts would inevitably go to people who were already purchasing their own insurances.

Nixon was well aware of the potential cost of insuring all Americans and the political opposition to raising taxes in order to do so. Mandating employers to provide coverage avoided an explicit tax increase. In the long term, most of the cost would be reflected in lower wages, but that was almost a hidden increase—one voters could not feel compared to raising income or withholding taxes. Since Nixon's presidency, every serious proposal for universal coverage has built upon the employer-sponsored insurance system.

Opposition from small business, the Chamber of Commerce, and conservative and libertarian groups was instrumental in defeating previous attempts at employer mandates. The Obama plan that was finally enacted (hereinafter called the "Obama plan") attempted to assuage the opposition by charging firms a relatively small penalty in place of issuing a mandate. It exempted businesses with less than fifty employees, and it created a program to provide subsidies to qualifying small businesses during the first two years they chose to provide insurance. Despite these provisions, the opposition continued, although it was not as vitriolic as it was under the Clinton plan.

## Insurance Reform

Private insurance companies have a number of underwriting practices that infuriate consumers. In spite of restrictions in HIPPA discussed previously, many individuals who have a preexisting medical condition find it difficult, if not impossible, to obtain coverage. If they do obtain coverage, their premiums are often painfully expensive. Insurance companies have been known to retroactively deny payment for care if they find that an individual had an undisclosed medical condition before they purchased coverage. They can place lifetime limits on coverage and can refuse to renew coverage to individuals or groups that have had expensive claims. Most privately insured individuals are covered under large group policies and do not encounter such restrictions. However, these practices present serious problems for individuals seeking coverage in the small group and individual markets. Underwriting restrictions are intended to prevent people from waiting until they are sick to purchase insurance. As we explained previously, insurance works because it spreads risk. It collects premiums from a wide group of people— both low and high risk—to pay claims for the small number of persons within the group who will contract an expensive illness. If those who are well do not purchase insurance until they actually get sick, insurance simply does not work.

Obama understood that putting an end to most of these underwriting practices was a crucial selling point for his health reform proposal. Such an action would be particularly salient for many of the 84 percent of Americans who already had insurance but were worried about losing it. He reassured them that they would always be able to get insurance, even with preexisting conditions, and that it could never be taken away. This was a powerful argument; much more powerful than asking their support to pay for those "others"—the 16 percent who were uninsured.

## Individual Mandate

Insurance reform thus became a basic part of Obama's health plan, but there was one caveat. As we discussed previously, insurers cannot forego their underwriting practices unless everyone is required to purchase insurance. Otherwise, those individuals who know they are likely to incur high medical costs will purchase insurance, while many of those who are healthy will postpone buying coverage until they become ill. Bill Clinton understood this when he introduced his plan, and even his moderate Republican opponents included an individual mandate in their alternative proposals. Even Harry Truman recognized the necessity to insure everyone in 1945. Aware of this, the congressional committees formulating their bills in the spring of 2009 included an individual mandate.

This was immediately problematic for Obama because Hillary Clinton and John Edwards criticized his campaign plan for lacking such a mandate (except for children). Debating Hillary Clinton, Obama asked her if she would jail people who chose not to obtain coverage. She answered that without a mandate this country could neither get close to universal coverage nor end many of the most unpopular underwriting practices of private insurance companies.

The president-elect was reluctant to change his position. Stuart Altman recalls that during the campaign, Obama worried about forcing relatively low-income individuals to buy expensive health plans. He also worried that forcing people to buy insurance would be unpopular and an easy political target. Republicans perceive a mandate as another increase in government control over individuals. Throughout the presidential campaign, they attacked the policy even though they had formerly supported it as a measure of individual responsibility. To his credit, Obama reversed his opposition after he became president, realizing that without a mandate he could not eliminate the health-underwriting practices consumers so disliked.

If the purchase of insurance is mandated, the government has to enforce the mandate by fines or other penalties. The severity of the penalties became a difficult policy issue. If the penalties were too large, people could rebel and seek to overturn the entire policy. However, if they were too small, some people might pay the penalty, waiting until they were sick before buying insurance. The latter problem occurred in Massachusetts, causing insurance companies to raise premiums in the small group and individual markets to make up for the losses they incurred in the early stages of reform. Some are now concerned that the penalties in the final Obama legislation are too small and could generate the same result. Given all of these considerations, the implementation of an individual mandate is challenging, but it is a prerequisite for insurance-underwriting reforms.

### Affordability: Government Subsidies, Medicaid Expansion, and Insurance Exchanges

If the purchase of insurance is mandated, it must be affordable. No plan will work if it tries to force people to buy coverage they cannot afford. The Obama plan includes a combination of tax credits, Medicaid expansions, and state-based insurance exchanges to lower the net cost to consumers. Like any government assistance, however, all of these initiatives raise other issues.

The Obama plan provides tax credits to purchase private insurance for individuals earning up to 400 percent of the federal poverty level ($88,200 for a family of four in 2010). These tax credits make the mandated purchase of insurance more affordable, but they are expensive and reduce tax revenues. Hence, they require unpopular offsets (taxes or spending cuts) to be budget neutral.

Expanding Medicaid is less expensive than subsidizing the purchase of private insurance because Medicaid pays lower fees to providers and has smaller administrative costs. For the first time, the Obama plan does away with the categorical requirements enacted at the inception of the Medicaid program in 1965. Under the final legislation, all individuals earning less than 133 (effectively 138) percent of the poverty level will qualify for Medicaid regardless of family or marital status.[5] Many states currently have more stringent income requirements and will have to raise them to the 133 percent level. As a result, nearly half of the newly insured under the program (sixteen out of thirty-two million) will be enrolled in the Medicaid and SCHIP programs.

Conservatives oppose such a large expansion of Medicaid because it increases public sector coverage and the role of government at the expense of private insurance. It also places a financial burden on the states, which share the cost of the program with the federal government. In order to reduce state concerns, the federal government agreed to assume most of the costs of the Medicaid expansion.

The Obama plan also includes the creation of state-based insurance exchanges to increase affordability. The large group market, primarily comprised of employer-provided insurance, is reasonably efficient and does not need an exchange. However, the individual and small group insurance markets are often problematic. In these markets, the high cost of administration and sales and the limited ability to spread risk make it difficult for insurance companies to be profitable. As a result, only one or two companies dominate many local markets (especially in rural areas), and they often employ strict underwriting practices and charge high prices. Insurance companies contend their practices are necessary for such types of insurance markets, but critics argue that their strategy is to select the best risks, avoid insuring unhealthy people, and profit from high prices and lack of competition.

The Obama plan creates insurance exchanges to make insurance in the individual and small group market more accessible and affordable. These exchanges are comprised of competing private companies that operate according to strict rules and specifications set forth by the exchange. Designed to simplify enrollment, they permit an easy comparison of the rates and benefits of competing private plans. The new exchanges are modeled after those in the Massachusetts health plan and have some similarities to those that were in the ill-fated Clinton plan.

In his original plan, Obama included a public option that would compete with private insurance. A public option was also included in the initial plan passed by the House of Representatives and by one of the committees in the Senate, but it was not included in the final plan. The merits of the public option and the intense debate on the issue are discussed at length in chapter 16.

Tax credits, Medicaid expansions and insurance exchanges all create their own issues and problems. Nevertheless, just as an individual mandate is necessary for insurance reform, affordability is a prerequisite for a mandate.

## Budget Neutrality

Obama repeatedly promised that his health reform proposal "would not add one penny to the deficit." The CBO is the final arbiter in scoring the legislation, and it estimated that the actual legislation would reduce the deficit by $138 billion over ten years. Obama achieved the surplus by a combination of spending cuts and tax increases that we discuss later.

## Cost Control

Obama's original proposal included a government-funded reinsurance system that would insure policies against high-cost patients. The idea was recommended by Stuart Altman, who had worked to include it in John Kerry's health care proposal in 2004. The campaign originally estimated it would lower insurance premiums by 4 percent. In addition to reinsurance, Obama claimed that a combination of his policies would reduce premiums by up to twenty-five hundred dollars per year. Those policies included increased insurance competition, reduced costs from the limits on insurance underwriting, chronic care treatment models, increased preventive care, investment in health information technologies (IT), and savings from universal coverage such as reduced uncompensated care.

Of course, all candidates claimed that their health programs would reduce costs. It was part of the normal puffery of campaign rhetoric. However, actually achieving such a large reduction was unlikely. In the final legislation, the reinsurance program was greatly reduced, and most other cost control efforts were included only as trials and demonstrations. In fact, it is fair to say that promises to "bend the cost curve" were mostly abandoned. Concerns remain that private insurance will still be very expensive for most Americans and that some aspects of the reform legislation could actually increase premiums.

History may tell whether Obama ever really intended to include serious cost control. Certainly the opposition of the health industry would have been intense. Possibly, he intended all along to campaign on cost control but not fight for it when it was eliminated in the final legislation. As we have stated several times, we do not believe it would have been politically possible to enact near universal coverage if the plan had included substantial cost control.

## Summary of the Obama Framework

These policies described above comprise the general framework of the Obama health plan:

- A near universal system
- An employer "mandate" (in the form of a monetary penalty)
- Insurance reform ending exclusions for preexisting conditions, refusals to issue, caps on lifetime benefits, and rescissions of coverage
- An individual mandate (originally limited to children)
- Medicaid expansion for low-income individuals
- Tax credits for low-income individuals and small business to buy private coverage
- State-run insurance exchanges for individuals and small business (originally including a national plan and a public option)
- Financing so that the program will not add to the federal deficit

Of course, this comprehensive reform plan has many other provisions, including the financing details that we address later. But it is important to recognize, aside from the bombastic rhetoric, that the basic structure is quite logical and builds on the existing system. Moreover, it is quite similar to the plan developed by Richard Nixon in the '70s, to the plans put forward by Republican Senators John Chafee and Robert Dole in the '90s, and to the universal health plan enacted by the state of Massachusetts under Republican Governor Mitt Romney in 2006.

There is no question that the details of the plan are complex. The legislation has a number of shortcomings (which we will discuss) and many regulations that will likely be controversial. Conservatives and libertarians had valid philosophical reasons to oppose the plan. In addition, the Republican Party had logical political reasons to try to defeat the effort. Nevertheless, the basic structure of the plan is an outgrowth of mainstream policies that have been recommended by both political parties for the past thirty-five years. The Obama reform legislation is a huge package of changes for the health care system, but viewed from a historical perspective, it is neither a radical government takeover nor a substantial departure from the piecemeal system that already exists.

# CHAPTER 12

# EARLY PLAYERS
# AND DONE DEALS

## Ted Kennedy and Strange Bedfellows

Dying from brain cancer, Ted Kennedy was determined to fight for universal health care to the very end. In the fall of 2008, before Barack Obama had assumed the presidency, Kennedy organized the "Workhorse Group." Comprised of corporate lobbyists and health care interest groups with a wide variety of political perspectives, the group conducted secret meetings in a Senate conference room. Kennedy, famous for his ability to reach across the aisle, had organized such stakeholder meetings in the past on issues such as civil rights and immigration.[1] The objective of the group was to reach a consensus among "strange bedfellows" on how to proceed with health care reform.

The members of the Workhorse Group were not just Democrats and liberals. Some of the largest employers in the country wanted to reform the system. The rising cost of providing health benefits was reducing their profits, diminishing their international competitiveness, and hampering their labor negotiations. In addition, the forty-six million uninsured represented lost potential revenue to drug companies, insurers, and health care providers, and they cost hospitals huge amounts of money in uncompensated care. A broad consensus was emerging that something needed to be done, and Kennedy's forum attracted some of the most vitriolic opponents of past health reform efforts. It included such previous naysayers as the NFIB, the Business Roundtable, the Chamber of Commerce, AHIP, the Pharmaceutical Research and Manufacturers of America (PhRMA), and the AMA.

Strange Bedfellow groups were not new to health reform. Ron Pollack, the founder and executive director of Families USA, was the dean of such efforts. As early as 2001, Pollack teamed with his ideological opponent, Chip Kahn—then the president of the HIAA—to form the first Strange Bedfellows health reform group. After the failure of the Clinton health plan, Pollack helped to organize such groups as "Divided We Fail" in 2007 and the "Health Reform Dialogue" in 2008.

However, the Workhorse Group had Ted Kennedy's imprimatur and the attention of the president and the Congress. Not all of those in attendance had the same goals. Some knew they probably would oppose the effort down the road, but they wanted to have input into a process that could influence the eventual outcome. A surprising amount of consensus emerged from the seemingly disparate group. Most wanted to build on the current, employer-based system, control costs, move toward universal coverage, expand Medicaid, and provide government subsidies and tax incentives to help people purchase insurance. Significantly, many of the participants favored an individual mandate with some kind of tax penalty on those who did not comply.[2] Possibly, their consensus influenced Obama to change his position.

How much impact the Workhorse Group had is hard to assess. But, by the time Barack Obama became president, the health reform train was well out of the station and following a familiar route. And why not? Since the time of Richard Nixon, it was clear that any serious proposal for universal health care would have to roll down the same track.

## Daschle Dashed

The two men sat in Tosca, a tony Italian restaurant in downtown Washington. It was shortly after the 2006 midterm elections. "Don't always think you will have another shot," Tom Daschle advised the junior senator from Illinois. Daschle had been the Democratic leader in the Senate for ten years, alternating between minority and majority leader, until his defeat in the 2004 election. He knew the workings of the Senate better than almost anyone. Briefly, he had entertained the idea of running for president, but then became one of the earliest supporters of Barack Obama. Now, meeting in his favorite restaurant, he was urging Obama to run.

On December 11, after Obama won the election, he announced that Daschle would assume a dual role in his administration. Not only would he become secretary of the Department of Health and Human Services

(DHHS), but he would also serve as director of the new White House Office of Health Reform. Pundits considered it a wise appointment. The president was a relative novice, having served less than one term in the Senate. Moving comprehensive health reform through the upper house was going to require consummate skill. Obama needed someone who knew the ins and outs, who understood the exercise of power, and who had the respect of members on both sides of the aisle. By appointing the former majority leader, the president was demonstrating just how serious he was about health care reform. The Democrats could not have been more delighted—except, possibly, for one senator from Montana, Max Baucus, the head of the powerful Senate Finance Committee.

It was well known that Baucus and Daschle did not like each other. Baucus was independent and did not always side with the Democrats on important issues. He was very close to Chuck Grassley, the ranking Republican on the Finance Committee and had often collaborated with Grassley, angering other Democrats. He had voted with Grassley to approve George W. Bush's first tax cut and had earned the enmity of liberals, who called him "Bad Max." When Daschle was majority leader, Baucus had helped the Republicans pass the Medicare Prescription Drug bill after they had excluded Daschle and the Democratic leadership from the conference committee. But Baucus had also won some important battles for the Democrats, and his independence and civil demeanor had earned him respect on both sides of the aisle. If Obama needed bipartisan support to pass health reform, Baucus and his Senate Finance Committee would be essential to the effort.

Having been the former majority leader, Daschle's nomination should have breezed through the Senate, but that did not happen. According to *Politico*, "Democratic aides complained that Baucus had slow-rolled the nomination."[3] On January 30, the Senate Finance Committee released a report disclosing that shortly after Obama was elected, Daschle paid the IRS $140,000 in back taxes for previously undisclosed income.

To be fair, Daschle's underpayment could have been an honest mistake. He failed to declare as income the use of a car and driver supplied by a client, and a Form 1099 supplied by the same client was in error and had omitted one month of income. Unfortunately for Daschle it was a bad time for sympathy. Obama had campaigned for high ethical standards and had railed against the influence of lobbyists. Yet already in his nascent administration, his nominee for commerce secretary, Bill Richardson, had withdrawn because of ethical problems, and his nominee for treasury secretary, Tim Geithner, had failed to pay thirty-four thousand dollars in back taxes. Daschle's own image was not helped by the fact that he had accepted a two-million-dollars-per-year position at a Washington lobbying firm shortly after leaving office. The Obama administration was reeling, and Daschle, who would have faced a bruising confirmation fight, was asked to withdraw his nomination.

The story is important because it changed the top players on Obama's health team. Kathleen Sebelius became the secretary of HHS and Nancy-Ann DeParle was appointed head of the White House Office of Health Reform. Both had exceptional qualifications. Losing Daschle, however, hurt the reform effort in two areas. First, having been majority and minority leader, Daschle was a much stronger force in the Senate. Without his presence, Max Baucus, a much more moderate and conciliatory person, became a considerably more important player. Second, Daschle was a public figure and articulate spokesman who could have helped sell the health reform plan to the American public. Neither Sebelius nor DeParle could compare with him in that area. And, despite his extraordinary speaking skills, Obama never seemed to connect with the public on the benefits of his health proposal. Without Tom Daschle, enacting health reform would be a good deal more difficult.

## Billy Tauzin: The Swamp Fox Makes a Drug Deal

Barack Obama was aware of how the opposition of key interest groups had helped defeat the Clinton health plan. Hence, one of his early initiatives was to try to bring potential opponents on board. On March 5, he held a health care summit, bringing together stakeholders from across the health care sector. Then, on May 11, speaking in the State Dining Room, Obama made a dramatic announcement. Major health industry stakeholders had pledged to reduce the rate of growth in health spending by 1.5 percentage points each year from 2010 to 2019. Such a reduction would yield a savings of over two trillion dollars. Impressively, the offers had come from some of the most important former opponents of health reform including the AMA, PhRMA, AHA, and AHIP, all of which had participated in the Workhorse Group. These pledges were not solemn commitments, but rather an agreement to work with the administration toward achieving that goal. The detailed commitments would require hard bargaining. They would require substantial quid pro quos. The White House would oversee these deals from behind the scenes, but they needed a point man to conduct the negotiations. With Tom Daschle gone, Max Baucus became their man.

Aside from being chair of the all-important Senate Finance Committee, Baucus was a good personal choice. He was a moderate who worked well with Republicans and had the respect of the business community, particularly the health industry, which had given more than $2.5 million to his campaign since 2005.[4] He began by negotiating a secret deal with Billy Tauzin, the chief lobbyist for the pharmaceutical industry. Tauzin was a likeable raconteur who relished sharing Cajun stories from his home state of Louisiana. His smooth manner ingratiated him with fellow members of Congress, but his fast dealing had earned him the nickname the "Swamp Fox." He was first elected to Congress as a Democrat in 1980 and rose to become assistant majority whip. Then, in 1995, after Newt Gingrich and the Republicans took control of Congress, Tauzin switched to the Republican Party. Not, however, before he had made a deal to retain his seniority. In short order, he became deputy majority whip, and the only person ever to hold House leadership positions in both major parties. In 2003, as chair of the Energy and Commerce Committee, he was instrumental in the deal that prevented Medicare from negotiating prices with drug companies—a provision in the Medicare Prescription Drug legislation that Democrats still decry. Then, only two months after the deal was consummated, Tauzin resigned from Congress and took a two-million-dollars-per-year salary as the chief lobbyist for PhRMA.

PhRMA, which had violently opposed the Clinton health plan and given generously to Republican candidates, had practically become an enemy of the Democratic Party. But in 2006, Tauzin reversed their position, giving support to a number of Democratic candidates and changing their long-standing opposition to health care reform. Perhaps he saw opportunity where others did not. But, when the Obama administration was looking to make a deal, the Swamp Fox had laid the groundwork.

This was quite remarkable considering the president's recent campaign. Obama had run a television campaign ad called "Billy," lambasting Tauzin for help making the prescription drug deal for PhRMA and then going to work for them for two million dollars. Obama had not only promised to end that kind of politics with lobbyists, but also promised to secure the ability for

Medicare to negotiate drug prices and to allow reimportation of drugs from other countries.

Yet, this was precisely what Baucus and the administration willingly surrendered to Tauzin to get PhRMA onboard. PhRMA agreed to provide eighty billion dollars in savings over ten years by partially filling the Medicare "donut hole." They would do that by giving 50 percent discounts on prescription drugs for people who fell within the "hole." Furthermore, they promised to spend $150 million on advertisements in support of health reform. In return, the administration agreed to block any congressional effort to negotiate Medicare drug prices and to prevent any reimportation of prescription drugs. The secret agreement negotiated with Baucus was cemented at a meeting in July in the Roosevelt Room of the White House.[5] The attendees included chief executives of Abbott Laboratories, Merck, and Pfizer, as well as Tauzin, Rahm Emanuel, and other White House aides.[6]

On July 31, however, the House Energy and Commerce Committee passed its version of reform, and it included a provision to allow Medicare to negotiate prices with drug companies. Tauzin and his board were furious because they had been secretly promised otherwise. In an attempt to hold the administration to its word, Tauzin went public with the deal. He told the press the administration had said, "We need somebody to come in first. If you come in first, you will have a rock solid deal."[7] With those words, the secret deal Tauzin promised the Obama administration was no longer secret.

Needless to say, the administration was embarrassed. Jim Messina initially confirmed the deal, but after a barrage of criticism, the White House backed away from affirming the details. The Republican leadership was livid. John Boehner sent a personal letter to Tauzin sharply criticizing the deal and accusing him of "appeasing a bully."[8] Liberals lambasted Obama for welshing on his campaign promises. Nevertheless, both sides substantially kept their promises throughout the legislative battle, although the administration secured some small, additional monetary concessions from PhRMA.

Billy Tauzin's employment with PhRMA did not last as long as his deal with Obama. After Scott Brown's election, when it appeared health reform would fail, there was much criticism that he struck an unnecessary deal. A particular sore spot was PhRMA's expenditure of over one hundred million dollars advertising support of the reform plan. Whether PhRMA became dissatisfied with Tauzin over the health deal or over his well-publicized behavior and demeanor—or both—is not clear. But on February 11, apparently pressured by the PhRMA board, the Swamp Fox announced his resignation.

## On the Bus or off the Bus?
## Karen Ignagni and America's Health Insurance Plans

George Magazine called her the twenty-first most powerful person in politics.[9] The *New York Times* wrote, "In a city teeming with health care lobbyists, Ms. Ignagni is widely considered one of the most effective."[10] But the organization Health Care for America Now gave her an award for the "Best Protector of Profits at the Expense of Our Health."[11] Karen Ignagni, president and CEO of AHIP, the health insurance industry's trade and lobbying organization, has been given many different labels by friends and foes. But one thing is certain: she accomplished something no other person in her industry had ever done. She convinced America's largest health insurance companies to support comprehensive health reform, including ending insurance-underwriting practices such as exclusions for preexisting conditions, rescissions of coverage, and pricing according to health status.

The health insurance industry had been intractable foes of the Clinton health plan. During that time, the industry had no reform plan of its own and simply opposed the administration's proposals. However, Ignagni had a broader view. She had worked on health care benefits for many years, starting as an analyst for the agency that became the Health Care Financing Administration (HCFA). She became a member of the Committee for National Health Insurance, the organization founded by Walter Reuther that we discussed in chapter 3. After HCFA, Ignagni became a staffer for the Senate Labor and Human Resources Committee under Senator Claiborne Pell (D-RI). Then, she began an eleven-year stint for the AFL-CIO, directing its department of employee benefits. When she left labor to become the president of the American Association of Health Plans (AAHP), some accused her of going over to the dark side. However, from Ignagni's perspective, it was a continuation of what she had done all along—providing people with health care benefits. In 2000, AAHP merged with HIAA and became AHIP.

AAHP was an association dominated by traditional health insurance companies with strong representation from large group practice plans like

Kaiser Permanente and the Health Insurance Company of Greater New York (HIP). In fact, it was the CEO of HIP, Tony Watson, who was instrumental in recruiting Ignagni to AAHP. HIAA, on the other hand, represented many small health insurers as well as large for-profit plans. It was HIAA and its president, Chip Kahn, that was in the forefront of the campaign to defeat the Clinton plan. When the merger occurred, Ignagni was selected to become the president and CEO of the new organization.

Ahead of most of her members, Ignagni realized that the current system had severe problems and her industry often received the blame. Early on, she joined some of the Strange Bedfellows groups seeking a broad consensus on how to reform health care. Then, while George W. Bush was president, she convinced her companies and board members to begin a three-year study and "listening tour" with the goal of formulating their own comprehensive health reform proposals.

Ignagni's member companies had a wide range of insurance practices and a variety of competing interests. Nevertheless, they were able to agree on specific proposals that included universal coverage, an individual mandate, and cost containment. Although there were important differences in details, AHIP's general framework was similar to Obama's and to nearly all the other serious proposals in the past to reform the health care system: universal coverage based on employer-provided private insurance, an individual mandate with government subsidies to assist the poor, and strict limits on insurance underwriting. The biggest difference was insurance company opposition to a public option.

On March 5, 2009, Ignagni appeared with Obama following a White House forum on health care reform. "You have our commitment to play," Ignagni told the president, "to contribute and to pass health reform this year."[12] However, that historic commitment was short-lived.

Shortly after the March forum, Ignagni and AHIP entered into negotiations with Max Baucus and his Senate Finance Committee. Similar to negotiations with Billy Tauzin who promised eighty billion dollars in savings, the Democrats wanted AHIP to commit to a certain level of savings that would be counterbalanced by increased business from the newly insured. AHIP agreed to such a negotiating framework in principle, but it disagreed with the Democrats' numbers. Ignagni insisted that AHIP had already put substantial money on the table by doing away with many insurance-underwriting practices and by committing to an expensive program of administrative simplification. On top of that, the organization was willing to save the government eighty billion dollars over ten years through reduced government payments to private Medicare Advantage plans. Ignagni argued that further concessions requested by the Democrats would cause financial losses and hurt her member companies.

The two sides were unable to reach an agreement. Liz Fowler, the chief health counsel for the Senate Finance Committee, insists that Democratic demands were reasonable.[13] The Finance Committee had hired a Wall Street analyst to estimate how much the industry would benefit from newly insured customers. Fowler points out that the committee was able to strike reasonable compromises with the other industry stakeholders, but not with AHIP. "The ideas they brought," she told us, "were always 'don't cut us.'"[14] Ignagni disagrees. She told us AHIP actuaries analyzed the estimates used by the Democrats and found they were simply wrong. The Democrats, she insisted, never put forth numbers that made business sense for the industry.[15]

History may eventually reveal which side is correct. Some on the left believe that Ignagni never intended to support the Democrats' health reform effort, but she pretended to play in an effort to influence the legislation. Others believe that the administration never wanted to make a deal with the insurance industry. Instead, it needed an enemy to help rally support for reform, and it chose the unpopular insurance industry as its whipping boy. Liberal Democrats were already unhappy about the drug deal, and Fowler admits a deal with insurance companies "probably would have hurt us politically."[16] Whether it was their intention from the beginning is not known, but by the end of July, the Democrats were openly attacking the insurance industry. On July 30, Nancy Pelosi referred to the industry as "immoral villains."[17]

Without a negotiated compromise, the legislation became less favorable to AHIP. Annual fees were assessed on the insurance industry, and they kept rising because other stakeholders had made their deals and their contributions were capped. More importantly, however, was a change in a key provision. Chuck Schumer and other liberal Democrats were concerned that the individual mandate would impose a financial hardship on lower-income individuals. Olympia Snowe (R-ME), the only Republican that seemed likely to support the Senate bill, had the same concern. Schumer and Snowe cosponsored an amendment that exempted anyone from the mandate if the cost of insurance exceeded 8 percent of his or her income. Previously, the exemption had been at 10 percent. Furthermore, the amendment reduced the penalty for noncompliance with the mandate. According to the amendment there would be no penalty in the first full year of the plan (then 2013) and a $200 penalty in the second year, which would gradually increase to $750 ($1,500/family) by 2017. Previously, the penalty had been $950 ($1,900/family) beginning in the first full year of the plan. Even that was a considerable reduction from the $3,800 penalty in Baucus's original draft. With support from the liberals and Olympia Snowe, the amendment easily carried. Ignagni and AHIP were livid. As we have explained throughout the text, insurance companies cannot dispense with underwriting practices unless everyone is required to be in the pool. Otherwise, healthy people will wait until they are sick to buy insurance. The penalties were reduced so much that CBO estimated two million fewer people would buy insurance.[18]

As congressional discussions continued, Ignagni and AHIP became more disenchanted with the plan. A provision required insurance plans to spend at least 85 percent of premiums on direct medical care (the medical loss ratio) when they insured large companies and 80 percent when they insured small companies. Liberals and consumer advocates believed this was a key provision to protect consumers and reduce insurance premiums. They considered its importance second only to the public option. However, the 80 percent requirement was a high threshold for companies that ensure many small firms and have to employ large numbers of outside brokers. It was also viewed as unnecessary government intrusion into the basic operations of private companies. Although the provision was strongly opposed by Republicans and by all sectors of the insurance industry, it was retained in the final legislation.

The insurance industry was also concerned about regulation of rating bands—the extra amount plans can charge older people relative to younger people (because older people cost more). Liberals and consumer advocates inserted a provision that reduced the maximum allowed difference between rates for the young and old from six-to-one to three-to-one. This is a particularly important issue in the individual and small group market. Insurance companies argued that the narrower bands would reduce premiums for older people but raise them for the young, causing many young people to drop out of the pool.

The legislation also included very little cost control, a key issue for insurance companies because it enables them to price premiums more affordably and, hence, sell more policies. Ignagni predicted that insurance premiums would rise, subsidies would become more expensive, and a major explosion in cost would occur. The day before the Senate vote, AHIP released a study it commissioned from Pricewaterhouse Coopers claiming that insurance premiums would rise 79 to 111 percent higher over ten years than they would have without reform. Although many analysts agreed that the legislation was likely to cause some increase in premiums, the report was attacked as being deceptive and highly exaggerated.

The report sent shock waves throughout the Congress and the health care industry. Members of the Senate Finance Committee were angry at both the timing and the content of the report. Shortly after the study was released, a Pricewaterhouse Coopers spokesperson "sent out an unexpected press release backing away from the analysis and blaming AHIP for its deficiencies."[19] After the report, AHIP and the Senate Democrats stopped working with each other. Liz Fowler told us, "that was sort of a fatal blow."[20]

For the rest of the legislative battle, AHIP worked in various ways to change a number of important components of the health reform effort. Three days before the final vote, Ignagni issued a press release detailing their strong dissatisfaction with numerous provisions of the bill.[21] In addition, several national for-profit insurance companies, using AHIP as a conduit, funneled support to the US Chamber of Commerce to underwrite tens of millions of dollars of television ads attacking the legislation.[22]

It did not have to be that way, and it is still impossible to fix the blame on one side or the other. Americans distrust private health insurance companies, and the industry made an easy target. However, Karen Ignagni brought the industry to a place it had never been before. She steered her members to adopt a program very close to Obama's, and she put realistic proposals on the table. Ron Pollack, the president of the liberal advocacy group Families USA, once said this about Ignagni: "Karen wants to get a 'yes' on meaningful health care reform. For those who care about universal coverage, she's been a very strong and effective advocate."[23]

## Hospitals: A Triumvirate Makes a Deal

The hospital industry had good reasons to support comprehensive health reform and universal coverage. Subject to the Emergency Medical Treatment and Active Labor Act (EMTALA), hospitals must treat and stabilize anyone who comes through their doors, regardless of his or her ability to pay. Largely because of the nation's forty-six million uninsured, hospitals incur significant losses providing uncompensated care, a measure that includes free care plus bad debt. In 2007, before the deep recession in 2008, uncompensated care at the nation's 4,897 registered community hospitals averaged 5.8 percent of total costs.[24] One study estimated that the Senate health reform bill (the final bill without reconciliation) would reduce the country's projected uncompensated care by sixty to ninety-four billion dollars just in the year 2019.[25] Hospitals currently recover much of these losses through federal and state programs and by charging higher prices to privately insured patients. Nevertheless, the addition of thirty-two million paying customers from the ranks of the uninsured would be a significant boost to the industry's bottom line.

In addition to the uninsured, many other issues in the health reform debate were crucial to hospitals. Hence, they were involved in discussions with the Obama administration from the very beginning, and it was to their advantage to negotiate as a united front. Three of the most important hospital associations, the AHA, the Federation of American Hospitals (FAH), and the Catholic Health Association (CHA), worked closely together throughout the legislative process to lobby for their members.

### The AHA—A Plethora of Issues

Only two weeks after Obama assumed the presidency, Richard Umbdenstock, the president and CEO of the AHA, was invited to the White House for his first meeting with the new administration. Over the next five months, he would have no less than eight more White House meetings. If Barack Obama's strategy of dealing with stakeholders was going to work, he had to have Umbdenstock and the AHA on board.

And no wonder. The AHA was by far the largest hospital association with nearly five thousand hospitals nationwide. In many localities across the country hospitals were the largest employers, and their board members were often the most politically connected and influential members of the community. However, because AHA's membership was functionally and geographically diverse, it had to satisfy a wide range of constituents, some of which had competing interests.

In concert with the other two hospital associations, the AHA began negotiating with the administration in the spring of 2009. Discussions were conducted through Baucus's Finance Committee, but the important decisions were ratified at the White House. Similar to the deal with Billy Tauzin and PhRMA, hospitals were asked to contribute to the cost of the health reform plan since they would benefit from newly insured patients. Again using data from Wall Street analysts, the administration asked the hospitals to contribute $200 billion in savings to government programs over ten years. The hospitals countered with $75 to $80 billion. They eventually settled on $155 billion, a figure that was predicated on the promise that the plan would insure 94 percent of American residents and 97 percent of citizens—an increase of about thirty-six million people. Approximately $100 billion would come from future reductions in the Medicare fee schedule and about $40 billion would come from reductions in disproportional share payments (payments Medicare makes to hospitals that provide large amounts of free care).

The bargain, however, did not affect all hospitals equally. Those with limited numbers of uninsured and/or large numbers of Medicare patients could lose more than they gained from the increased numbers of insured people. In addition, the AHA had many rural hospital members who were upset about Medicare payment levels. Hospitals in low-cost, rural areas believed they were being penalized relative to high-cost, urban areas and wanted Medicare payments to be readjusted to reflect the disparity. Of course, urban hospitals opposed any readjustment that might lower their fee schedule. Many of the rural hospitals were represented by Blue Dog Democrats who, in the health reform debate, often held the balance of power within the Democratic caucus.

Along with the other two associations, the AHA was opposed to the proposed Independent Payment Advisory Board. The IPAB, as it was called, would have a fifteen-member board that would have considerable power over Medicare payment rates. In any year after 2014, if Medicare spending growth exceeded a target amount, the IPAB would make recommendations to reduce spending.

The hospitals had two problems with the IPAB proposal. First, they had already promised $155 billion in revenue reductions. That was a larger give-back than any other player in the health care industry, and they were determined to keep that as an upper limit. If the IPAB was to reduce health spending, it had few choices aside from lowering Medicare payments to hospitals and doctors. Lower payments meant revenue reductions for hospitals beyond the negotiated limit.

The second problem was the nature of the IPAB's recommendations:

they were not merely recommendations. They would automatically become law unless Congress passed an alternative with at least the same amount of savings. The hospitals, as well as many moderate and conservative members of Congress, were wary of creating a commission with so much power that would be accountable to no one except the president who appointed them. Congress had the responsibility to set Medicare rates, and members did not want to relinquish that power. Likewise, the hospital lobby did not want to cede the lobbying power over the issue that they had with members of Congress.

The public option was another important issue. Hospitals feared that a powerful public option would enable the government to set payment rates rather than having rates determined through a competitive market. Already having to accept rates that were below their costs for Medicaid and Medicare patients, hospitals did not want to risk further potential losses from a public option.

Yet another issue was the strength of the individual mandate. A mandate with strong penalties and few exemptions would help ensure that the goal of insuring thirty-six million additional people would be achieved. However, if the mandate was weakened, fewer people would purchase insurance and hospitals would not receive the additional business for which they traded $155 billion in future revenue.

Numerous issues of a more technical nature were important to the industry, and with so many matters unresolved, the AHA could not provide an early endorsement of health reform. While PhRMA and the AMA announced their support early, the AHA withheld approval until the fall of 2010, continuing to negotiate on behalf of its members. The other two members of the triumvirate, with far fewer players and a more homogenous membership, were less constrained.

## Former Opponents Become Supporters: A Chip off the Old Bloc

Chip Kahn, a life-long Republican, was the man who engineered the Harry and Louise ads that helped kill the Clinton health plan. On March 5, 2009, as president of the FAH, Kahn was on the other side. "From my standpoint," he told *Newsweek*, "we're all on this train together, and I expect to ride it all the way into a signing ceremony."[26]

Chip Kahn began his political career in the '70s when he managed Newt

Gingrich's first two campaigns for Congress. Since that time he has become one of the most highly respected health experts in the country, having served on Capitol Hill as Health Subcommittee staff director and as minority health counsel for the House Ways and Means Committee. During the Clinton health reform battle, Kahn was the executive vice president of the HIAA. The Clinton health plan would have been detrimental to HIAA member companies, and Kahn became, perhaps, its most effective opponent. Yet, paradoxically, he has always been open to reform. "On the one hand, I felt the country missed [dodged] a bullet (by defeating the Clinton proposals)," he told *Newsweek*. "On the other hand, I thought there were compromises that could have been wrought that would have been really helpful to people."[27] Since the Clinton plan, Kahn participated in several bipartisan efforts to find common ground on health reform. Even when he was still president of HIAA in 2001, he had joined one of Ron Pollack's first Strange Bedfellows groups and published a joint proposal for comprehensive reform.

In 2001, Kahn switched from the insurance to the hospital industry, becoming president of the FAH, the trade association representing for-profit hospitals. FAH had been a staunch opponent of the Clinton health plan. This time, it was different. The federation's board, although conservative in nature, understood the business sense of universal coverage and health care reform, and it encouraged Kahn (who was already like-minded) to produce a proposal for comprehensive reform.[28] The basic structure of Kahn's proposal was similar to Obama's, except it had less regulation, no tax financing, and no public option.

The FAH, with a much smaller and less diverse membership, did not have the internal conflicts of the AHA. As a result, it was easier for Kahn to work with his board, and he could be more nimble in making decisions. Their positions on most of the important issues were similar. However, the difference in rural and urban Medicare payments, a major sticking point for the AHA, was not as important to the federation. The federation's more unified position on the issues enabled Kahn to be a strong force in the negotiations.

On the one hand, Kahn must have been pleased that the basic framework to achieve universal coverage in the final legislation closely resembled the plan he crafted for the federation's board several years before. On the other hand, as a lifetime Republican, he would have preferred a different bill. A plan with fewer taxes, fewer regulations, and fewer mandates on small employers would have been more consistent with his philosophy. Under

Kahn's leadership, the FAH achieved most of its negotiating objectives, but in supporting the Democratic initiative, Chip Kahn may have lost a few Republican friends.

## One Courageous Nun

She may only represent 642 hospitals compared to Richard Umbdenstock's five thousand, but Sister Carol Keehan had fifteen meetings on health reform at the Obama White House, including seven with the president himself. Sister Carol is the president and CEO of the CHA. In 2007, the trade publication *Modern Healthcare* voted her the number one most powerful person in health care.[29] Both the president and the magazine's editors were prescient. An early and ardent supporter of the Obama health reform effort, Sister Carol played a crucial role in its passage. Robert Casey, the pro-life Democratic senator from Pennsylvania, stated, "I can say without any hesitation that if the CHA were not involved in this effort, it's highly likely we wouldn't be able to pass the bill."[30]

The CHA worked closely with the AHA and the FAH to negotiate an agreement with the administration. For the most part, the three organizations had similar positions on the issues, although the CHA did not oppose the public option. Like the FAH, the CHA was smaller and its member hospitals were much more homogenous than those in the AHA. With fewer differences, it was easier for its members to establish a unified position of support for health reform. However, the CHA had to confront an additional problem. The legislative language regarding abortion erupted into a difficult controversy within the Catholic hierarchy.

Historically, the Catholic Church had always been a strong supporter of universal health care as part of its charitable mission to care for the poor and disadvantaged. However, the US Conference of Catholic Bishops opposed the Senate version of the health reform bill because of its language regarding abortion. Sister Carol and the bishops did not differ on moral questions. Neither would have supported any legislation that allowed federal funds to be used for abortion. However, Sister Carol and the CHA concluded that the law forbade such funding. The bishops disagreed.

As we explain in a later chapter, differences over abortion nearly caused the defeat of health reform. The bishops lobbied feverishly against the language in the Senate bill. They instructed every Catholic Church throughout the country to urge its parishioners to oppose the legislation.[31] In the face of such unbending opposition from the highest Catholic authority in the country, it was no small matter for Sister Carol and the nuns to support the other side. Sister Carol was resolute. As a sister of charity, she believed the legislation would help millions of the poor and uninsured.

Shortly before the legislation was passed, Sister Carol met with Francis Cardinal George, the president of the US Conference of Catholic Bishops, in an attempt to reach a mutual accord on the divisive issue. They discussed a possible agreement on a position paper she had drafted for the meeting. However, after she left, the cardinal never responded to her repeated efforts to contact him in regard to the agreement, and she subsequently announced her support of the health reform legislation.[32]

The nun's assurances about the abortion language gave both comfort and cover to many members of Congress who were sincerely torn by the issue, and the ensuing compromise paved the way for final passage of the bill. Chip Kahn told us, "I would say that there is only one profile in courage in all of health reform—it is Sister Carol."[33]

As of this writing, the bishops and Sister Carol have not reconciled their differences. On June 17, 2010, Cardinal George blamed "Sister Carol and her colleagues" for what he called the "proabortion" legislation. Nevertheless, *La Civilta Cattolica*, a Rome-based Catholic journal that undergoes prepublication review by the Vatican secretary of state, had a different view. It praised the health care legislation, stating that it marked "a needed and long-awaited beginning . . . to introduce measures that aim for greater justice for all citizens and, in particular, for the most vulnerable."[34]

## The Hospitals Make a Deal

By banding together, the three hospital associations achieved many of their goals. A number of Medicare payment adjustments were specified that would benefit rural hospitals, and the secretary of HHS was required to analyze new methods to account for geographical differences in payments.

The individual mandate became weaker as the Democrats tried to hold their caucus together. The estimated number of newly insured dropped from 97 to 94 percent of residents. Chip Kahn had lambasted the administration for not fulfilling the terms of their negotiation. On October 1, he told the press, "They have not yet met the standard of our deal."[35] The hospitals were able to restore some of the strength of the mandate in the final bill, albeit not as much as they would have liked.

The public option was discarded. Although it was a priority in negotiations, the administration never promised to make that concession to the hospitals. However, the hospitals had correctly anticipated that there would not be enough support in the Senate to retain the controversial policy.

In a significant victory for the hospitals, they won a ten-year exemption from any cuts prescribed by the IPAB. Karen Ignagni, already unhappy about the lack of cost control, was furious. The hospitals were the largest cost center, representing about one third of health care spending. Exempting them from the IPAB, she told us, would undermine its effectiveness to reduce costs.[36] Michael Maves, the new president of the AMA, called the exemption a serious inequity. But the hospitals insisted that they would not go beyond their $155 billion cap, and they were largely successful in preserving that limit.

Two powerful lobbies, the pharmaceutical industry and the hospitals, had come over to the other side. Now it was the turn of the most powerful and long-standing opponent of reform—the AMA.

## The AMA Changes Sides

For twenty-six years, no president of the United States had addressed the AMA. Yet, with nearly 250,000 members, it was the most powerful lobby in health care. It had opposed Medicare and every attempt at universal coverage including proposals by Harry Truman, Richard Nixon, John Kennedy, Lyndon Johnson, and Bill Clinton. In the first half of 2009, it had already spent $8.1 million lobbying to influence the health reform debate. It was, indeed, a force to be reckoned with, and Barack Obama needed its support.

On June 15, 2009, the president returned to his native Chicago to address the AMA's House of Delegates. This time around, the doctors' organization appeared more open to comprehensive reform. The AMA had participated in the Health Reform Dialogue Group and in Ted Kennedy's Workhorse Group. However, it would not be an easy audience for the president. Differences on a number of outstanding issues were impediments to the organization's support. By far the most important issue was the Medicare sustainable growth rate formula (SGR). Every year since 2000, the formula had dictated a reduction in Medicare fees paid to doctors, and every year Congress had postponed part or all of the reduction. By the time Obama addressed the AMA, the cumulative backlog required a reduction in the fee schedule of 21 percent—a totally undoable number. Already, in 2009, Medicare paid doctors 20 percent less than it paid private insurance companies, and it paid hospitals, on average, only 94 percent of their costs.[37] Further cuts could reduce access to care for seniors as well as earn the enmity of the powerful lobby. The AMA wanted the SGR repealed, and the Democrats were sympathetic. However, repeal would add over $200 billion to the health care proposal and make budget neutrality nearly impossible.

The SGR was not the only issue that stood between the AMA and the Democratic proposals. Malpractice reform had been at the top of the doctors' agenda for many years, and the Republican Party's support of tort reform had won them favor from the AMA. In contrast, the Democrats generally opposed capping damage awards to individuals, a view that was in concert with the Trial Lawyers Association, a key Democratic support group.

The public option was also an issue. Similar to hospitals, doctors believed a powerful public option could fix prices at rates resembling those of Medicare and Medicaid. They had similar concerns about the proposed IPAB, which allowed an administrative board to reduce government payments if the rate of health expenditures increased above a target amount.

The AMA delegates expressed appreciation for Obama's appearance, but they did not receive the commitments they wanted, and their reactions were mixed. The president told them he would postpone the current year's scheduled fee reduction of 21 percent, but he did not promise repeal. Of course, that is what every administration had done for years, since the cost of a one-year delay paled in comparison to total repeal. He promised to "curb" malpractice lawsuits, but told them he would not support capping damage awards. He also affirmed his support for the public option, telling the delegates that the "public option was their friend."[38]

James Rohack became the president of AMA shortly after Obama's speech. Logs indicate he visited the White House numerous times during the debate, but Rohack and the AMA were unable to get the concessions they wanted. Nevertheless, they delivered important support. On November 5, the AMA provided a crucial endorsement for the Affordable Health Care for America Act, the final House bill that narrowly passed on November 7. It gave its support despite the fact that the House bill included a public option and did not repeal the SGR. The House leadership had promised to pass a separate bill repealing the SGR—which it did, but the repeal bill never passed the Senate.

As the House was considering its reform bill, the AMA was also lobbying the Senate. After Max Baucus issued his markup of the Senate bill, the AMA sent a letter with a positive tone but withheld its endorsement. Again, it was concerned about the SGR and IPAB, as well as other issues.

Senate Democrats needed the AMA endorsement but did not have the leeway to budge on several important issues. Finally, late in September, Harry Reid called for a meeting with the AMA and other prominent physician groups. Reid promised to call up separate legislation to repeal the SGR, even though it would cost over $200 billion. He also promised to increase the doctors' fee schedule by .5 percent in 2010. In return, the doctors were told that the administration "needed and expected their support."[39] Attending the beginning of the meeting were White House Chief of Staff Rahm Emanuel and OMB Director Peter Orszag—a signal that the White House was backing the deal.[40]

Although the AMA did not get much of what it wanted, it had no place to go. Shortly before Christmas, when it appeared likely that reform would pass the Senate, the AMA finally delivered its endorsement of the Senate bill. It was clear that the SGR would not be repealed without Democratic support, so the organization had little choice but to offer its support and rely on Democratic promises. Its endorsement made it clear that it expected a repeal bill as well as several other matters to be worked out in the House–Senate conference.

Of course, it turned out that there was no conference. In the end, some items on its list were granted. Primary care and general surgeons were given a fee hike that was not counterbalanced by other fee reductions. An annual doctors' Medicare fee was eliminated, as was a tax on cosmetic surgery. And the public option was no longer part of the reform legislation. However, the freeze on the SGR reduction was only extended for two months. A weakened Democratic Party with a huge budget deficit was going to be hard-pressed to enact repeal. Malpractice reform was absent, and potential payment reductions from the IPAB were still a serious concern. The AMA had won nearly every battle it undertook during all the years it opposed reform. Now that it changed sides, the outcome of this battle was very much in doubt.

# CHAPTER 13

# BAUCUS, GRASSLEY, AND THE GANG OF SIX

T hey were their party's ranking members on the Senate Finance Committee and had alternated as chair for the past nine years, depending on whose party had the majority. Unlike others in these times of political division, Max Baucus and Chuck Grassley had worked closely together, attempting to forge bipartisan agreements. In fact, since 2001 they had met every Tuesday at 5:00 p.m. in Baucus's conference room. The best chance for a bipartisan health reform bill resided in the ability of these two men to come to terms.

The president, learning from Bill Clinton's mistakes, had outlined his general framework for health reform and had purposely deferred to Congress to work out the details. Tom Daschle was no longer an official player after withdrawing his nomination as secretary of HHS. Ted Kennedy was too ill to lead the Senate maneuverings. And Harry Reid, the Senate majority leader, was a strong believer in delegating power to his committee chairs. Hence, the power and responsibility devolved to Max Baucus, who insisted he could work with Chuck Grassley to produce a bipartisan bill.

Health reform had so many issues and complexities that the committee needed an efficient vehicle to address all the moving parts. Baucus and Grassley created the "gang of six" to undertake the task. Beginning on June 17, six Senators, three from each party, often met twice a day in Baucus's office, attending a morning session from 10:00 a.m. until noon, breaking for lunch, and assembling again at 2:30 p.m.

Each of the six players brought his or her own issues and attitudes to the bargaining table.[1] On the Democratic side, Baucus represented the center. He was a probusiness moderate and cared more about reaching a bipartisan agreement than insisting on almost any detail of the bill. Kent Conrad, a moderate from North Dakota, was chair of the Senate Budget Committee and known as a deficit hawk. Conrad was concerned about spending and was an opponent of the public option. It was Conrad who proposed nonprofit, member-owned cooperatives as a compromise alternative. Jeff Bingaman from New Mexico was the most liberal member of the gang. He supported the public option but let it be known he was open to compromise. Considering the left-leaning mainstream of the Democratic Party, the three constituted quite a moderate group.

Chuck Grassley was the most important member on the Republican side. From the very beginning, Grassley insisted that he favored reform, but only if the bill was bipartisan. He made it clear he would not go it alone, but would need at least three or four other Republicans on board. Grassley strongly opposed a public option and an employer mandate. He wanted to ensure there would be no rationing or other interference with the doctor–patient relationship. He also favored malpractice reform.

Olympia Snowe was a moderate from Maine who often broke with the Republican Party on social policy issues. She had been one of three Republicans who voted for Obama's stimulus package, earning her the disparaging label of "RINO"—Republican In Name Only. Snowe was considered the most likely Republican to support health reform. She opposed the public option, but had suggested a "trigger" whereby a public option would be instituted if the rate of cost growth exceeded a specified target. Snowe was concerned about affordability for people who were mandated to purchase insurance, and she favored cost control initiatives.

The final member of the gang was Mike Enzi, a conservative from Wyoming. Enzi was a curious choice because it was not clear if he actually supported comprehensive reform. He had voted against the health bill that was passed by Kennedy's Health, Education, Labor, and Pensions Committee. Enzi insisted that any bill had to have seventy-five to eighty votes, a seemingly unattainable goal. He opposed any tax increases or reduction in Medicare spending to pay for the bill. He was also strongly opposed to the public option.

Despite the differences about individual items, the group seemed to agree on the general framework of reform. Baucus felt that if the gang of six could reach a compromise, his committee could report out a bipartisan bill. Attempting to find common ground on the outstanding issues, the group began working on three papers that would yield multiple policy options in the areas of cost, coverage, and financing. With that strategy, Baucus embarked on a negotiating process that he hoped would yield a consensus before the August recess.

It was not to be. Republican senators came under intense pressure from their leadership not to reach any compromise with Democrats. Mitch McConnell's strategy seemed to mimic that of Newt Gingrich fifteen years before: to deny the Democrats a victory from enacting health reform regardless of the content of the legislation. Chuck Grassley would not stand alone against his party's leadership. He would need the support of several Republicans and would not go forward if he only had the support of Olympia Snowe. As Baucus offered a compromise in one area the ground kept shifting, and he could not tie up an agreement. On July 13, at a White House meeting with Obama, Reid, and Pelosi, he was pressured to report out a bill, but he stuck to his strategy, still striving for bipartisanship. On August 6, the president met with all six participants, but there would be no agreement before the summer recess.

Max Baucus ran out of time. In the first week of September, just after returning from the August recess, he announced a draft of his plan and said he would push it through the committee even if there was no bipartisan support. A determined Max Baucus, an intense man who had once completed a fifty-mile ultramarathon, still held out hope for an agreement. He released his plan on September 9, but called it a draft for discussion rather than the traditional "chairman's mark."

To the chagrin of liberals, he had removed the public option. Instead, he inserted Kent Conrad's proposal for member-controlled, nonprofit, state-run cooperatives. He had avoided an employer mandate. Instead, he assessed firms with over fifty employees a charge equivalent to any subsidies the government would have to pay to the firm's workers who bought their own insurance (limited to a maximum of four hundred dollars per worker). He had avoided any income or payroll tax increase. Instead, he assessed a "Cadillac tax" on expensive health plans.

During the following two weeks, he listened to the recommendations and criticisms of his committee members. Hoping to draw support, he added a number of amendments to his original proposals. The major changes related to affordability, a chief concern of Olympia Snowe. Subsidies were increased for lower-income people and penalties for not complying with the mandate were reduced. He also satisfied the president's two requirements: total spending for the bill was less than $900 billion, and it did not add to the deficit.

Baucus introduced his chairman's mark on September 22 and held a full committee vote on October 13. The bill passed the committee 14–9, capturing only one Republican vote—that of Olympia Snowe. Even the moderate Snowe made it clear that she might not support the bill when it came before the full Senate. Opposition came from both liberals and conservatives. Howard Dean said, "The Baucus bill is the worst piece of health care legislation I've seen in thirty years."[2] Kevin Brady (R-TX), delivering the Republican's weekly radio address, stated, "The massive health care plans being crafted behind closed doors in Washington will ultimately allow the government to decide what doctors we can see, what treatments the government thinks you deserve, and what medicines you can receive."[3]

The Baucus bill was too far to the right for liberals and too far to the left for conservatives. Democrats castigated Baucus for wasting so much time. Republicans skewered him for rushing the proposal to Congress before a full discussion. Despite the derision, however, the Baucus bill would turn out to be very close to what eventually became law. And, in September of 2009, Max Baucus had little room for maneuver—not after the "Summer of Death Panels."

# CHAPTER 14

# THE SUMMER OF DEATH PANELS

## An Angry Public

On August 6, 2009, fifteen hundred people tried to jam themselves in to a town hall meeting on health reform in Tampa, Florida.[1] Angry protestors who could not fit in the room banged on doors and knocked on windows of the Hillsborough County Children's Board building. A near riot erupted as protestors yelling "tyranny, tyranny" and "forty million illegals" drowned out the speakers. US Representative Kathy Castor (D-FL) had to be escorted out of the hall by local police.

Elsewhere throughout the country, protestors furious about health care reform confronted members of Congress attending traditional town hall meetings during the annual August recess. In Lebanon, Pennsylvania, over one thousand people showed up at a town hall meeting with 250 seats to protest Arlen Specter's support of health reform. Protests occurred in Missouri, Michigan, Colorado, Maryland, North Carolina, New York, and many other areas of the country. Signs with swastikas comparing Obama to Hitler were not uncommon, as were claims of socialism, death panels, and euthanasia. No one had expected the level of passion and vitriol that members of Congress encountered.

An undercurrent of anger had been brewing in the country for some time. The unemployment rate was hovering close to 10 percent, millions of Americans were losing their homes to foreclosures, and many had cancelled or postponed their hopes of retirement after the stock market plunge decimated their savings. People were mad! In the face of the banking crisis and a possible depression, the president had tried to avert disaster by continuing the bank bailouts initiated by President Bush, enacting an $800 billion economic "stimulus package," and bailing out two of the three major US auto-mobile manufacturers. The economy began to recover, but at a meager pace. Few people felt better, and Americans found little satisfaction in the fact that things could have been worse. Meanwhile, the administration's actions had been hugely expensive, adding to the budget deficit, and seemingly injecting government into all aspects of the economy.

Health reform could hardly have come at a worse time. The Democrats' program would cost close to a trillion dollars over ten years, and nearly half of that would be raised by increasing taxes and fees. It was another big gov-ernment program, and who felt they had the money to pay for it? Moreover, parts of the program were decidedly unpopular. Seniors worried about cuts in future Medicare payments. Small business worried about an employer mandate. Individuals disliked the idea of government forcing them to buy insurance, and some worried they would not be able to afford the premiums.

Although there were many legitimate issues, most of the debate did not focus on substance. Many honest differences were obscured by misinforma-tion and misunderstanding, and some by outright lies. By the end of the summer recess, the negative publicity had taken its toll, and public support for the Democrat's health reform effort began a steady decline.

## The Truth, the Part Truth, and Nothing Like the Truth

Some of the protests against the health reform proposals focused on true problems. The program was expensive, taxes would be raised, insurance pre-miums were likely to rise, government would play a larger role, individuals would be required to buy insurance coverage, and people who already had insurance would have to pay more money on behalf of people who were uninsured. Tea Party members were particularly focused on the amount of spending and the additional intrusion by the federal government.

Some of the claims had a kernel of truth but were clearly exaggerated. It was not accurate to call any of the congressional proposals a government takeover of health care. True, the government role would increase. There was fairly heavy-handed regulation of insurance, more people would be enrolled in Medicaid, and the state-run exchanges would have to conform to federal guidelines. Individuals would be required to purchase, and most employers would be required to offer, insurance or else pay a fine. But it hardly resembled an actual government-run system. It was based on the existing private insurance market in which most people received private insurance benefits from private employers. Hospitals and other care institutions were private, not owned by the government. Doctors were private, not employed by the government. Drugs, pharmacies, device manufacturers, nurses, home-health aides, and the like, all were private. Prices, except in the case of Medicare and Medicaid, were determined in the market. Except for insurance reforms such as the ban on preexisting conditions and lifetime benefit caps, the majority of Americans would feel little effect from reform.

It was an exaggeration to imply that most people would have to change their insurances. A small number of people who worked for small firms and had employer-provided insurance might have to purchase their insurance from the exchanges instead. Some seniors enrolled in Medicare Advantage plans would have to change back to traditional Medicare. Notwithstanding, the great majority of insured Americans would simply keep the insurances they had.

It was also an exaggeration that seniors would lose Medicare benefits because of future cuts in payments. Future payments to doctors would still increase, but at a slower rate. There were no provisions to cut benefits and no evidence that slowing the increase in payments would cause any significant reduction in access to doctors' services. The one exception was the Medicare Advantage program in which some seniors would lose extra services (only services beyond those provided by traditional Medicare). Although the number of Medicare beneficiaries enrolled in Medicare Advantage plans had grown to twelve million (about 25 percent of the Medicare population), it was difficult to argue that the government should keep paying private insurance plans 15 percent more on average for the exact same services provided by traditional Medicare.

Some claims were simply untrue. This was not socialized medicine. Undocumented immigrants would not receive any government subsidies or benefits under the plan. In fact, the protests about immigrants receiving benefits were so strong that the final legislation forbade illegal immigrants from purchasing health insurance on the state exchanges even if they paid entirely with their own money. This was unfortunate, since hospitals would have to provide uncompensated care to some who might have otherwise purchased insurance, and taxpayers and privately insured individuals would have to foot that bill. Of all the false claims made by opponents of reform, the one that reverberated the loudest was the existence of death panels.

## Death Panels

"My parents or my baby with Down Syndrome will have to stand in front of Obama's 'death panel' so his bureaucrats can decide, based on a subjective judgment of their 'level of productivity in society,' whether they are worthy of health care." Those were the exact words of Sarah Palin, posted on her Facebook page on August 7, 2009.

They were not true. Although they have no basis in fact, the persistent claims of death panels can be traced to two particular legislative policies: Medicare payments to doctors for end-of-life counseling and CER.

### Reimbursing Doctors for Voluntary End-of-Life Counseling

The major source of worry about death panels related to end-of-life counseling. The Medicare fee schedule did not always pay doctors for the time they devoted to provide end-of-life counseling voluntarily requested by their patients.

The capabilities of modern medicine have greatly expanded treatment options and have enabled doctors to sustain peoples' lives even if their qualities of life are poor. Some people may wish to utilize every possible life-sustaining treatment until the moment they die. Others do not want to die in an ICU with tubes and monitors permeating their bodies and would prefer palliative or hospice care and dying at home in the presence of their loved ones. Modern medicine provides many treatment options, but few people have the clinical knowledge to understand all of those options or their implications.

In April of 2009, a bipartisan bill was introduced that would allow Medicare to pay doctors if patients voluntarily requested advice about end-of-life choices and if doctors devoted time providing such counseling. The bill was introduced by Earl Blumenauer (D-OR) and cosponsored by Charles Boustany (R-LA), Patrick Tiberi (R-OH), and Geoff David (R-KY).[2] Provisions of the bill were later included in one of the House bills (HR 3200) and were debated in the Senate.

The head of Gundersen Lutheran Health system, the largest hospital system in Wisconsin, came to Washington to testify. He explained how Gunderson had developed a successful counseling program to ensure that patients received end-of-life care that was humane and consistent with their wishes and beliefs. Despite support from such middle-American institutions and Republican cosponsors, opposition to the policy by conservatives and Tea Party members was virulent. In town hall meetings all over the country, members of Congress were confronted with angry claims of government death panels. The protests did not simply emanate from the grass roots. Aside from Sarah Palin, protesters were encouraged by Republican Party leaders. Chuck Grassley stated, "We should not have a government-run program that determines if you're going to pull the plug on grandma."[3] John Boehner said the legislation would "start us down the path to government-encouraged euthanasia."[4]

Such statements by Republican leaders were startling because the need for such legislation had been recognized by both political parties for some time. In 2003, the MMA provided coverage for terminally ill patients considering hospice care. Doctors affiliated with hospices would be paid for "counseling the beneficiary with respect to end-of-life issues and care options, and advising the beneficiary regarding advanced care planning." The only significant difference in the 2003 bill is that it applied only to terminally ill patients considering hospice care. In the 2009 proposals, patients could request such information before they were considered terminally ill; 204 Republican House members and 42 Republican Senators voted for the 2003 bill. Among those who voted in favor were Grassley and Boehner.

Rather than embroil reform legislation in controversy, Democrats removed the provisions from both the House and Senate bills. It was clear, however, that the issue had been demagogued. It also became painfully clear after his comments that Chuck Grassley had decided not to support health reform.

### Comparative Effectiveness Research

A second source of concern about death panels was associated with funding for CER. The Institute of Medicine defines CER as follows:

> CER is the generation and synthesis of evidence that compares the benefits and harms of alternative methods to prevent, diagnose, treat, and monitor a clinical condition, or to improve the delivery of care. The purpose of CER is to assist consumers, clinicians, purchasers, and policy makers to make informed decisions that will improve health care at both the individual and population levels.[5]

With the proliferation of new pharmaceuticals and the ever-increasing number of new technologies and methods to treat illnesses, doctors, patients, and others could benefit from independent studies that compare different treatment regimens and indicate which constitute best practices. CER might compare one drug to another or indicate whether an illness is best treated by surgery or medication.

Why would people get upset about such research? There are several possible sources of concern, but none of them comport with what was actually contained in the legislation. The major concern was that CER would prevent people from getting certain treatments because the research indicated it was too expensive or the likely outcome did not justify the cost. This was the source of the erroneous claims that death panels would decide the cost to treat grandma was not worth the benefit. However, the actual legislation explicitly barred any consideration of cost. The purpose was simply to identify the best treatment.

A second concern was that patients' choices would be reduced because the research would recommend one drug or procedure and doctors might not provide, or insurers might not cover, other alternatives. Arguably, it might be a good policy to recommend or cover only the best treatment, but those kinds of restrictions were forbidden in the legislation. The final bill stated that the research findings "could not be construed as mandates for practice guidelines, coverage recommendations, payment, or policy recommendations."[6] The legislation also specifically acknowledged that research should focus on both the population and individual levels because different treatments sometimes work better for different people.

A third concern was that government would intrude on the doctor–patient relationship and bureaucrats would make decisions instead of physicians. However, the legislation created a nongovernment entity to conduct the research called the Patient-Centered Outcomes Research Institute (PCORI). The members would include representatives from consumers, patients, hospitals, industry, nurses, payers, physicians, researchers, surgeons, and the leaders of the National Institutes of Health and the Agency for Healthcare Research and Quality.[7] The institute would be funded by a tax on insurance companies (approximately two dollars per insured) and would receive approximately $500 million per year by the year 2015.

Fears that CER would lead to death panels and rationing did not simply emerge from individuals. Some drug and device manufacturers opposed the policy. When a $1.1 billion appropriation for CER was included in the Obama administration's stimulus bill, these companies hired the well-known public relations and lobbying firm Barbour, Griffith, and Rogers to portray the policy as the first step toward rationing.[8] The drug and device companies worried that if CER determined that their products were not the most effective, purchasers would not buy them and insurers would not cover them. Manufacturers market many "me too" drugs that are similar to others on the market but possibly could be rated less effective. These companies also feared that once CER was instituted, the next step would be cost effectiveness analysis. As previously mentioned, however, consideration of cost was prohibited under the legislation. There was simply nothing in the CER legislation that could be associated with death panels.

# CHAPTER 15

# THE SPEAKER CARRIES THE DAY

## The Path Through the Forest

I ronically, as the mood of the country turned against health care reform, Congress moved closer than ever before to passing a bill. After the summer protests and the October vote in Senate Finance, all five congressional committees, three in the House and two in the Senate, had passed comprehensive health reform bills. The path through the forest now seemed clearer. Speaker Pelosi would combine the three House bills into one and vote in early November. Following that, Majority Leader Reid would combine the two Senate bills, which he could successfully pass with his sixty-vote super majority. Then, a Democrat-controlled conference committee would iron out the differences and bring the bill to the floor of each house for a final vote. If all went smoothly, Barack Obama could sign the historic legislation before Christmas.

To Nancy Pelosi, the path did not appear quite so easy. The Democrats controlled the House by a margin of 258–177. Regardless of the content of the legislation, she did not expect to get one Republican vote. Hence, she could afford to lose up to forty members of her own caucus and still squeak by 218–217. The problem was that her caucus was ideologically and geographically diverse. She had single-payer liberals and Blue Dog conservatives, members who were pro-life and pro-choice, those who were prolabor and those who were probusiness. She had members from highly paid Medicare states and those from states where payments were much lower. Somehow, she had to find enough middle ground to hold 218 of them together.

## The Issues

The public option was the issue that was most prominent in the public spotlight. Although Max Baucus had removed it from his Senate bill, all three House committees supported the policy. Pelosi had gone on record insisting that the final House bill would have a public option. Furthermore, many liberals who hated insurance companies, and would have preferred to do away with them in a single-payer system, threatened to oppose any bill without a public option.

Unfortunately, for Pelosi, there were fifty-four members of the Blue Dog Coalition, and many had issues with the public option. For one thing, the conservative Blue Dogs were probusiness and anti–big government. Therefore, they were philosophically opposed to a powerful government-run public option. More specifically, many of the Blue Dogs were from rural areas where Medicare payment rates were relatively low. Hence, they strongly opposed any public option that tied payment rates to Medicare.

The Speaker's bill contained a compromise position. The bill would have a public option, but payment rates would be negotiated rather than pegged to Medicare rates. The CBO estimated that under such a policy, the public option would cost more than private plans and would enroll only six million people. Most liberals reluctantly accepted the compromise, likely figuring that once a public option was instituted it could later be expanded.

Differences in Medicare payments between high-cost and low-cost states divided the Democratic caucus. This was a long-standing problem that we previously discussed in relation to Medicare Advantage plans. Although press reports paid scant attention to the issue, it proved difficult to resolve. Part of the reason was its zero-sum nature. If rural areas were to be paid relatively more, then urban areas would receive relatively less. The Speaker's bill required the Institute of Medicine to study the problem and propose new payment methodologies. However, when the House later had to accept the Senate bill, no such provision was included. Low-cost states did get some favorable adjustments in the final bill.

Financing was also a divisive issue. The Senate Finance bill employed a tax on "Cadillac insurance plans" to finance a significant portion of its bill. However, labor unions strongly opposed the policy because, in many cases, they had bargained away wages to secure those benefits. Liberals also complained that the tax would impact many people who worked in government or high-risk industries that had expensive health policies but low or moderate wage levels. Instead of a Cadillac tax, Pelosi included a "millionaires tax"; a 5.4 percent tax surcharge on individuals earning over $500,000 or families earning over one million.

Liberals and conservatives also differed over the employer mandate. The Senate Finance Committee had technically avoided a mandate by not requiring employers to provide coverage but charging them if their employees received government subsidies to purchase insurance. The more liberal house members insisted on a mandate in which all but small employers would pay 8 percent of payroll if they did not comply. Conservatives argued that such a charge would hurt small business. Pelosi's compromise was to exempt all firms with a payroll less than $500,000, a figure that was twice as high as the original threshold. As a result, 86 percent of small firms would be exempt from the mandate.

The more liberal House members agreed on a number of provisions that differed from the bill that would be passed by Senate Finance. They expanded Medicaid eligibility to 150 percent of poverty (it was effectively 138 percent in Finance). They reduced the penalty on individuals for not complying with the mandate, and they lowered the maximum percent of earnings people would be required to pay for coverage (thus exempting people from the mandate who had to pay more than the threshold percentage). Subsidy payments were also increased. Those provisions made insurance more affordable for low- and middle-income people, but angered providers and insurance companies that sought a robust individual mandate. The House also provided for a national exchange as opposed to the fifty separate state exchanges specified in the Senate bill.

Nancy Pelosi had scheduled a vote by the full House on Saturday, November 7. She had cobbled together a set of policies and compromises that could have been sufficient to hold enough of her diverse caucus together to pass a bill. Except it wasn't. One outstanding issue still threatened to kill the legislation: abortion!

## Abortion Politics: A Bitter Pill for the Speaker

Nancy Pelosi was a pro-choice Catholic who had hoped to avoid the abortion controversy. Liberal members of her caucus were ardent supporters of abortion rights. However, a block of about forty pro-life Democrats threatened to oppose the bill unless there was a further compromise on abortion. On Monday morning, five days before the vote in the House, Pelosi still lacked a majority unless she could get both sides of the abortion issue to compromise.

Abortion became legal in the United States in 1973, when the Supreme Court handed down a 7–2 decision in the famous case of *Roe v. Wade*. Since that time, the courts have narrowed abortion rights but have never overturned the decision. In 1976, Congress passed the Hyde Amendment, named after Congressman Henry Hyde (R-IL). The Hyde Amendment is actually a rider that has been attached to annual appropriation bills every year since 1976. It forbids the use of most federal funds to pay for abortions (except in cases of rape, incest, or danger to the life of the mother). Although its scope has varied over the years, it has always applied to annual appropriations for the DHHS, which include all federal funding for Medicaid. It has also been applied to Native Americans, federal employees and their dependents, military personnel and their dependents, Peace Corps volunteers, federal prisoners, disabled women receiving Medicare, and young women in the Children's Health Insurance Program.[1]

Barack Obama and the Democratic leadership had hoped to avoid any controversy about abortion by producing a health plan that complied with the intent of the Hyde Amendment and did not change the legal status quo. The Senate Finance Committee had agreed on a compromise whereby individuals who received subsidies from the federal government would be required to pay with personal funds for any part of an insurance policy that covered abortion. The payment for abortion coverage would be remitted separately and remain distinct from other premium payments. Even if payments were due monthly, a separate check or other form of payment would have to be remitted each month to cover insurance for abortion services.

However, that compromise did not satisfy pro-life members of the House of Representatives nor the US Conference of Catholic Bishops. Their problem focused on subsidized plans that provided abortions including those plans in the new insurance exchanges. Low-income individuals enrolled in those plans would receive federal subsidies to help purchase health insurance. If such health insurance policies included coverage for abortion, opponents argued, the subsidies would constitute the use of federal funds for abortion and violate the spirit of the Hyde Amendment.

A forceful effort by the Roman Catholic Church rallied pro-life supporters in the House to reject a compromise similar to the one in the Senate. The bishops rejected the use of segregated funds on the grounds that money was fungible, and whether some came from one source and some from another, it was only an accounting gimmick, and the subsidy still helped pay the same amount toward a policy that included abortion. Democrats were stung by the bishops' opposition, having expected the Catholic Church to support universal health coverage as they had for several decades. Instead, the bishops waged an intense campaign demanding that their letter of opposition be read at all masses throughout the country and urging their priests and parishioners to write letters and pressure members of Congress.[2]

By Friday morning, one day before the vote, Pelosi had only 205 supporters. The president was scheduled to speak to the Democratic House caucus and rally support, but with Pelosi involved in frantic negotiations, he postponed his meeting until the next morning. Bart Stupak (D-MI) was the leader of the Democratic pro-life forces, and he controlled enough votes to decide the fate of the bill. Stupak had offered an amendment that was supported by the Catholic bishops and pro-life forces. The amendment forbade any insurer that wanted to participate in the insurance exchange from including abortion coverage in its health plans because some of the purchasers might be receiving government subsidies. Abortion rights groups were incensed. Low- and moderate-income women could still purchase a separate abortion policy with their own money, but who would do that? No one planned to have an abortion. Who would buy insurance for something they didn't want and didn't expect to need? And what insurance company would market a policy for women who didn't expect to need it? The likely effect of the amendment would be that millions of low- and moderate-income women who purchased insurance through the exchange would not be able to purchase a policy that covered abortion.

On Friday, Pelosi met separately with members of the pro-choice caucus, the pro-life coalition, and the bishops' conference. The representatives of the pro-life coalition were Bart Stupak, Mike Doyle from Pennsylvania, and Brad Ellsworth from Indiana. Ellsworth's previous effort to reach a compromise reveals the extent of passion from abortion opponents. A stalwart opponent of abortion, Ellsworth had proposed an amendment slightly stronger than the Senate solution. Under his proposal, not only would funds be segregated, but a private contractor would receive all the funds and ensure that no subsidized funds were used to pay for abortion coverage.

Ellsworth was immediately castigated by pro-life groups. Doug Johnson, the legislative director of the National Right to Life Committee stated, "It was a bayonet in the back from someone who said he was one of us."[3] The bishops and a core group of Stupak supporters rejected Ellsworth's amendment. But the repercussions went further. The Susan B. Anthony List identified Ellsworth as one of six "tier one" Democrats they would target for defeat in 2010.[4] As it turned out, the group happily applauded the election results when Ellsworth lost his House seat.

Pelosi and Stupak finally struck a compromise on Friday night. Abortion coverage would be prohibited in the public option, but would be subject to an annual vote on the health insurance exchange.[5] Late Friday night, Stupak phoned his supporters and obtained their support for the compromise. Pelosi, however, was less successful. The pro-choice Democrats refused to accept the compromise as part of the bill. If it had to be considered, they insisted on a separate amendment. That way they could express their opposition and possibly even defeat the amendment. When Stupak was told that the compromise language would not be included in the bill, however, he decided that the agreement had been breached, and the amendment would have to contain his original language.

With no other options, Pelosi was forced to make a wrenching personal decision. She would allow the Stupak amendment to be introduced for a vote on the House floor. She would attempt to convince her pro-choice members to accept the amendment they so detested.

On Saturday morning, the president addressed the Democratic House caucus and urged them to "answer the call of history." Shortly afterward, the House bill, the Affordable Health Care for America Act, was introduced on the House floor. In the House of Representatives, the majority was able to exercise tight control of the proceedings. Pelosi allowed only two amendments to come to the floor. One was the House Republican proposal for health care reform. It contained a number of state-based initiatives for the small group and individual insurance market, and a $250,000 cap on noneconomic malpractice awards. However, it was an incremental as opposed to a comprehensive reform proposal, and it did not aspire to universal coverage. The CBO estimated the plan would cover an additional three million people out of the forty-six million uninsured. Everyone understood that the amendment would be rejected by the Democratic-controlled House.

Pelosi also allowed a vote on the Stupak amendment. It was a painful decision for many pro-choice Democrats. It would be the largest setback to pro-choice forces since the ban on partial-birth abortions was enacted six years before. However, without the amendment, everyone knew the bill would die. Liberal Democrats held their noses and voted for the amendment, which passed 240–194. "The people who voted for the bill were voting to advance the ball down the field," Pelosi explained. "We could not allow it to take down the bill. We have to defer that conversation for when we go to the table."[6] "The table," in Pelosi's parlance, was the House–Senate conference. Of course, unbeknownst to the Speaker and her caucus, the conference would never occur.

The Stupak amendment passed at 10:30 p.m. on Saturday night. Shortly afterward, the House approved the Affordable Health Care for America Act by a vote of 220–215. Thirty-nine Democrats voted against the bill, and one Republican voted in favor. That Republican was Anh Cao, an American of Vietnamese descent who defeated William Jefferson in the 2008 election. Readers may recall Mr. Jefferson from chapter 2 when he pressured President Clinton to freeze the tobacco tax and was subsequently convicted of corruption after ninety thousand dollars in cash was found in his freezer.

The House bill would cost $1.05 trillion over ten years and insure an additional thirty-six million Americans. It had substantial differences with the bill still being formulated in the Senate, including the public option, the manner of financing, a more generous provision of subsidies, and the Stupak amendment. Yet Nancy Pelosi had overcome monumental challenges to hold her caucus together. It was an impressive accomplishment for the Speaker and a huge step forward for the president's health reform effort. Beaming in the Rose Garden the day after the vote, Barack Obama urged the Senate to "Take up the baton and bring this effort to the finish line."[7] The president still hoped to sign a health reform bill before Christmas. It was going to be a lot harder than he thought.

# CHAPTER 16

# THE SENATE AND THE
# CHRISTMAS EVE HEALTH BILL

## Maneuvering Through the Blizzard

It was the largest December snowstorm ever recorded in Washington history. Roaring up the coast from the Gulf of Mexico, it shut down the Capitol by Saturday morning. Public transportation was suspended, airports were closed, and a state of emergency was declared. By Saturday evening, 16.3 inches of snow blanketed Reagan Airport, and twenty-three inches piled up elsewhere in the region—more snow than the Capitol usually gets in an entire winter. County Executive Jack Johnson said, "We have too many people on the highway. People are not to leave home. No matter where they are, we are going to have them go back. The conditions are too awful."[1]

Nevertheless, early Saturday morning, in the brunt of the giant storm, a certain group of one hundred people had to get to work. Senator Barbara Mikulski (D-MD), nursing a broken ankle, left her home in Baltimore at 7:30 a.m. It took her driver two hours to reach the Capitol, whereupon he helped her negotiate her walker over the accumulated snow. Other senators were chauffeured through the snow-covered roads in Chevrolet® Suburbans®. For one senator it was exceptionally difficult. Robert Byrd, ninety-two years old and in failing health, was the longest serving senator in the country's history. Byrd was president pro tempore of the senate, the third in line for succession to the presidency. As such, he had a round-the-clock security detail that could assist the wheelchair-bound senator in getting to his Capitol Hill office from his home in McLean, Virginia. In and out of the hospital, Byrd had missed 40 percent of the roll call votes in 2009 because of his health. He was determined not to miss this one. His party was depending on him. In fact, both parties were depending on each and every senator to make his or her way through the gathering storm.

The date was December 19, 2009. Barack Obama and the Democratic caucus were desperately trying to get their health reform plan through the Senate before the Christmas recess. The president had wanted the Senate to finish by Thanksgiving so he could sign the bill by Christmas. That window had closed, but if both houses of Congress enacted bills before the holiday, the House–Senate conference could still produce a bill that could be signed early the next year. It would be a historic achievement for Barack Obama. For nearly one hundred years, every other attempt to enact comprehensive health reform and universal coverage had failed. The president had expended enormous political capital on this near-universal bill. Its enactment would be a landmark event, but its failure could be a death knell for the Obama presidency and the Democratic majority.

Democrats held fifty-eight seats in the Senate. Two independents who caucused with them and supported health care reform gave them a sixty-vote, filibuster-proof majority. However, the Republican Party adamantly opposed the legislation, and many lawmakers had valid substantive objections. The most glaring was its high cost: nearly one trillion dollars over ten years. Taxes would have to be raised to pay for the bill, and many believed that it would increase the budget deficit. Republicans disliked the expanded role of the federal government. The bill would substantially increase the amount of federal regulation and would add millions of people to the public sector Medicaid program.

There were those in the Republican Party, particularly in the leadership, who opposed the bill purely for political reasons, regardless of its content. No matter what role the Republicans played, they believed, Obama and the Democrats would likely receive all the credit. Moreover, party leaders remembered how the failure to enact health reform wounded the Clinton administration and precipitated the Republican takeover of the 104th Congress. Many Republicans sought a repeat of that scenario.

In addition, Republicans were angry about the process. They claimed that their minority party had no say in the crucial parts of the legislation even though the Democrats had trumpeted bipartisanship. Furthermore, they were appalled that such a comprehensive bill, affecting more than one-sixth of the economy, could be rammed through the Congress on a strictly partisan, party-line vote. As a result, the health reform debate became angry and bitter, and the Republican leadership vowed to derail the legislation by any means, including attempts to delay and filibuster every vote. Since sixty votes were required to terminate a filibuster (cloture), the Democrats needed the vote of every member in their caucus.

Waiting on the senatorial agenda was the $600 billion Defense Appropriations bill. The measure included $130 million to fund the ongoing wars in Afghanistan and Iraq. With American soldiers in harm's way, nearly every senator supported the measure. However, the Senate calendar was dominated by health reform. Harry Reid, the Democratic majority leader, agreed to call up the bill on December 17. Reid thought he had assurances from several Republicans that they would support his efforts. Nevertheless, when he called the bill to the floor, the Republicans initiated a filibuster. It had nothing to do with the defense bill. They simply wanted to delay the health reform vote until after the Christmas recess.

Earlier that day, Bernie Sanders (Ind-VT) had agreed to an earlier vote on his single-payer amendment so that Reid could bring up the defense bill. Sanders was a socialist and a long-time supporter of a single-payer health system. He knew his amendment had no chance to be adopted, but, in its entire history, Congress had never taken an up-or-down vote on single-payer. Sanders wanted the opportunity to force a vote on his amendment, and Reid granted it, needing his support. As soon as Sanders introduced the amendment, Tom Coburn (R-OK) insisted that the entire 767-page proposal be read into the record. After Senate aides spent three hours reading to an empty chamber, Sanders gave up and withdrew his amendment without a vote.

Reid felt angry and double-crossed, first by the action of Coburn and then by the filibuster of the defense bill. He scheduled a cloture vote on the defense bill for 1:00 a.m. on Friday, December 18, the earliest time allowed under Senate rules. Possibly needing every vote in his caucus, Reid prevailed on the liberal senator Russ Feingold for support. Feingold opposed the Iraq and Afghanistan wars and resolutely voted against every authorization of funds. However, Feingold also wanted health reform, and, against his conscience, he reluctantly promised Reid his vote. Reid also needed the vote of the ailing Robert Byrd, who was wheeled in to the Senate chamber at 1:00 a.m. The Democrats won the cloture vote 63–33, enabling Reid to end the filibuster and schedule a final vote on the defense bill for Saturday morning. He had not anticipated the ferocity of the storm.

Reid knew that Republicans would use parliamentary procedures on Saturday morning in an attempt to delay the bill. If they succeeded, the health bill would be doomed for the session. Every Democrat had to overcome the drifted snow and blocked roadways to reach the Senate chamber. Police were reporting traffic backups of up to seven miles in Virginia and motorists stuck in their vehicles for up to twelve hours.

Early Saturday morning, senators from both parties had fought through the storm and were gathered on the Senate floor. Suddenly, an ovation erupted among the Democratic caucus. The ailing Robert Byrd, confined to his wheelchair, but resplendent in a dark blue suit and red, white, and blue tie, was wheeled into the chamber. The Democrats overcame the procedural motion by a vote of 63–33. Then, when it was clear that the Democrats had the votes, all but nine Republicans reversed their positions and the defense bill passed easily by a vote of 88–10. With Reid no longer needing his vote, Russ Feingold was able to satisfy his conscience and vote "nay."

The Senate calendar was finally clear to begin debate on the health care bill. But until that morning, there was no bill. All the time Harry Reid was trying to pass the defense appropriations bill, he still lacked the votes to pass health reform. He was still trying to cobble together his manager's amendment, a combination of policies that were acceptable to every Democratic and independent member, a package that could finally garner the necessary sixty votes to overcome republican filibusters.

We will examine some of the issues facing Harry Reid before returning to the debate in Washington.

## The Senate Bill: Policy Decisions, Compromises, and Payoffs in Harry Reid's Manager's Amendment

Addressing shivering crowds in Chicago and snow-covered rallies in New Hampshire, Barack Obama first outlined his health plan in the 2008 campaign. It was pushed, pulled, manipulated, and finessed by three House and two Senate committees. As the winter snowstorms began to head east in the week before Christmas, the Senate version sat on Harry Reid's desk. Somehow, Reid, Obama, and the Democratic leadership had to amend the proposal to get sixty supporters onboard.

Final negotiations on major legislation are not pretty. Members of Congress all know how to play the game. Knowing their votes are needed, they can hold out for something in return. Sometimes that something is a substantive improvement or a reasonable compromise that improves the legislation. Sometimes it is to defend a conscientious belief. But other times, it is simply to bargain for federal largesse to benefit the member's district or an influential constituent. As Harry Reid put together his manager's amendment, he had to deal with all of the above.

## The Louisiana Purchase

Mary Landrieu (D-LA) had been relatively easy. Reid had needed her vote on November 21, when Republicans filibustered the motion to begin debate on health reform. Elected from a southern state, Landrieu faced intense pressure from both sides of the aisle and had withheld her support of health reform. She needed a reason to tell her constituents she would vote to end the filibuster. Reid promised to insert an amendment providing one hundred million dollars of federal Medicaid subsidies for "certain states recovering from a major disaster." Louisiana, although never mentioned by name, was the only state that met the two-page definition of what constituted "certain states." Reid had engineered less-publicized deals with other wavering senators including Ron Wyden (D-OR) and Blanche Lincoln (D-AR). Landrieu made it clear that she still opposed the public option and was not promising to support the final bill. Reid knew that future concessions would be necessary. For now, however, he had secured her wavering vote. On November 21, the Senate had voted 60–39 to end the filibuster, enabling it to begin the historic debate on health care reform. The so-called Louisiana Purchase became part of Reid's manager's amendment.

## The Public Option—It's Much More Complicated than You Think

Of all the provisions in Obama's health plan, the public option drew the most press coverage and public controversy. The concept of a public option first appeared in California in 2001–2002. The basic idea was to include a publicly run insurance plan (i.e., a government-run plan such as Medicare) in an insurance exchange comprised of competing private plans. Consumers could choose among the competing plans, selecting either the public option or any one of the private plans. The primary goals of a public option are to reduce the price of health insurance premiums by providing more competition, lowering administrative costs, and, under most proposals, paying providers less for medical services. Whether a public option can achieve those goals, and what the consequences would be to the health care market, is uncertain and largely dependent upon how it is structured.

There are two primary concerns in creating a public option: the mechanism used to set payment amounts for providers and the rules governing eligibility to enroll in the plan. Unlike private plans, a public plan can use the power of government to fix the prices it pays doctors and hospitals for services. Government entities usually do not negotiate payment rates with individual providers. They set rates through legislation or regulation and require providers to accept those rates in order to participate in the program. This is the case with Medicare and Medicaid, which pay much lower rates than private insurers. A powerful public plan could set lower rates, reduce its costs, and charge lower premium prices.

At first glance, this might seem like a good idea, but it can have several negative consequences. Doctors and hospitals currently lose money providing services to Medicare, Medicaid, and the uninsured. They recoup those losses by charging higher premiums to private patients (known as cross-subsidizing or cost shifting). If some private patients began to pay lower rates through a public plan, providers may seek higher payments from other private patients or refuse to treat public-plan patients at all. Worse still, if enrollment in the public plan is so large that providers need to participate and cannot shift costs to private patients, it will substantially reduce their revenues and force considerable changes in the entire delivery system.

Eligibility is the second major issue. If eligibility is not restricted, enrollment will be large—especially if the public plan sets lower provider payment rates than private insurers. Large enrollment could not only force out private competition but also could seriously undermine the current employer-provided insurance system as more companies and employees opt for the public plan. This would change the way most Americans purchase insurance and throw many people into the individual market.

However, if eligibility is too restricted, or the public plan pays providers similar rates as private insurers, enrollment may be too small. Since the public plan is likely to enroll more high-risk individuals, it needs to balance its risk by attracting a sufficient number of healthy enrollees. Otherwise it could become a dumping ground for private insurance plans. Private plans could increase profits by marketing to young, healthy patients and letting others enroll in the public plan.

Can a public plan be structured to garner the advantages of increased competition and lower administrative costs while avoiding the concerns enumerated above? That question caused a number of different proposals as Democratic members of Congress tried to recommend public plan structures that would alleviate the negative concerns and attract political support. Hence, the range of proposed pricing mechanisms included fixing provider reimbursement levels at Medicare rates, fixing them at Medicare rates plus 5 or 10 percent, or requiring "negotiated rates." In simple terms, negotiated rates meant tying prices to a standard such as the average of private rates within each region. Most proposals initially limited eligibility to those individuals who could not get employer-based insurance, Medicare, Medicaid, or military coverage; and to small businesses with less than twenty-five employees. However, many proposals allowed considerable expansion of eligibility over time. Proposals also differed on whether public plans would be national or state-based, with similar concerns about the size and market power of the public plans.

The variations in the public plan resulted in huge differences in projected enrollment. The bill passed by the House of Representatives in November 2009 specified negotiated rates and limited eligibility. The CBO estimated that under those conditions six million people would be enrolled in the plan by 2019, a relatively modest number. However, the Lewin Group estimated that if the public plan paid Medicare rates and there were no restrictions on enrollment, 131 million people would enroll in the plan. If that occurred, the private market would wither, and a government-run, single-payer system would result.

The long debate about the public option, however, did not focus on policy alternatives and substance. Instead, it was about the role and the size of government in people's lives. Those issues fell right on the fault line of the explosive political divisions characterizing American politics in 2009.

Liberals saw the public option as a means for government to provide a vital social service where the private insurance market had failed. Many on the left disliked and distrusted health insurance companies. They thought the public option would, at a minimum, provide competition and keep insurance companies more honest. They pointed out that many health markets had few competitors, and increased competition from a low-cost public plan would force private insurers to reduce their premium rates. Advocates of the public option publicly downplayed the risks and difficulties of trying to create a level playing field with both private and government competitors. At the same time, however, many liberals did not want a level playing field. They hoped that a public option would eventually force private insurers out of the market and create a single-payer resembling Medicare—a goal they had pursued for many years. John Edwards actually gave voice to that sentiment during the presidential campaign. Edwards commented that a public option could be a "potential transition to a single-payer," and stated, "I'm not opposed to that."[2]

That sentiment is precisely what conservatives and many moderates—even those in the Democratic Party—feared the most. They believed that once a public option was adopted, even if it was initially restrictive, it would be under constant pressure to lower reimbursement to providers and expand eligibility to individuals and businesses. For similar reasons, doctors, hospitals, other providers, and insurance companies opposed the public option. They believed that once a public option was in place, government would always be under pressure to reduce cost by reducing reimbursement to providers. Hence, even though initial price and enrollment restrictions for some proposals were quite stringent, many believed those could change considerably in the future.

Conservatives and some moderates also saw the pubic option as an intrusion by government into the private market. They believed an insurance exchange comprised of private companies could increase competition without the need for a government-run entity. Furthermore, they argued that much of the projected savings from a public option were illusory because the reduced cost to the government from setting low rates would simply be cost-shifted to other payers.

With such wide differences in beliefs about complex details, it is not surprising that the rhetoric descended to political sound bites. Democrats and liberals blasted private insurance companies and maintained that a public option was necessary to keep them honest. Republicans and conservatives argued that a public option was just more big government and big spending and would lead to a government takeover of health care.

What was Harry Reid to do? The president had committed his support for the public option since the nominating campaign, when all three Democratic candidates supported similar versions of the policy. His support continued throughout the beginning of the health care debate, although he later hinted that if the policy was excluded it might not be a deal breaker. Nancy Pelosi and liberal members of the House insisted on a public option and included it in the final plan passed by the House. A number of liberal Democrats publicly stated they would not support a bill without a public option. However, Democrats had tried and failed throughout the spring to find enough support in the Senate.

For several months, Reid had watched as Max Baucus attempted to attract conservative Democrats and a few moderate Republicans to the concept. Olympia Snowe (R-ME) had proposed a trigger in which a public option would be instituted only if insurance rates rose at more than a specified rate. Others proposed a public option that would allow any state to opt out. By the time the summer recess began, however, Baucus had failed to find any variation that would win Republican votes. More importantly, there were several members of his own caucus that would not support reform if it included a public option.

Exactly when Reid and Obama realized that the public option had no chance of passing the Senate is not known. Some believe that Obama knew all along and was only using the policy as a negotiating tool—something he could concede at the end of the negotiations to get the last crucial votes. It appears likely that he genuinely favored the policy, but he must have known for quite some time that it had no chance. Nevertheless, he was unwilling to state unequivocally that he would accept a reform proposal without it, apparently wary of losing liberal support.

Once the Senate began debate on the health bill in November, Reid was looking for a compromise position. On December 9, he gamely announced that he had a deal. In place of a public option, Reid proposed that people between the ages of fifty-five and sixty-four (the "near-elderly") could buy into Medicare. It was a policy first proposed by the Clinton administration, and one that was dear to the hearts of liberals. The near-elderly needed more medical care than any other age group except those who were eligible for Medicare. Accounting for this, private insurance companies charged high premium rates to this age group and, in some cases, avoided issuing nongroup insurance at all. A Medicare buy-in would not only alleviate the health insurance access problem for the near-elderly, but would also expand the single-payer Medicare system, a goal that liberals had sought since Medicare's inception in 1965.

By announcing the deal—before he really had a deal—Reid thought he could force Joe Lieberman to accept the package. Lieberman opposed the public option but had publicly supported a Medicare buy-in when he ran on the presidential ticket with Al Gore. With this new alternative to a public option and Lieberman's support, Reid was gambling that liberals would be appeased and moderate Democratic holdouts like Ben Nelson and Mary Landrieu would likely go along.

Lieberman, however, was not to be had so easily. Coming from the insurance-rich state of Connecticut, he was not going to support a policy that removed an entire ten-year age group from the private insurance market. Angering many Democrats, Lieberman went on CBS television and announced he would support a filibuster of any bill that included either a Medicare buy-in or a public option.

Although the press generally blamed Lieberman for the failure of the Medicare buy-in, other powerful forces were just as important. It was not only insurance companies that would lose money from the buy-in. Doctors and hospitals would have to accept lower Medicare reimbursement rates when they treated near-elderly patients, a group that was a lucrative source of income. Hence, the AMA and the AHA lobbied strongly against the policy. Aware of the opposition, even the AARP declined to offer its support. Having made previous deals to win the endorsement of these organizations, the administration could hardly risk alienating them, even if it had Lieberman's support.

In the end, Harry Reid did what he had to do and what Barack Obama may have intended for some time. He agreed to give up the public option (and the Medicare buy-in) in return for the support of Lieberman and other holdouts. Instead, the manager's amendment included a multistate exchange, similar to FEHBP that would include at least one consumer operated non-profit insurance plan called a Consumer Operated and Oriented Plan (CO-OP). On December 21, after a year and a half of bitter debate, Reid presented his manager's amendment to the Senate. There was no public option.

The adamant stance taken by some liberals is difficult to reconcile. For nearly one hundred years, it was a liberal objective to shore up the social safety net by providing universal health care. Yet, they threatened to oppose a bill that would insure over thirty million Americans because it did not have a public option—a policy that had never been tried, would be difficult to implement, and would enroll only six million people (under the House plan). It was reminiscent of when liberals rejected Richard Nixon's universal health plan in 1974 because it was not a single-payer. In the end, liberals accepted the inevitable and supported the compromise, but their insistence polarized both sides and dominated the public debate at the expense of other issues.

Perhaps, their insistence had an unintended effect. Chip Kahn cites the debate over the public option as one of the primary reasons for the passage of health care reform. In his analysis, the heated debate consumed the media coverage and kept opponents from focusing on their strongest arguments—the cost of the bill, the budget deficit, increased taxes, and a larger role for government in people's health care. Equally important, it erected a huge straw man for the Democrats, which they could hold out and then finally trade away to secure the last crucial votes for health care reform.

### Financing the Senate Bill: How Much Will It Cost, and Who Will Pay?

Barack Obama had insisted that health care reform could not add one dollar to the federal budget deficit. It had to be budget neutral. Somehow, the Democratic leadership would have to find $871 billion to pay for the plan. Every dollar of savings would be a reduction in someone's income. Every dollar of revenue would come out of someone's pocket. Yet Harry Reid had to hold every Democratic and independent vote. As he struggled with the last details of his manager's amendment, he seemed to have a nearly impossible task. What combination of spending cuts, tax increases, and industry surcharges could raise all that money and not alienate a single senator?

The following table provides a condensed summary of how Democratic senators and Harry Reid paid for the health reform plan. These projections pertain to the Senate bill as modified by the manager's amendment and are taken from CBO estimates.[3] This is the bill that actually became law, except some provisions were later superseded by the bill enacted under reconciliation. The projections for the final bill (including reconciliation) are shown in the last column.

### Medicare: Funding about 50 Percent of the Total Plan

The largest source of financing came from the Medicare program. All of the Democratic health proposals depended on a reduction in the projected growth of Medicare spending to pay for a substantial portion of the plan. In part, this was necessary because of the way legislative proposals are scored. Only savings in federal spending count toward paying for the plan. Thus sav-

Table 16.1

| Condensed Summary of Financing for the Senate Bill with Manager's Amendment before and after Reconciliation ($ Billions, Cost over Ten-Year Period) | | |
|---|---|---|
| Source of Funds | Before Reconciliation | After Reconciliation |
| Reductions in Projected Medicare Spending | | |
| Annual FFS Updates | 186 | 196 |
| Medicare Advantage | 118 | 136 |
| Disproportionate Share Payments | 43 | 36 |
| Other | 91 | 87 |
| Subtotal Medicare Reductions | 438 | 455 |
| Medicare Withholding Tax | 87 | 210 |
| Tax on Cadillac Plans | 149 | 32 |
| Industry Fees | 101 | 107 |
| Mandate Penalties (28 employer and 15 individual in Senate bill) | 43 | 65 |
| Other Taxes | 62 | 89 |
| Other | 123 | 120 |
| Total Sources of Funds | 1003 | 1078 |
| Total Cost of Legislation | 871 | 940 |
| Reduction in Deficit | 132 | 138 |

Source: Authors' calculations from legislation.

ings to the private sector, in terms of lower health costs, do not receive any consideration. In addition, Congress was mindful that if Medicare spending was not reduced (or Medicare taxes increased) a segment of the program was projected to go bankrupt by 2017. With little opposition from his own party, Reid left the bill before the Senate largely unchanged. It funded $438 billion out of $871 billion—about one half of the total cost of the plan.

Over 40 percent of the projected reduction in Medicare spending growth ($186 billion) came from reductions in future government reimbursement rates to medical providers. It is important to understand that this was not a reduction in absolute dollar terms, but a reduction in the annual projected increases in payments to fee-for-service providers. As we discussed earlier, the major provider groups accepted the reduction in payments because they anticipated increased revenues from over thirty million people who were previously uninsured. Republican opponents repeatedly warned the elderly that the reductions would reduce benefits and "cripple Medicare." This was ironic considering Republicans had consistently proposed to reduce the growth of Medicare spending in the past and had enacted the largest reductions ever under Newt Gingrich in the Balanced Budget Act of 1997.

Some would have preferred reforms that reduced spending by improving the underlying efficiency of the health delivery system (i.e., bending the cost curve). Instead, the plan simply reduced the level of payments but did not attack the forces that made those payments increase. Significant changes to the delivery system would have encountered powerful political opposition, and, unlike Bill Clinton, Obama made a political decision to avoid such changes. Notwithstanding, the plan contained numerous pilot programs and demonstrations such as bundled payments, capitation, care coordination models, and accountable health organizations that could point the way toward future savings without encountering current opposition.

Nearly a quarter of Medicare reductions came from the Medicare Advantage program (MA). Readers will recall that MA plans are private, often for-profit, Medicare insurance plans that compete with the traditional government-run plan. Medicare pays private plans a fixed amount per person, per year. Originally, the payment rates were supposed to approximate the cost of treating a patient in traditional Medicare who lived in the same county. Hence, MA plans in rural areas and some cities (mostly in the Pacific Northwest) received lower per capita payment rates because Medicare costs per capita were lower in those areas. Conversely, payment rates in large cities (such as in the Northeast and California) were higher. Congressional delegations from low payment areas strongly opposed the differential payments. They argued lower reimbursement rates were unfair because it penalized those areas that were more efficient and had lower costs. In addition, it was more difficult to create sustainable networks of providers in areas with low population densities. Their lobbying efforts were ultimately successful, and beginning in 1997 (when private Medicare plans were called Medicare + Choice), they received several rate increases. The largest occurred in 2003 when some members of Congress, who otherwise would have opposed the increases, acquiesced because they were included in the bill that created the Medicare prescription drug benefit. As a result, by 2009, the government paid MA plans 15 percent more on average than it paid traditional Medicare and up to 30 percent more in some areas of the country.

Although the biggest gap between payments to MA and traditional Medicare plans occurred in low-cost regions, a differential existed even in high spending areas. Republicans had supported the increases because they wanted to encourage the creation of private plans that would compete with traditional Medicare. They believed private plans would be innovative in the way they organized care and would ultimately produce higher quality care at a lower cost. Most Democrats had never liked the program, suspecting the primary intent was to weaken the government-run Medicare program rather than to provide a more competitive market. They believed elimination of the extra payments would cause little harm and be a major source of funding for health reform.

Despite the Democrats' dissatisfaction, the MA program had become popular because the extra government payments allowed plans to provide additional benefits without charging higher premiums. Indeed, the most popular plans received such a high payment from the government that they charged enrollees no premium at all. By 2009, about twelve million individuals (approximately 25 percent of Medicare beneficiaries) were enrolled in private MA plans. If most of the subsidies were phased out, premiums would increase, zero-premium plans would probably disappear, and many MA plans would likely go out of business. As a result, many seniors would have to change their insurances, an outcome Republicans warned about but Democrats denied. On the other hand, Democrats argued it was wasteful and unfair for Medicare to pay for extra benefits only because a beneficiary enrolled in private coverage instead of remaining in the traditional Medicare program. Under the Senate bill, the per capita payments would gradually be reduced and would save the government an estimated $118 billion over ten years.[4]

### Tax Increases: Funding about 30 Percent of the Plan

With approximately half the funds coming from the Medicare program, the next largest source of revenue, about 30 percent of the cost of the plan, came from increased taxes. This was a much more controversial area and generated a number of different proposals. Barack Obama first proposed reducing the rate of taxable deductions for the wealthiest earners. Individuals and families in the top tax brackets would only be able to deduct 28 percent of their tax-deductible expenses instead of the current 33 to 35 percent.[5] He argued that deductions should not be worth more to the wealthy than they are to those with lower incomes. Under his proposal, the reduced rates would be the same as they were under Ronald Reagan and would only affect 1.4 percent of American households. The proposal would have raised an estimated $267 billion over ten years.

The tax proposal drew immediate opposition. Charities, universities and other nonprofit groups feared that contributions to their organizations would be reduced if the after-tax cost of charitable giving was increased. States with high costs and incomes such as New York argued that the change would impact their taxpayers disproportionately. Construction and real estate businesses were opposed because the after-tax cost of home mortgage payments would increase.

The House of Representatives had pursued a simpler and much more liberal track. Nancy Pelosi's final bill included the "millionaire's tax," an income tax surcharge of 5.4 percent on individuals earning more than $500,000 or families earning more than one million dollars. The tax would raise $460 billion over ten years and affect only .3 percent of tax filers. One might guess there would have been support among the 99.7 percent of taxpayers who would be unaffected. That was not the case, however, as widespread opposition existed to any rise in income tax rates.

Although there was little support in the Senate for raising the income tax, an increase in the Medicare withholding tax drew much less opposition, possibly because it was related directly to health care as opposed to general revenues. It would also help stabilize the Medicare Trust Fund. The bill before the Senate included an increase in the Medicare withholding tax for individuals earning over $200,000 and households earning more than $250,000. It raised the withholding tax from 1.45 percent to 1.95 percent (for employers and employees), an increase of .5 percent. Here was where Harry Reid took his most aggressive action. In his manager's amendment, Reid nearly doubled the increase in the original bill, raising withholding rates for high earners by .9 percent to 2.35 percent. Unlike the Social Security tax, which stops at a specified level of income ($106,800 in 2010), the Medicare tax has no maximum cap. Therefore, the tax increase is significant for the very wealthy.

When Barack Obama first suggested raising revenues by lowering the rate of tax deductions for the wealthy, the leaders of the Senate Finance Committee rejected the idea. The chair, Max Baucus, was still attempting to reach an accord with Chuck Grassley. At that time, both wanted all the financing to come from the health sector. Instead of reducing the rate of tax deductions, they wanted to tax expensive Cadillac health plans. As we discussed way back in chapter 1, Republicans, conservatives, and many health policy experts had long been dissatisfied with the tax deduction for health insurance. Currently, the cost of health insurance is a deductible expense for employers and is not included as a taxable benefit for employees. The result is that the net (after tax) cost of health insurance is artificially low, and employers and employees buy more comprehensive health insurance policies than they need. Such policies offer small deductibles and copayments and may include first-dollar coverage. As a result, the insured have little incentive to be cost-conscious because they do not have to spend their own money. Furthermore, the highest wage earners usually have the most comprehensive policies, and they derive the most benefit from each dollar of tax deduction (because they are in a higher tax bracket), while the poor and uninsured receive no benefit at all. A huge amount could be saved by eliminating the deduction. The estimated cost of the deduction to the federal government from 2010–2014 is $924 billion, nearly enough to finance the entire health care proposal.[6] However, supporters of the deduction fear that a total elimination could cause employers to stop providing insurance, increasing the number of uninsured and throwing millions of people into the more expensive individual market. Unions oppose any reduction in deductibility because they negotiated contracts in which they traded pay increases for more comprehensive health benefits.

Baucus and Grassley avoided the more extreme option of eliminating the tax deduction altogether. Instead, they proposed taxing only very expensive plans which became known as "Cadillac" plans—those that provided the most comprehensive benefits. The tax would not only raise money, but, as a consequence, employers would issue fewer such policies, and employees would be more cost-conscious and demand fewer medical services. The president and many other Democrats supported the policy.

Nevertheless, labor unions were adamantly opposed to limiting the tax deduction and lobbied against it throughout the health reform debate. Many Republicans, reversing their long-held positions, said the policy would hurt middle-class Americans and would violate Obama's promise not to raise taxes on anyone earning less than $200,000. Although the Cadillac tax was supposed to target high wage earners, the tax also would have impacted union employees in manufacturing and state employees who had substituted benefit increases for higher wages. Furthermore, the tax would be based on the cost of the plan (not the benefits covered), so it would disproportionately affect states with high medical costs. Here was a policy that appeared to make sense to most policy analysts, but one that angered labor unions and some of the Democrats' closest allies in large urban areas.

Of course, Grassley never came to an agreement with Baucus, and after months of negotiation within their own party, Democrats agreed on their own version of the tax. The Cadillac tax would levy a 40 percent excise tax on any policy with an annual cost of more than $8,500 for an individual or $23,000 for a family. It would raise $149 billion over ten years. In his manager's amendment, Harry Reid left the policy basically unchanged, but he would be forced to renegotiate with the unions at a later date.

### Other Provisions and Summary of Funding

Several other items were notable in the manager's amendment. Harry Reid increased the penalty individuals would have to pay if they did not comply with the mandate to purchase insurance. He increased tax credits for small businesses that were newly offering insurance benefits. He included annual fees on health sector companies that would benefit from increased insurance enrollment. Reid also included a controversial requirement for insurance companies to issue rebates to enrollees if they failed to spend at least a specified percent of premiums directly on health care (as opposed to administration, marketing, etc.). In the end, he managed to mollify most of his caucus while complying with the two markers laid down by the president: the package cost less than $950 billion and yielded more than $100 billion in deficit reduction.

### The Senate Bill: Abortion Politics and the Cornhusker Kickback

We return to the debate in Washington on December 18, one day before the Senate vote on the Defense Appropriations bill.

Chuck Schumer (D-NY) had been in Harry Reid's office for over twelve hours. The final vote on the defense bill was scheduled for early the next morning. Since the filibuster had been broken, the Democrats needed only a simple majority, and Schumer knew they would prevail. Then it would be time for Harry Reid to introduce his manager's amendment. After the Senate voted to consider a bill, its rules required a minimum of thirty hours before a vote could be taken. If all went according to plan and the Democrats could hold on to their sixty votes to defeat upcoming procedural filibusters, the Senate could still pass the health reform bill on Christmas Eve. They might have to schedule votes in the middle of the night, but there were just enough hours to get it done. If Reid's amendment was delayed, however, health reform was dead until after the Christmas recess and probably for Obama's presidency. There was just one remaining obstacle: the Democrats had only fifty-nine votes.

At one end of Reid's office suite was Ben Nelson (D-NE), unwilling to support the bill without further restrictions on abortion rights.[7] At the other end were Barbara Boxer (D-CA) and Patricia Murray (D-WA), both abortion rights supporters. Unless a compromise with Nelson satisfied the two female lawmakers, health reform would not pass the Senate. Boxer had been in one end of Reid's office suite for over seven hours, but had not even ventured into the same room as Nelson. Rahm Emanuel was monitoring the negotiations from a dinner in Georgetown. White House aides were camped in Reid's office, offering their advice. Reminiscent of Henry Kissinger, an exhausted Chuck Schumer had been shuttling back and forth, desperately trying to make a deal before the next morning. The heavy snow had already begun to fall, and Obama's health plan hung in the balance.

Less than two months earlier, Nancy Pelosi had been caught in a similar predicament and was forced to compromise by accepting the Stupak amendment. Now pro-life members in the Senate, backed by pressure from the Catholic bishops, wanted the Senate to adopt the same language. However, the Stupak amendment was a nonstarter in the Democratic caucus, and time was running out for a solution. Finally, at 10:30 p.m. on Friday night, December 18, they struck a deal. Nelson agreed to the compromise rejected by the House requiring strict segregation of government and personal funds to pay for abortion services that were included in any policy purchased through the insurance exchange. Furthermore, Nelson added a clause giving any state the option to exclude all abortion coverage from exchanges in its own state.

A wily player, however, Nelson exacted a price for his compromise. The Obama health plan would add millions of people to state Medicaid programs, and, although the federal government would pay the lion's share of the additional cost, the states would still have to pay for a portion of the shared federal-state program. Nelson obtained a concession from Democrats promising the federal government would give Nebraska (and only Nebraska) full and permanent reimbursement for any increase in Medicaid costs as a result of the bill. It was a plum worth over one hundred million dollars.

Ben Nelson and Barbara Boxer, having spent seven hours at opposite ends of Harry Reid's offices, approached each other and embraced. Chuck Schumer was near exhaustion. A happy Rahm Emanuel received the news by telephone. Barack Obama was informed of the deal aboard Air Force One on his way back from a summit on global warming. Planned Parenthood, the National Organization of Women, and the National Abortion Rights Action League immediately announced their opposition to the compromise. The US Conference of Catholic Bishops denounced the agreement and said it would oppose the bill. Republicans were livid, labeling the one-hundred-million-dollar concession to Nelson "the Cornhusker Kickback." But Harry Reid tucked the agreement into his manager's amendment, hoping that at long last he had the elusive sixty votes.

### Christmas in Washington

Harry Reid had secured the final two votes. He gave up the public option and the Medicare buy-in to win over Joe Lieberman. Then, in day-long negotiations with Ben Nelson, he agreed to more stringent abortion language and the Cornhusker Kickback. He had made special deals with Mary Landrieu, Bernie Sanders, Carl Levin, John Kerry, and Patrick Leahy. On Saturday morning, December 19, all fifty-eight Democrats and two independents battled a ferocious blizzard to pass the Defense Appropriations bill. Now, not a day too soon, he had his manager's amendment, which he finally brought to the Senate floor.

As soon as Reid introduced his amendment, Republican Minority Leader Mitch McConnell required that the entire amendment be read to the chamber. At 8:30 a.m., Senate aides began to read the 383-page document, a process that would take seven hours.

McConnell had stated in a press conference the day before that he would do everything possible to slow down the bill. Republicans were furious that the process was moving ahead despite their unanimous opposition. Orrin Hatch (R-UT) accused the Democrats of securing their sixty votes with "a grab bag of backroom, Chicago-style buyoffs."[8] They particularly acted incensed by the deals with Ben Nelson and Mary Landrieu, claiming they would cost taxpayers in other states. Harry Reid defended the bill, telling reporters, "there are one hundred senators here, and I don't know that there's a senator that doesn't have something in this bill that isn't important to them. If they don't have something in it important to them, then it doesn't speak well of them."[9] Reid also pointed out that the smaller $600 billion defense bill, enacted by a large majority earlier in the day, had 1,700 earmarks. Orrin Hatch's description was an exaggeration, but there was much truth in his assessment. Harry Reid's assessment was also correct. Washington policy had been made in that fashion throughout American history, and the current battle was no different.

Immediately after the manager's amendment was read to the Senate on Saturday, the Republicans initiated a filibuster. Reid scheduled a cloture vote for Monday at 1:00 a.m. It was the first of six procedural votes that Republicans had planned to delay the process, and each time the Democrats would have to muster all sixty votes. Nevertheless, Harry Reid had managed to stay just within his timetable. If all went according to schedule, a final vote on the Senate bill would take place on Christmas Eve. The 1:00 a.m. vote on Monday morning, December 21, was the key vote. If sixty senators would vote for cloture on the manager's amendment, those same sixty were highly likely to maintain their support through all the other motions—unless, of course, one of them was unable to show up.

And that was the last hope of Republicans who were bitter that such a huge piece of legislation could be rammed through by the majority without a single Republican vote. The process, which had become acrimonious, was about to get even more ugly. The Senate had almost always been known to conduct its debates with dignity and respect for fellow members, even during periods of intense disagreement. On Sunday afternoon, however, nine hours before the vote, Tom Coburn (R-OK) took the Senate floor and urged the American people to pray for personal harm to befall one of his Senate colleagues. "What the American people should pray," Coburn said, "is that somebody can't make the vote. That's what they ought to pray."[10] It seemed likely that Coburn had the ailing ninety-two-year-old Robert Byrd in his thoughts. The wheelchair-bound senator would have to travel through the snow and ice-covered streets for the 1:00 a.m. vote. A request by Democrats to schedule an earlier vote because of Byrd's health status had been denied.

It was not the first time that Republicans had urged divine intervention to defeat the health care bill. The previous Wednesday, December 16, Republicans conducted an online "prayer-cast" featuring Senators Jim DeMint (R-SC) and Sam Brownback (R-KS).[11] Lew Engel, the pastor who conducted the meeting, prayed for God to rule in the Senate. "We dare to believe today that you overthrow, overrule keys, that you actually rule in the Senate debates even as we pray." James Dobson of Focus on the Family addressed the gathering by telephone. "Heavenly Father," he prayed, "the principles of righteousness that you taught us are just being abandoned now by our governmental leaders. And if they prevail in the measures that they're now considering, even more babies will die. More than fifty million already have. And in other measures, the institution of marriage itself will be destroyed."

It is difficult to find anything in the health bill that would destroy the institution of marriage, but hyperbole and Godly intervention were not the exclusive domains of Republicans. Senator Sheldon Whitehouse (D-RI) compared the fervent Republican opposition to Nazis on Kristallnacht and lynching in the South. Whitehouse warned that Republicans would face a "day of judgment" and "a day of reckoning."[12]

With passions high on both sides of the aisle, senators began to convene after midnight on December 21 for the all-important vote. Shortly before 1:00 a.m. Robert Byrd, sitting in his plaid wheelchair and "bundled in a coat, scarf, and hat," was wheeled into the chamber.[13]

Dana Milbank describes the scene in the *Washington Post*: "Byrd was wheeled in, dabbing his eyes and nose with tissues, his complexion pale. When his name was called, Byrd shot his right index finger into the air as he shouted 'aye,' then pumped his fist in defiance."[14] The motion to close debate on the manager's amendment passed with a vote of 60–40, the bare minimum margin. Harry Reid's caucus had held together. Opponents recognized it was probably just a matter of time.

Despite the bleak outlook, Republicans continued their determined opposition. The next procedural vote was held at 7:00 a.m. on Tuesday, the twenty-third day of debate, and the Democrats prevailed 60–39. Then on Wednesday, Harry Reid was finally able to introduce a motion to end debate. Robert Byrd, dressed in a navy blue suit, was wheeled into the chamber for the third straight day, and the Democratic coalition held. Facing certain defeat, Republicans finally agreed to advance the final vote for early the next day, December 24, so members could be with their families on Christmas Eve.

It was the first time the Senate had convened on Christmas Eve day since 1895. The vote on the Patient Protection and Affordable Care Act began at 7:05 a.m. with Vice President Joe Biden presiding. When it came time for Harry Reid to vote, he was so exhausted that he initially voted "nay." Realizing his mistake, he quickly corrected himself, drawing the only bipartisan laughter of the proceedings.

It is customary in Senate roll-call votes for members simply to raise their hand and state "aye" or "nay." But when it came time for Robert Byrd to vote, he broke with tradition. Thrusting his long arm in the air and holding up one finger, Byrd exclaimed, "This is for my friend Ted Kennedy—aye."

The final vote was 60–39. Jim Bunning (R-KY) did not vote. It was a huge victory for Barack Obama, and the Democrats were triumphant. The president said that after the House and Senate bills were reconciled in conference, "this will be the most important piece of social legislation since the Social Security Act passed in the 1930s, and the most important reform of our health-care system since Medicare passed in the 1960s."[15]

However, the House–Senate conference was no small matter. There were important differences between the House and Senate bills. House members were still insisting on a public option. Bart Stupak and the prolife contingent of the Democratic House had already rejected the segregated funds abortion solution passed by the Senate. The millionaire's tax was still the chief source of financing for the House bill while the Senate chose a combination of increased Medicare withholding and a tax on Cadillac plans. The House insisted on small penalties for individuals who did not comply with the mandate, while the Senate had raised the penalty to 2 percent of income. The House wanted to extract more money from the pharmaceutical industry, but the Senate felt obligated to uphold its part of the negotiated agreement.

Departing for Christmas recess, Democrats from both chambers understood they would face difficult negotiations upon their return. Little did they expect, during their brief aftertaste of victory, that the political calculus was about to change. How many of them had even heard of a relatively unknown state senator from Massachusetts by the name of Scott Brown?

# CHAPTER 17

# SUCCESS AT LAST

## "We'll Go Through the Gates"

The first signs of trouble may have come from the *Cook Political Report* early in January 2010. Analyzing the special election for Ted Kennedy's Senate seat, Cook changed the status of the race from "Solid Democratic" to "Leaning Democratic." Massachusetts Attorney General Martha Coakley had easily won the Democratic primary on December 8, and she was running against a little known state senator, Scott Brown. In the bluest of blue states, it was almost inconceivable that a Republican could win the Senate seat held by Kennedy for nearly forty-seven years.

On January 11, just eight days before the race, the *Boston Globe* still showed Coakley clinging to a fifteen-point lead, but other polls claimed the race was tighter. Sensing a possibility for a game-changing upset, Republicans began to pour millions of dollars into the campaign. Scott Brown was soon all over the media, wearing his signature brown barn jacket and storming around the state in his pickup truck. An attractive-looking candidate, Brown had done semi-nude modeling when he was a college student. More importantly, however, he held himself out to be the candidate to defeat Obama's health plan. In the state where Ted Kennedy made universal health care the issue of his life, Brown vowed to be the forty-first vote to kill health reform.

By January 15, a Suffolk University/Channel 7 News poll showed Brown with a shocking four-point lead. The Democrats were in panic mode. The Friday before the election, Bill Clinton campaigned for Coakley, and on Sunday, the president himself flew up to Boston in a last-ditch effort to save Coakley's floundering campaign. It was too late. In a stunning upset, Brown performed a reverse Harris Wofford, using his opposition to health reform to easily defeat Martha Coakley and to end the Democrats' sixty-vote veto-proof majority.

Before Brown's election, Democrats understood that compromises between the House and Senate versions of the bill were going to be difficult. Shortly after returning from Christmas recess, they made a stunning announcement. Instead of the traditional House–Senate conference committee normally employed to reconcile bills from the two chambers, Democrats would exclude Republicans from the process and conduct negotiations within their own caucus. They had made up their minds to go it alone. Convinced that they could not attract any Republican support, they feared Republicans would use the conference committee to propose endless amendments and delay the process. By themselves, they would quietly be able to work out the compromises that would satisfy their members in both chambers. Then, when they brought the final bill to the Senate, they would still have their sixty-vote super majority. Not anymore!

In the weeks that followed, Democrats were in disarray. The pundits speculated that Obama would give up on comprehensive health reform and settle for an incremental bill. Perhaps he would propose something limited, such as health coverage expansions for families with children—something modest that could attract a few Republican votes. That was what Rahm Emanuel was advising. Just as he had done a year before, he counseled the president to scale down his proposal to something they could get through the Congress—"to put some points on the board."

In the last week of January, there was speculation that the president was wavering, undecided whether to scale back his plan. But one person was not wavering at all. Nancy Pelosi was steadfast, deriding Obama's lesser options as "Kiddie Care."[1] In a determined speech, for someone not known to be an orator, she exhorted her colleagues to continue the fight. "We'll go through the gate," she exclaimed. "If the gate's closed, we'll go over the fence. If the fence is too high, we'll pole vault in. If that doesn't work, we'll parachute in, but we're going to get health care reform passed for the American people."

One way to pass health reform was for the House simply to pass the Senate bill. If that happened, the whole battle would be over. The Senate had already approved the bill and, if the House voted for it, Obama would simply have to sign it in to law. On January 19, anticipating Brown's victory, Obama met with Reid and Pelosi in the Oval Office to discuss that and other alternatives.[2] Pelosi told the president that the Senate bill was a "nonstarter" in the House. A few days later, she told the press that there were not sufficient votes in the House to pass the Senate bill in its present form.

However, Rahm Emanuel and White House Advisor Jim Messina had another strategy. The House could pass the Senate bill and then file a new "budget reconciliation bill," superseding some of the provisions in the Senate bill that they opposed. Under budget reconciliation, there could be no filibusters. Only provisions that had budgetary consequences could be included in the bill, but Democrats would only need a simple majority of fifty votes. Such a process would infuriate Republicans and open Democrats to a barrage of criticism. Yet the same process had been used several times by Republicans—most recently by George W. Bush to enact his tax cuts.

Nancy Pelosi began to sound out the members of her caucus while the president borrowed a strategy from the Clinton administration. He invited members of Congress to partake in a televised, bipartisan summit on health care. Republicans agreed to participate, and the upcoming event generated substantial publicity. Republicans wanted the discussions to start from scratch, but Obama insisted the starting point would be the bills already passed by the House and Senate. Moderating the discussion on his own terms, with a thorough command of the issues, Obama made a strong case for his plan. Some observers, including Chip Kahn, believe that this was a key turning point in the battle. The president, after being criticized for not taking command of the negotiations, began to exercise forceful leadership. After the summit, he traveled to several cities to rally support for reform. Events had started to turn his way.

An inadvertent boost had come from Anthem Blue Cross in California when they announced premium hikes of up to 39 percent in the first week in February. Outrage over the price hikes was widespread in the media. In response, Henry Waxman, chairman of the House Energy and Commerce Committee, required company executives to appear before Congress. Testimony revealed that Anthem had recorded $4.2 billion in profits the previous year and had spent twenty-seven million dollars in 2007 and 2008 on company retreats to lavish resorts.[3]

After the dim prospects of January following Scott Brown's election, momentum had suddenly begun to shift. Nancy Pelosi, one of the best vote counters ever to hold the Speaker's gavel, was picking up votes. Then, on March 3, Obama delivered a key speech from the East Room of the White House. Headlines reported his call for an up-or-down vote on health care reform, but that was not the crucial part of his speech. Obama gave the final confirmation that the Democrats would use reconciliation to pass the health bill. "I believe the United States Congress owes the American people a final vote on health care reform," the president said. "We have debated this issue thoroughly, not just for a year, but for decades. Reform has already passed the House with a majority. It has already passed the Senate with a supermajority of sixty votes. And now it deserves the same kind of up-or-down vote that was cast on welfare reform, the Children's Health Insurance Program, COBRA health coverage for the unemployed, and both Bush tax cuts—all of which had to pass Congress with nothing more than a simple majority."[4] The die was cast. Now the fate of health care reform depended on two eventualities: first, whether the Democrats could agree among themselves; and second, whether they could successfully employ the reconciliation strategy. The president had correctly recalled the times reconciliation had been used in the past, but it had never been used, or intended to be used, as a "pas de deux" to pass and then alter another piece of legislation.

## Who is Alan Frumin?

The *Seattle Times* described Alan Frumin as "a man you wouldn't recognize in a job you've never heard of."[5] Judd Gregg (R-NH) stated, "He's basically the defense, the prosecution, the judge, the jury, and the hangman in this scenario."[6] The scenario Gregg was referring to was the process of reconciliation to pass health care legislation. Whether and how that process could be used was up to one man, the Senate parliamentarian, an otherwise obscure political appointee by the name of Alan Frumin.

The United States Senate operates according to customs and precedents almost as much as it does by official rules. Procedural customs have been accumulating for over two hundred years, and few people in the Congress, or in the entire country, have a grasp of the arcane minutiae that governs the senior legislative body. As a result, in 1935, the Senate created the position of parliamentarian: the person who decides what procedures are allowed according to the rules and customs of the Senate.

Alan Frumin, a graduate of Georgetown Law, began working in the parliamentarian's office in 1977. He was appointed Senate parliamentarian in 1987 by Robert Byrd. When Republicans gained control of the Senate in

1995, they appointed his predecessor, Robert Dove, to the head position, and Frumin became the assistant parliamentarian. However, in 2001, the Republican majority leader, Trent Lott, wanted to add five billion dollars to the budget as a contingency fund for natural disasters. Dove disallowed the measure under the rules of reconciliation, undiplomatically labeling the leader's appropriation a "slush fund." Trent Lott immediately fired Dove and reappointed Frumin to the top spot. Only three other people preceded the combined twenty-nine-year tenure of Frumin and Dove, but Frumin is the only person ever appointed by both political parties.

The parliamentarian's office has been fiercely independent and has maintained a reputation for political fairness. As the sole arbiter of Senate procedure, it has also become quite powerful. Those characteristics much resemble the Congressional Budget Office, except that the director of the CBO cannot easily be fired. In the debate over health care and reconciliation in 2010, Alan Frumin's position was much like Robert Reischauer's in 2004. He was bound to make one side unhappy.

Neither the Democrats nor the Republicans considered Frumin an ally. Frumin had worried the Democrats when he told Kent Conrad (R-NC) that health care legislation "passed through the reconciliation process may end up looking like 'swiss cheese,' because certain provisions of a bill may survive while others are stricken."[7] However, he had also infuriated Tom Coburn and the Republicans during the Christmas debate in the Senate. As we earlier reported, when Coburn insisted that Bernie Sanders's entire 767-page single-payer amendment be read out loud, Sanders gave up and withdrew his amendment. Coburn then protested that the whole document still had to be read, even if Sanders wanted it withdrawn. Frumin ruled against him and was accused by Jim DeMint of being "clearly biased." Angering both sides, Frumin, like Reischauer in the CBO, had built a reputation for fairness. Robert Dove stated, "He's a very good man. He will call it straight. He will make all kinds of enemies."[8]

Reconciliation is governed by the Byrd Rule, which we explained in detail in chapter 2. Provisions under the Byrd Rule require only a fifty-one-vote majority. Every measure under reconciliation must directly impact the budget and be more germane to the budget than to policy. Debate is limited to twenty hours. After that time, an unlimited number of amendments may be introduced and put to a vote, but they cannot be debated.

Democrats were concerned about a number of procedural issues. Members in the House did not like a number of provisions in the Senate bill and had little trust that their Senate colleagues could guarantee a reconciliation bill would pass. They worried that if they voted for the Senate bill first, the Senate might then fail to pass the reconciliation bill, and they would be stuck with provisions they opposed. Hence, they wanted to pass the reconciliation bill before voting on the Senate bill. However, that could not be done.[9] Democrats also feared that if any provision was deemed improper under the Byrd Rule, the Senate would have to vote on the bill without the excised provision. If that occurred, the altered bill would have to go back to the House to undergo another close vote, a danger and delay Democrats wanted to avoid. Hence, leading up to the vote, Democrats had numerous meetings with Frumin, discussing the eligibility of various provisions. Those kind of prevote discussions are called "Byrd Baths," and any provisions that are stricken are called "Byrd Droppings."

Intending to challenge any measure that might be ruled improper, Republicans focused on the delay in implementing the Cadillac tax. Labor unions hated the tax and threatened to withdraw their support unless the tax was scaled back by the reconciliation bill. House members negotiated an agreement with their Senate counterparts to postpone the tax until 2018—a substantial compromise that reduced the ten-year proceeds of the tax from $149 billion to only $32 billion. If Alan Frumin labeled the provision a "Byrd Dropping," opposition from labor could kill the health care bill. However, Frumin ruled that the provision complied.

Another hurdle for the Democrats in the reconciliation process was the intention of Republicans to offer unlimited amendments. Although none could be debated, each amendment would require a vote and would delay the process. Such a delaying tactic is called "vote-o-rama," and Alan Frumin judged that its use was consistent with Senate rules. After the twenty hours of debate ended on Wednesday night, March 24, Republicans began to offer repeated amendments.

Some amendments were clearly intended to embarrass Democratic lawmakers. Tom Coburn introduced an amendment to bar the use of federal funds to cover the cost of erectile dysfunction drugs for convicted sex offenders. Such drugs are covered under most formularies without regard to the background of each insured individual. If Democratic senators approved the amendment, the reconciliation bill would have to go back to the House. If they rejected it, Coburn claimed, they would be forcing taxpayers to give convicted rapists and pedophiles erectile dysfunction medicine. Democrats held their nose and rejected the amendment by a vote of 57–42. Sharron Angle subsequently approved a television ad criticizing Harry Reid's vote on the amendment in her unsuccessful campaign to unseat him in the 2010 midterm election.

In the end, Frumin ruled two provisions out of order. However, they were both related to Pell Grants and education, not health reform, and although the reconciliation bill had to go back to the House, members approved it in short order.

## The President's Trifecta

After Obama's March 3 speech and their commitment to use reconciliation, the Democrats continued to gain momentum. On March 12, Nancy Pelosi met with the House Democratic caucus and predicted that health reform would pass within the next ten days. The president postponed a trip to Indonesia and Australia to help garner the final votes. The White House and the Democratic leadership were negotiating deals and bringing heavy pressure on their members to fall into line.

Meanwhile, the opposition was furious. Mitch McConnell accused the Democrats of "twisting themselves into pretzels" trying to pass a health reform bill that people hated. Republicans and their allies funded a multi-million dollar advertising campaign targeting forty House Democrats whose vote to support health reform might hurt their chances for reelection. A coalition led by the Chamber of Commerce had already spent eleven million dollars in the month of March and was expected to spend thirty million dollars by the end of the month.[10]

With victory seemingly within their grasp, Democrats and their supporters fought back. Continuing to beat up on insurance companies, they repeatedly used the message, "If insurance companies win, you lose." The pharmaceutical industry spent twelve million dollars on advertisements to support reform. Where Democrats could not afford to advertise, they used every available method of arm-twisting and persuasion. A New Jersey congressman, John Adler, had previously voted against the health bill. Supporters of reform organized a group of twelve clergy to meet with Adler's Rabbi, who promised to speak to Adler about his vote.[11]

The president was constantly active, meeting and telephoning wavering members. On March 15, he flew to Ohio to campaign in the districts of two wavering congressmen, Dennis Kucinich and John Boccieri. Kucinich, a leading liberal voice, was a single-payer advocate who had opposed the Obama version of health reform. The president invited Kucinich to travel with him on Air Force One for the flight to Ohio. Obama not only sought to convince the liberal lawmaker on the merits of the health bill, but also explained the danger to his presidency and the Democratic Party if the initiative was to fail. Barack Obama, in full campaign mode, was making an all-out, make-or-break effort to salvage health care reform.

On Wednesday, March 17, the president hit the trifecta. First, Dennis Kucinich reversed his position and announced his support of the bill. "We have to be very careful that the potential of President Obama's presidency not be destroyed by this debate," Kucinich stated. "Something is better than nothing.... If my vote is to be counted, let it count now for passage of the bill, hopefully in the direction of comprehensive health care reform."[12]

A second boost came from a broad coalition of Catholic nuns comprised of more than fifty Catholic women's orders and organizations. The coalition, claiming to represent over fifty-nine thousand nuns in the United States, sent a letter to Congress urging them to support the Senate bill. Referring to the bill's provisions to help the uninsured and pregnant women, the letter stated, "This is the real pro-life stance and we as Catholics are all for it."[13] A week earlier, Sister Carol Keehan, the president and CEO of the CHA, had also delivered a crucial endorsement. "This is a historic opportunity to make great improvements in the lives of so many Americans," she wrote.[14] Both endorsements were in direct contradiction to the US Conference of Catholic Bishops, which reaffirmed its opposition over the abortion language in the Senate bill and urged Congress to vote against the bill. Numerous pro-life Democrats had still been withholding support for the bill, and the nuns' support was a major event. Shortly after the letter was made public, Dale Kildee (D-MI), a key holdout on abortion, announced his support of the bill.

The third winner for Obama on March 18 was the much-anticipated report of the Congressional Budget Office. The CBO concluded that the Senate bill, together with the reconciliation bill, would reduce the deficit by $138 billion over ten years. That compared to a reduction of $118 billion in the original Senate bill. The figures were music to the ears of the Democratic leaders who were still negotiating with Blue Dog holdouts concerned about the bill's cost. Within a day of the announcement, two Blue Dogs, Bart Gordon (D-TN) and Betsy Markey (D-CO), announced their support of the bill.

The Democrats had overcome three big hurdles. Almost all the liberal holdouts, following Dennis Kucinich, were prepared to accept a bill that was less than they wanted. Pro-life Democrats remained split, but with endorsements from the nuns and the CHA, a number of former opponents had switched sides. And several budget-conscious Blue Dogs were sufficiently pleased with the CBO budget projections to voice their support.

Having confirmation from the CBO that their package would meet the president's budgetary requirements, Democrats finalized the reconciliation bill and introduced it on Thursday, March 19. Under House rules, debate on the bill could begin in seventy-two hours. The Democrats' long-sought vote on health reform would finally take place on Sunday, March 22. There was just one problem: the Democrats were still about six votes short.

## Bad for Bart

Once again, abortion rights became the deciding issue. Bart Stupak had delivered the final crucial House votes in November when the Democratic leadership accepted his restrictive amendment on abortion. Then, the Christmas Eve Senate vote was secured when Ben Nelson made his last minute compromise at an all-day negotiating session in Harry Reid's office. Now it was Stupak again who was withholding his support of the Senate bill. Stupak claimed to have ten or eleven prolife Democrats who would vote with him on the divisive issue. He may have lost a few after the nuns' endorsement, but Nancy Pelosi was not confident she had enough votes without his support.

Bart Stupak was going to be vilified either way. He told CBS News on March 18 that his life had become "a living hell."[15] He had stopped answering his telephone because of obscene calls and violent threats. Supporters of health reform, including devout Catholics, were telling him that the Senate bill ensured that no federal money could be used for elective abortions. Opponents were telling him the opposite, urging him to hold out for the language he had originally secured for the House bill. A century of effort to provide universal health care to Americans rested on his shoulders. Caught in the middle, and torn by conscience one day before the historic vote, Stupak finally agreed to a compromise position. The president would issue an executive order declaring that no federal money could be used for abortions (except in the case of rape, incest, or danger to the life of the mother), and Stupak would support the Senate bill.

Bart Stupak's support virtually assured passage of health care reform, but it essentially ended the congressman's political career. When he addressed the House during the final debate on Sunday, Randy Neugebauer (R-TX), shouting from the House floor, called him a "baby killer." Following the vote, he received numerous death threats and obscene phone calls. Recordings of bitter calls, such as the following, were made publicly available by CBS News: "Congressman Stupak, you baby-killing mother f—er…I hope you bleed out your a—, got cancer and die, you mother f—er," one man said in a message to Stupak.[16]

If Stupak ran for reelection, he would face challenges from both the Left and Right. The National Abortion Rights Action league promised to support his Democratic primary opponent. The Tea Party express began a $250,000 advertising campaign against him. On April 9, less than three weeks after the House vote, Bart Stupak, a nine-term congressman, announced he would retire at the end of his term.

## Polarized and Angry

For several months, polls had revealed that a slight majority of Americans opposed the health reform bill. Republicans claimed that the Democrats were not only subverting the will of the people, but doing so in a completely partisan manner without one Republican vote. Moreover, they were using the procedural budget tool of reconciliation, never intended to enact major legislation, to accomplish their goal. After government bailouts of the financial and auto industries and the huge economic stimulus package, conservatives were aghast that the Democrats were further expanding the role of government in the face of a huge impending budget deficit.

Despite their complaints, however, the Republican leadership saw their chances of stopping the huge health reform bill slipping away, and their reaction was angry. They continually derided the reform package as a government takeover of health care that the American people did not want. It was being shoved down their throats, Republicans claimed, by a party out of touch with the American people.

March of 2010 was a time when there was much anger and anxiety throughout the country. The recovery from the severe economic recession was achingly slow, and the unemployment rate still hovered around 10 percent. Many Americans had lost a good deal of their life savings as a result of the financial crisis, and homes were being foreclosed at a record pace. For some time, the anger emanating from the president's opponents in Washington had been resonating with anxious and dissatisfied citizens throughout the country and had spawned the nascent Tea Party movement. A grass roots movement, the Tea Party's core issues were mainstream: less government and lower taxes. The movement had no formal hierarchy, but the dominant voices came from conservative talk radio personalities such as Glenn Beck and Republican politicians such as Sarah Palin. The giant health reform package came to represent the kind of big government Tea Partiers adamantly opposed, and they came to Washington in droves to protest the legislation.

Like many protest movements, including those on the left, there was an angry fringe to the Tea Party protests. Signs could be seen around the Capitol reading "I didn't vote for the socialist," and "If Brown can't stop it, a Browning can," depicting a Browning handgun. On Saturday, one day before the vote, demonstrators derided Democratic House members on their way to a meeting with the president. Walking toward the Longworth House Office Building, Emanuel Cleaver (D-MO) was spit on and called a nigger. John Lewis (D-GA), a hero of the civil rights movement, also was called a nigger by angry protestors. Earlier, Barney Frank, the openly gay congressman from Massachusetts, had been subject to homophobic epithets.

There was some truth to Republican claims that were fueling the anger. Polls *did* show about half the American public opposed the legislation. The Democrats *were* using their majority and the reconciliation process to force through a bill that had no bipartisan support. The bill *did* represent a larger role for the government in health care, and it *would* be partially supported by higher taxes.

However, the Democrats saw it differently. They were convinced that opposition to the bill had been fueled by misinformation. Claims of death panels, socialized medicine, a government takeover of health care, a threat to seniors' Medicare benefits, and a huge addition to the deficit were all claims that were simply not true. They all had a kernel of truth, but they misrepresented the true nature of the bill. Furthermore, the Democrats believed that the real partisanship could be attributed to the minority. The Republicans, they argued, simply wanted to deny Democrats a victory for political reasons and would not have agreed to comprehensive reform regardless of the substance. With support from the representatives of doctors, hospitals, drug manufacturers, consumers, and the elderly, it was hardly believable that every single Republican opposed the bill for substantive reasons. Democrats believed they had formulated a mainstream bill that simply was being blocked by a politically motivated, filibustering minority. Rarely in recent American history had a political debate become so polarized.

## Success at Last

After Bart Stupak announced his support of the bill on Sunday, March 21, everyone knew that the battle was essentially over. Nancy Pelosi was sufficiently assured of her margin of victory that the only question was which Democrats she would permit to vote against the bill in order to help them with their reelections. Following the allowed two hours of debate, the House voted 219–212 to pass the bill that the Senate had approved on Christmas Eve. The Patient Protection and Affordable Care Act passed without a single Republican vote. Thirty-four Democrats voted nay. The act was the largest and most important piece of social legislation since Medicare and Medicaid were enacted in 1965.

Republicans were not about to cease their opposition. John Boehner (R-OH) said, "the American people are angry. This body moves forward against their will. Shame on us."[17] Virginia Foxx (R-NC) called the legislation "one of the most offensive pieces of social engineering legislation in the history of the United States."[18] Immediately after passage, the Republicans began to speak of repeal.

Democrats, on the other hand, were jubilant. For many, this was the culmination of nearly a century of effort. For the president, who had invested a huge amount of political capital, it was a historic achievement. On the evening of the vote, with Joe Biden by his side in the East Room of the White House, he spoke about the significance of the accomplishment to the American people: "In the end, what this day represents is another stone firmly laid in the foundation of the American dream. Tonight, we answered the call of history as so many generations of Americans have before us. When faced with crisis, we did not shrink from our challenge—we overcame it. We did not avoid our responsibility—we embraced it. We did not fear our future—we shaped it."[19]

After the House passed the Senate bill, it immediately passed its own reconciliation bill by a similar 220–211 vote. The Senate had to approve the reconciliation bill with a fifty-one-vote majority, and, as described earlier, Republicans utilized challenges and a series of amendments to block and/or delay the bill. Nevertheless, the health reform bill would be the law of the land whether or not the reconciliation bill was approved. In the end, Congress approved the bill, even though it had to go back to the House with minor changes.

On Tuesday, March 23, Barack Obama signed the bill into law. A crowd of nearly three hundred people attended the signing ceremony in the East Room of the White House. The president signed the legislation with twenty-two pens. Most went to congressional and executive branch supporters, but two were reserved for nongovernment individuals. Victoria Reggie Kennedy, the wife of the late senator, and Sister Carol Keehan of the CHA both received commemorative pens. The historic signing ceremony was marred by only one glitch, when a microphone recorded the vice president whispering in Barack Obama's ear, "Mr. President, this is a big f—ing deal."[20] The comment circulated immediately over the Internet and elicited a Twitter response from White House Press Secretary Robert Gibbs: "Yes, Mr. Vice President, you're right!"[21]

## The House–Senate Compromise—
## How Reconciliation Changed the Senate Bill

House Democrats had a comfortable majority, and they did not have to contend with the filibuster like their Senate colleagues. As a result, the leadership did not need to win over every member of its conservative branch, and the liberals exercised greater control. Their predilection would have been to finance a larger part of the health bill by taxing the rich, to increase subsidies to the poor to protect them from the individual mandate, and to curtail the power of private insurance companies. However, in their negotiations with the Senate, they had to confront two realities. First, only items directly impacting the budget could be included in reconciliation; and second, the Senate, which had to get every single one of its members to pass the bill, was not going to allow changes that would anger those who had reluctantly supported the bill at their own peril.

Speaker Pelosi had to walk a tight line. There were concessions she would have to get in order to assemble her 216-vote majority. At the same time, she knew she could not push the Senate too hard. But one thing was working in her favor. Democratic members of Congress knew they had to come to an agreement. If they failed, their majority, their committee chairmanships, and, perhaps, their careers were at stake.

The final legislation—the Senate bill combined with the reconciliation bill—raised the ten-year cost of the reform package from $871 to $940 billion. The CBO estimated that the combined package would reduce the deficit by $138 billion compared to a reduction of $132 billion under the Senate bill. Under the combined package, the CBO estimated that thirty-two million additional people would have health insurance, raising the percentage of legal nonelderly insured from 83 to 94 percent. This would leave about twenty-three million nonelderly residents uninsured—of which approximately one-third would be illegal immigrants. These coverage estimates are approximately the same as in the Senate bill. Following is a brief summary of the most important provisions of HR-4872, the Health Care and Education Reconciliation Act.

## Medicare Withholding Tax

The largest source of revenue for the increased cost of the bill came from raising and broadening the Medicare withholding tax. Max Baucus had raised the tax to 3.8 percent (1.9 percent each for employer and employee) in his manager's amendment. The withholding tax had always been confined to earned income, but the reconciliation bill broadened the tax to include unearned income (i.e., interest, dividends, annuities, and royalties). As in the Senate bill, only individual taxpayers earning over $200,000 or families earning over $250,000 are subject to the tax and only income above the threshold is taxed at those rates. Because it is generally wealthier people who have sources of unearned income, this tax change falls very heavily on the rich. With this provision, an estimated 74 percent of the tax proceeds supporting the bill will come from households earning over one million dollars and 91 percent from households earning over $500,000.[22] About 2.6 percent of households will pay the higher tax while 97.4 percent will be unaffected.[23] Indeed, the total impact of the president's health reform bill is strongly redistributive. Much of it is financed by the wealthy and much of the benefit accrues to the poor and uninsured. Proceeds from the Medicare withholding tax increase will yield $210 billion compared to $87 billion under the Senate bill.

## Medicare Advantage Plans[24]

The reconciliation bill derives sixteen billion dollars of additional savings from Medicare Advantage (MA) plans, bringing the total savings from lower MA payments to $136 billion. Reimbursement to MA plans will vary from 95 percent of the cost of traditional Medicare plans in high-cost areas to 115 percent in low-cost areas. The bill also requires MA plans to spend at least 80 to 85 percent of premiums on direct medical care. These provisions will reduce the competitiveness of MA plans, which had been generously subsidized, and will require some beneficiaries to switch from private MA plans to traditional Medicare.

## Donut Hole

The donut hole for Medicare prescription drugs will be closed by 2020. At that time Medicare beneficiaries will pay a 25 percent copayment for brand-name and generic drugs and Medicare will pay the balance. Beginning in 2011, drug companies will provide a 50 percent discount on brand-name drugs for those who fall into the donut hole. In 2010 a rebate of up to $250 was available to those who entered the donut hole.

## Cadillac Tax

One provision that reduces revenue is the Cadillac tax. Under pressure from unions, public employees, high-risk employers, and high-cost states, the Democrats agreed to postpone the tax until 2018. That reduces the ten-year proceeds from $149 billion to thirty-two billion dollars. The democrats did manage to keep the 40 percent tax relatively intact, but whether it will ever take effect remains to be seen.

## Industry Fees

Increased fees are required from pharmaceutical manufacturers, device manufacturers, and health insurance providers. The fees will provide $107 billion compared to $101 billion under the Senate plan.

## Subsidies and Tax Credits

The reconciliation bill provides increased tax credits for individuals earning up to 400 percent of poverty and increased subsidies in the insurance exchanges for those earning less than 250 percent of poverty. The definition of income is modified for the purposes of eligibility for Medicaid, premium subsidies, and tax credits. The modification effectively changes the national eligibility threshold for Medicaid from 133 to 138 percent of poverty.

## Employer and Individual Mandates

Employers' penalty for not providing insurance is increased to $2,000 per employee from the greater of $750 or 2 percent of wages. However, in an effort to help small businesses, the first thirty full-time employees are exempted (so a firm with fifty employees could be penalized only for twenty of them).

Penalties for noncompliance with the individual mandate were modified by reconciliation. The fixed dollar amounts of the penalties are reduced from $495 in 2015 and $750 in 2016 to $325 and $695, respectively. However, under the Senate bill, the penalty was the greater of the fixed amount or 2 percent of income. The reconciliation bill gradually increases that percentage to 2.5 percent. The overall effect is to make the penalties more progressive.

## Medicaid

The federal government will reimburse the states for 100 percent of their costs of providing services to individuals newly insured under the legislation for the years 2014–2016. Then, the reimbursement rate will gradually decline to 90 percent by 2020 and remain at that rate thereafter. The "Cornhusker Kickback" was expunged from the bill.

## Dependent Children

Beginning six months after enactment, adult children will be eligible for family coverage up to age twenty-six. Underwriting practices for this age group, such as lifetime limits and rescissions of coverage, will be prohibited.

# CHAPTER 18

# HOW HE DID IT
## A POLITICAL STRATEGY
## LEARNED FROM HISTORY

Make no mistake. Without a significant Democratic majority in Congress, Barack Obama would not have passed comprehensive health care reform. It was easier for Republicans, who could always attract some Democratic support. Yet Republicans were often divided because the public perceived health reform as a Democratic issue. Hence, Richard Nixon's universal health proposals attracted many Democrats, but not a sufficient number to overcome opposition within his own party. When Ronald Reagan enacted Medicare Catastrophic and George W. Bush added Medicare prescription drugs, there were enough Democratic votes to prevail over Republican opponents. FDR had huge majorities in 1935, but not enough to propose universal health care and risk his Social Security program. Truman also had majorities, but both FDR and Truman had to contend with the southern wing of their own party that feared health reform would force them to integrate southern hospitals. Medicare was defeated for six consecutive years and would have failed again if LBJ had not run up huge Democratic majorities with his lopsided defeat of Barry Goldwater. Bill Clinton had substantial majorities, but with fifty-seven senators, he could not overcome Republican filibusters, and his health plan never garnered bipartisan support. With a filibuster-proof majority, Obama had to contend only with his own caucus. However, that only made success exceedingly difficult instead of virtually impossible.

It seemed so unlikely that Obama could overcome all these obstacles that our working title when we began this book was "Failure Again." Yet the president learned many lessons from the successes and failures of his predecessors. He crafted a strategy that seemed questionable at times and doomed on more than one occasion, but he ultimately prevailed. We now examine the major elements of his political strategy.

## Strike Early

Lyndon Johnson believed that the height of his power would occur immediately after his election, and after that, it would only decline. As we reported, Medicare was at the top of his domestic agenda, and he instructed his team to move quickly. Bill Clinton intended to copy LBJ's example but ended up doing just the opposite. The timeline for the Clinton health reform effort was pushed back repeatedly as Ira Magaziner drew up an extremely complex plan. Clinton also let other issues intervene, such as gays in the military and tax increases to eliminate the deficit. By the time Clinton introduced his bill, his presidency had been weakened by scandal and controversy.

Obama's goal was to have congressional votes on health reform before his first summer recess. He had the benefit of an early start because the primary campaign required him to outline his basic plan. Congressional and industry groups began working on reform plans prior to his inauguration. However, like Clinton, he was delayed by intervening events: the financial crisis, the bank bailout, and the subsequent stimulus bill. He also experienced lengthy delays by congressional committees as they tried to craft compromise legislation and gain bipartisan support. Several deadlines were missed, and the chances for success deteriorated as opposition groups coalesced. Nevertheless, had he not started the process immediately after his nomination, the delays likely would have been worse. Despite a number of setbacks, he was able to pass bills through both houses of Congress before his first Christmas recess. Had that process been postponed at all—even until Congress reconvened in January—it is quite likely the effort would have failed.

## Get Congressional Buy-in

Lyndon Johnson, a former Senate majority leader, was a master at manipulating the Congress. As we saw in chapter 5, he knew his biggest hurdle was Wilbur Mills and the House Ways and Means Committee. Johnson encouraged Mills to take all the credit for Medicare, calling the legislation the Mills bill, and telling the congressman that it would be the signature achievement of his career. Bill Clinton, again, did the opposite. Formulating his complex health proposal in the White House instead of developing it within the Congress was a fatal mistake. Not only did Congress fail to buy in to his plan, but there was resentment from members of his own party who felt excluded from the process.

In contrast to Clinton, Obama outlined his general principles and let five congressional committees formulate their own bills. Throughout most of 2009 he was criticized by many for weak leadership, letting congressional debate drag on for many months instead of taking charge and setting forth the details he wanted. One can certainly make a case that he could have pushed the congressional leadership to act more quickly. Nevertheless, when the final votes were needed, both Speaker Pelosi and Majority Leader Reid had worked through the committee process and built strong coalitions. The Democratic Congress held together tighter than almost anyone predicted and eked out an unlikely victory.

## Maintain Flexibility and the Ability to Compromise

Throughout the long battle, Obama stubbornly refused to be tied down to specific positions. Both wings of his party pushed him to take a position on the public option, but by staying vague, he did not alienate either side. When his initial financing plan was rejected, he accepted other alternatives. When it became clear that he needed to support an individual mandate in order to get insurance reform, he publicly abandoned the well-publicized position he had defended during the primary campaign.

Ronald Reagan inspired people with his principles, but rarely got bogged down in details. When Reagan needed to pass Medicare Catastrophic, he made large concessions to the Democrats. By contrast, again, Bill Clinton stuck too long to a specific plan that many people did not like.

By avoiding a commitment to specific positions, Obama was able to make the compromises he needed to garner sufficient support. Some criticized his lack of specificity as an example of weak leadership. Yet LBJ, whose strength of leadership was never questioned, was confident enough to quietly exercise his power behind the scenes and let Wilbur Mills and Congress determine the details of Medicare and Medicaid.

## Build on the Current System and Minimize Change

If there was one clear lesson from the failure of the Clinton plan, this was it. Powerful interests built on the status quo are apt to be threatened by change.

And people who are satisfied and familiar with their current arrangements are bound to resist the new and unfamiliar. We saw how Clinton's managed competition plan would have made profound changes in the industry and would have changed the way virtually every individual would purchase insurance or receive medical care. In contrast, Obama's plan minimized the amount of change. It built on the employer-based system and the private market for health insurance, supplemented by existing public programs such as Medicare and Medicaid. Many recommended substantial changes in the delivery system to make the system more efficient and cost effective. Obama acknowledged those ideas, but wisely chose less far-reaching reforms by funding trials and demonstrations. Obama stated repeatedly, "If you like the insurance you have, you can keep it." The claim was a slight exaggeration, but the great majority of insured Americans will likely keep their existing coverage.

## Work with Stakeholders and Special Interests

Special interests had been the bane of health policy proposals for nearly a century. We saw how the AMA opposed universal insurance as early as Teddy Roosevelt and gave tacit support for smoking in an attempt to derail Medicare. Insurance companies campaigned against every comprehensive reform proposal, as did most business groups. Other health interests, such as pharmaceutical companies, device manufacturers, and hospitals, helped defeat a number of reform initiatives. Conservative political groups opposed nearly any proposal that increased the government role in health care, whereas liberals and labor unions opposed universal proposals that were not single-payer.

Perhaps the key element in the Obama strategy was to bring all the interest groups to the table and to make compromises and deals that would gain their support. Obama knew how the "Harry and Louise" campaign and other interest group strategies had helped defeat the Clinton plan. He also observed how George W. Bush, under different circumstances, had promulgated generous deals with interest groups to help pass the Medicare prescription drug benefit.

## Do Not Attempt to Expand Access and Cut Costs at the Same Time

In a perfect world, a comprehensive health reform proposal would focus on controlling costs as well as expanding access. The Obama plan has been severely criticized for focusing almost exclusively on access and providing only small initiatives to "bend the cost curve." The criticism is undoubtedly valid, but, of course, we do not live in a perfect world. Every dollar of reduced cost is a dollar of reduction in somebody's income. That somebody's organization will lobby against the plan, often spending considerable resources to fund the opposition. When Bill Clinton's managed competition morphed into managed competition within a global budget, it threatened to limit revenues across the health system and was opposed throughout the industry.

Ultimately, one has to decide whether his or her preferred approach, which might be politically impossible, is better or worse than a less ideal alternative that is more likely doable. John McDonough, one of the organizers of Kennedy's Workhorse Group, was a long-time advocate of single-payer until he realized that all of his efforts had "not succeeded in getting health insurance to a single person."[1] McDonough later became one of the architects of Massachusetts's universal health plan, on which the Obama plan was largely based. Massachusetts made the politically expedient decision to expand access first and deal with cost control later. The access initiative was an unparalleled success, insuring over 97 percent of the state's residents. As of this writing, the state has not yet developed a program of cost control, although several commissions have recommended substantial changes in both the payment and delivery of health care services.

There is no correct answer as to whether Obama's strategy to largely avoid cost control was preferable even though it certainly was less than ideal. It is the opinion of these authors that comprehensive health reform and near-universal coverage would have been impossible to enact if substantial cost control were included. Given the political realities, we believe Obama's strategy was necessary. Nevertheless, there is a clear and evident danger. If Obama, or a subsequent administration, cannot follow up with a reasonably effective way to control cost, the system could fail and his apparent success will have been short-lived.

## Employ All Available Tools—Reconciliation

The president and the Democratic Party expected there would be Republican opposition to health care reform and that opponents might use the filibuster to defeat legislation. Realizing they might not be able to commandeer sixty votes to break a filibuster, they considered a fallback option: using budget reconciliation to help enact health reform.

As you may recall, the Clinton administration wanted to use reconciliation for health reform, but there was formidable opposition—including that of Robert Byrd. Since that time, however, George W. Bush used the tactic on several occasions, including both tax cuts. Many considered those uses improper, since the tax cuts were not paid for, and the purpose of reconciliation was to make it easier to enact legislation that reduced the budget deficit.

President Bush's use (or abuse, as some would say) of reconciliation made it politically more acceptable for Obama to reserve the option—particularly since his health bill would reduce the budget deficit. In order for a bill to be brought to the floor under reconciliation, it must first be specified in the president's budget resolution. Obama took a firm stand early in his presidency and included reconciliation in his first budget resolution. It was an early indication that he was willing to engage in tough partisan politics to fight for health care reform. The budget resolution for fiscal 2010 was passed by both houses of Congress in April 2009 without a single Republican vote.

## Public Relations Matters: Hone Your Message to the Majority and the Middle Class

Barack Obama understood that he had to focus his appeal to the public's self-interest. The 85 percent of the people who had health insurance were not going to support comprehensive reform only to help the 15 percent who were uninsured. Polls showed that most people favored universal coverage, but not if they incurred a personal cost. The majority was simply not that altruistic. Maybe in war. Possibly in some national emergency. But not to pass expensive and complex health legislation. And not when opponents were warning of death panels and a government takeover of medical care.

The president had to give them reasons why his health initiative would help them, the majority who were already insured. Hence, his speeches rarely focused on covering the uninsured. He knew insured people were afraid of losing their coverage if they became sick, unemployed, or changed jobs. Therefore, he honed his message to assuage those fears. He promised that insurance companies could no longer refuse to cover preexisting conditions, could no longer cap the amounts of coverage, and could no longer terminate coverage except in the case of fraud. Keeping in mind Bill Clinton's popular phrase, "insurance that can never be taken away," he repeatedly reassured people that if they liked their coverage they would be able to keep it.

## Maintain Determination and Commitment

Every political battle has its own unique characteristics and challenges. How much of Obama's strategies can be applied to future legislative efforts is not known. Nevertheless, there is one distinguishing characteristic of this epic political battle: the president never wavered in his commitment and determination to enact a comprehensive bill.

At numerous junctures, his closest advisors urged him to abandon or scale back the effort. Rahm Emanuel and Joe Biden warned him from the beginning that a protracted battle for health care reform could destroy the rest of his agenda. Emanuel urged him to propose incremental reforms that could be pushed quickly through Congress "to put points on the board."

The president understood that his determination exposed him to enormous political risk. He was constantly reminded how the failure of the Clinton plan led to the Republican takeover of Congress. Many observers contended that if the health care initiative failed, the Democrats would be defeated in the midterm elections and Obama would be a one-term president. As the battle went on through the summer of 2010, the polls turned against him. With the pundits predicting almost certain defeat, Obama held firm and renewed his efforts. Repeating a strategy employed by Bill Clinton, he called for a joint session of Congress on September 9 to deliver a rousing speech on his health care proposal.

> I understand that the politically safe move would be to kick the can further down the road—to defer reform one more year, or one more election, or one more term. But that's not what the moment calls for. That's not what we came here to do. We did not come here to fear the future. We came here to shape it.[2]

Then, after January 19, when Scott Brown stunned the Democrats by winning Ted Kennedy's seat and ending the Democrats' veto-proof majority, the pundits predicted the battle was over. The odds against success seemed virtually insurmountable. Rahm Emanuel again advised the president to cut his losses—to settle for an incremental package of reforms. Yet again, the president persevered. In his State of the Union message eight days later, Obama reiterated his commitment to comprehensive reform:

> Here's what I ask Congress, though: Don't walk away from reform. Not now. Not when we are so close. Let us find a way to come together and finish the job for the American people. Let's get it done. Let's get it done.[3]

Reasonable people can differ about the pros and cons of Obama's political strategy. In the end, however, he accomplished what like-minded Democrats had failed to do for one hundred years. Few can argue that his absolute commitment and dogged determination were not crucial factors in his eventual success.

# CHAPTER 19

# THE FUTURE IS COST CONTROL

## Changing the Systems for Health Care Delivery and Finance

The passage of the Obama Plan is a major step in reforming the US health care system. However, cost and affordability still loom as major challenges. Government, private employers, and individuals will rebel against the increasing costs of health care if further reform is not forthcoming. Health care premiums for employer-based insurance already costs over 18 percent of family income, and, at current trends, will consume 24 percent by 2020.[1]

Although the Obama health plan largely avoided measures that would "bend the cost curve," there were a number of initiatives that could reduce spending growth over time. Some of those that involved significant changes in health care delivery and finance were in the form of demonstration projects. Such programs provided a way for the administration to experiment with system change without incurring opposition from consumers or from the health care industry. The Obama plan creates a federal innovation center that will award demonstration grants to develop innovative new forms of health care financing and delivery. The center is authorized to spend up to one billion dollars per year over the next ten years. In addition to demonstration projects, some regulatory changes were instituted that may reduce cost growth, but might also encounter strong political opposition. We briefly explore the most important initiatives.

### Primary Care and Prevention

The Obama plan includes a number of provisions that will experiment with more integrated and coordinated systems of care. The focus of these provisions is to organize care around primary care doctors who coordinate their patients' entire range of health care services. These models emphasize prevention, wellness, and the use of evidence-based medicine.

Currently, the US health care system is not coordinated around primary care and does not provide sufficient incentives for doctors to practice primary care medicine. Primary care is among the lowest paid specialties in the country. The earnings of specialists averaged almost $340,000 in 2008, whereas primary care doctors had average earnings of $186,000.[2] As a result, there is a serious shortage of primary care physicians. The Obama plan includes $168 million to train five hundred new primary care physicians by 2015. However, this is only a small down payment to ameliorate the shortage of 33,100 primary care physicians.[3] The plan also includes a 10 percent bonus for five years for primary care Medicare providers and increased pay for primary care Medicaid providers in 2013 and 2014.

Most primary care physicians are paid on a fee-for-service basis. Consequently, they are not paid for coordinating care among other providers, a critical element in managing chronic care. Estimates suggest that 95 percent of Medicare spending is for chronic care patients.[4] As we noted in previous chapters, policy experts have recommended replacing fee-for-service with capitated systems of payment since 1915. President Nixon encouraged the creation of Health Maintenance Organizations and enacted the HMO Act in 1973. Under a capitated system, health insurance plans are responsible (at their own financial risk) for all of a patient's health needs, and they do not generate increased income by providing more services. They also have an incentive to provide preventive services and well-care to keep patients healthy.

The Obama plan links primary care incentives with increased funding for preventive services. It eliminates cost sharing for proven preventive services for all insurance plans, both public and private. It also establishes a public health investment fund to provide grants to state and local governments, community based organizations, and employer wellness programs for preventive health initiatives.

Aware that capitated managed care plans produced a consumer backlash in the '90s, the Obama administration sought to avoid some of the practices that were unpopular. Hence, in the two initiatives that follow, patients are not limited to a closed network of doctors, and payment options include "shared savings" as well as partial capitation.

## Patient-Centered Medical Home (PCMH)

The idea of a patient-centered medical home has been around for many
years. The American Academy of Pediatrics introduced the term "medical
home" in 1967.[5] It builds on the concept that each patient should have access
to a primary care physician and a system that provides all necessary and
appropriate care in a coordinated and efficient manner. Such care should
emphasize preventive services supported by up-to-date and complete medical information. Research studies have demonstrated that such an approach
used in other countries, and in a limited number of places in the United
States, increases patient satisfaction, health, and longevity.[6] There is also evidence that increased use of primary care results in reduced hospitalizations
and specialist's services and improvements in morbidity and mortality rates.[7]
Most primary care in the United States does not meet the criteria to qualify
as a PCMH. Research indicates that each year an average Medicare beneficiary sees two primary care physicians and five specialists working in four different practices.

## Accountable Care Organizations (ACOs)

The CMS define an ACO as "an organization of health care providers that
agrees to be accountable for the quality, cost, and overall care of Medicare
beneficiaries who are enrolled in the traditional fee-for-service program."[8]
Ideally, ACOs will be organized around primary care providers, but multi-
specialty physician groups, hospital-based physicians, and community
hospitals can all contract and qualify as ACOs. Regardless of form, such
organizations will develop mechanisms to coordinate and integrate all types
of services including primary, specialty, hospital, and posthospital care. Such
integration can be accomplished through a single organization that has the
capacity to provide all needed care or through some form of virtual integration where separate groups work together to coordinate all patient services. Regardless of structure, however, patients will be able to choose any
provider and not be limited to those in the ACO; thus avoiding one of the
flashpoints that produced the managed care backlash.

The government will provide financial incentives for ACOs to provide
all of a patient's health needs but will avoid capitation, which also caused
consumer dissatisfaction in the '90s. Instead, it will pay providers on a fee-

for-service basis that is supplemented by a "shared savings" program. If the ACO spends less than a regional benchmark, all members of the organization will share in a portion of the savings. If, on the other hand, an ACO fails to generate the expected savings, providers will earn less. The amount of shared savings will also depend on an ACO's performance in meeting designated quality measures. Such a structure will remove the incentive to reduce cost by lowering quality. As opposed to capitation, the shared savings approach minimizes the downside losses if a group fails to achieve its benchmark, but it also limits the upside potential. Some analysts question whether the financial incentives of the shared savings approach will be sufficient to attract independent physicians and other providers.[9] Unlike many initiatives in the Obama plan, the ACO option is already authorized by legislation and is not simply a demonstration program. The legislation also permits the government to experiment with other payment approaches, such as partial capitation. Some provider groups would accept the greater risk of partial capitation for the possibility of earning greater returns. Although ACOs have many similarities to the managed care organizations of the '90s, a major difference is that they are organized around doctors and do not involve an insurance company intermediary.

### Regulatory Measures

The Obama plan includes several regulatory measures that we have previously mentioned, all of which have the potential to reduce the rate of increase in health spending. Three of the most important initiatives are the tax on high-deductible health plans, the requirement that insurance plans spend a minimum proportion of premiums on direct patient care (medical loss ratio), and the Independent Payment Advisory Board (IPAB). All three initiatives are controversial, opposed by numerous stakeholders, and a target of the Republican Congress as we go to press.

The reconciliation bill postponed the tax on high cost Cadillac health plans due to labor union and political opposition. Many economists favor the proposal, although it might be more effective if it were based on the benefit package instead of the cost. Currently delayed until 2018, the survival of this policy is uncertain.

Regulating the medical loss ratio has encountered strong opposition from the insurance industry. It is also seen as one of the most intrusive federal regulations of private business. Strong stakeholder opposition could water down or eliminate the regulation.

The IPAB is the strongest tool in the Obama health plan to limit cost increases. It establishes the Medicare target growth spending rate in 2018 as the average previous five-year increase in GDP plus one percentage point. For example, if GDP grows at an average of 3 percent, the target will be 4 percent. If Medicare spending growth exceeds the target, which it has over much of the last ten years, the board will issue recommendations to reduce the growth rate down to the target or cut it by a minimum of 1.5 percentage points.

Budget hawks see IPAB as an effective mechanism to slow health care spending. Peter Orszag, the former director of Obama's OMB, suggested that IPAB could become one of the most important components of the health reform law.[10] However, many conservatives attack IPAB as another expansion of government control of the health sector. James Capretta, a fellow at the Ethics and Public Policy Center in Washington, DC, called it "government-driven managed care."[11] Capretta argues that the IPAB will mostly employ cuts in payment rates to providers, a tool that Congress has generally been reluctant to impose for any length of time.

Some liberals also oppose the policy. They contend it will take the power of overseeing the Medicare program away from Congress and the president. Moreover, they fear that the mandated reductions will ultimately lead to a deterioration of Medicare services. Most medical provider groups share this concern. As we noted earlier, hospitals, which are the largest cost center in the health care industry, were able to secure a ten-year exemption from IPAB payment reductions. At this time, the implementation and potential impact of the IPAB is uncertain.

All of the initiatives described in this chapter constitute a fairly ambitious agenda to experiment with change without forcing large-scale, untried policies on the entire system. This is a reasonable course of action considering the political obstacles and the fact that no one has a proven strategy to reduce health care cost growth. Nevertheless, even if all these strategies bear fruit, they are not enough, in themselves, to sufficiently alter the long-term growth trend in health care spending.

# EPILOGUE

The historical development of the American health care system reflects the political culture of the country. Unlike many industrial countries in Europe and other parts of the world, Americans place a high value on the private marketplace, insist on limited government, and support a pluralistic society that tolerates a wide range of political and industrial interest groups. As a result, America's health care system is built upon the private market. Doctors, hospitals, health insurance plans, pharmaceutical companies, and medical device and supply companies are nearly all private and are powerful political and economic players.

Health care, however, is not like other commercial products. Any country's private health system needs substantial government involvement, if only to provide access to care for over a quarter of a typical population that includes the aged, poor, disabled, and mentally ill. As the capabilities and the cost of medicine advanced in the twentieth century, the gaps in our private, insurance-based system became more apparent. Hence, we added the Hill–Burton requirements in the '40s and Medicaid in the '60s to care for the poor. We added Medicare in the '60s to care for the aged and disabled, and we added the SCHIP program in 1997 to care for children. When the capabilities and cost of pharmaceuticals advanced in the latter part of the twentieth century, we added a prescription drug benefit to Medicare. When kidney dialysis and retroviral drug treatments became available, we added coverage for end-stage renal disease and AIDS.

The result was a piecemeal system that divided care along age and income, along inpatient and outpatient settings, and divided insurance coverage among private companies, the states, and the federal government. This piecemeal growth made it difficult to enact universal health insurance and nearly impossible to control costs.

By the time Barack Obama was elected president, the United States was the only industrialized country in the world that failed to provide universal health care to all of its citizens. At the same time, it was, by far, the costliest health care system in the world. Amidst much controversy, President Obama finally succeeded in the century-long struggle to enact universal (actually, near-universal) health care. Despite rhetoric to the contrary, the framework of the Obama plan is built on the same mainstream policies that have been proposed by Democrats and Republicans since Richard Nixon. America was not going to enact a government-controlled, single-payer system, and no one has ever constructed a system based on tax credits that would achieve universality.

The cost of the Obama plan is close to one trillion dollars over ten years. Indeed, this is a substantial amount of money. However, it is necessary to consider the total amount of US health spending and the size of the US economy to have any perspective on that number. Because most of the cost of the legislation will be financed by reductions in future spending increases from various parts of the health care industry (not premiums, nor taxes, nor out-of-pocket spending by individuals), the net increase in health spending from the Obama plan will be about $300 billion over ten years. Over that ten-year period, spending is expected to increase only two-tenths of one percent faster than it would have without the plan.[1]

However, those numbers obscure the looming crisis. It is not the increased spending from the Obama plan that is the major problem—it is the amount the United States will spend on health care exclusive of the plan that demands our attention. Government spending for health is a particular concern. Health spending already accounts for about 20 percent of the entire federal budget, higher than Social Security or defense. Unless major changes are made, spending for health will continue to grow faster than GDP and crowd out other national priorities. However, the powerful forces that drive health care spending will continue with or without the Obama health plan.

Experts agree that the largest factors driving health costs are advances in technology and the ever-increasing capabilities of modern medicine. We will spend money to cure the diseases of tomorrow with capabilities that we can barely imagine today. Government and private insurance will continue to shield consumers from the full cost of the services they receive, and, like people anywhere, consumers will want access to the new and costly treatments that will sustain their health and prolong their lives. And we will continue to be a wealthy society. Wealthy countries, like wealthy individuals, will choose to devote a substantial portion of income to keep their citizens alive and well. However, even wealthy countries have their limits. Many Americans may not accept the sacrifices that are inevitable when health care consumes over 20 percent of our national income.

As a result, the future of health care policy will be all about controlling cost. The Obama plan is only a first, small step in experimenting with various ways to alter our systems of health care delivery and finance. As we reported, the '70s and early '80s was a period in which the United States attempted to control health costs through regulation. Then, in the mid-1980s and much of the '90s, policy makers encouraged market competition. Both methods yielded early successes, but were eventually overrun by the relentless pressures for more complex and more expensive health care. Throughout those attempts, liberals favored regulatory controls by government, and conservatives favored competition in the private market. In the future, we will need both.

After a century of attempts, we have joined the rest of the industrialized world in providing access to health care for nearly all of our citizens. Now it is incumbent upon us to join together as a nation and lead the world in discovering an equitable, humane, and efficient way to contain health care costs.

# ENDNOTES

## Introduction

1. Office of News and Public Information, News from the National Academies, "Health Insurance Essential for Health and Well-Being, Report Says; Action Urgently Needed from President and Congress to Solve Crisis of the Uninsured," February 24, 2009, http://www8.nationalacademies.org/onpinews/newsitem.aspx?RecordID=12511 (accessed December 28, 2010).

2. Jack Hadley, "Sicker and Poorer: The Consequences of Being Uninsured," *Report Prepared for the Kaiser Commission on Medicaid and the Uninsured*, May 2002, http://www.kff.org/uninsured/upload/Sicker-and-Poorer-The-Consequences-of-Being-Uninsured-Executive-Summary.pdf (accessed December 28, 2010).

3. Rasmussen Reports, "On Health Care, 51% Fear Government *More Than Insurance Companies*" (emphasis mine), August 10, 2009, http://www.rasmussenreports.com/public_content/politics/current_events/healthcare/august_2009/on_health_care_51_fear_government_more_than_insurance_companies# (accessed August 20, 2009).

## Prologue

1. World Health Organization, "The World Health Organization's Ranking of the World's Health Systems," 2000, http://www.photius.com/rankings/healthranks.html (accessed April 8, 2010).

2. A robust risk pool is a characteristic of insurance markets that we discuss in chapter 1.

# PART I: THE HARD ROAD TO SUCCESS

## Chapter 1: Nixon Comes Close

1. Flint Wainess, "The Ways and Means of National Health Care Reform, 1974 and Beyond," *Journal of Health Politics, Policy and Law* 24, no. 2 (1999): 310.

2. David Blumenthal and James Morone, *The Heart of Power: Health and Politics in the Oval Office* (Berkeley: University of California Press, 2009), p. 242.

3. Richard D. Lyons, "A Legislative Goal that Has No Foes Stalled by Differences in Approach," *New York Times*, August 27, 1974.

4. Stan Jones, telephone interview by the authors, August 19, 2009.

5. Ibid.

6. Jill Quadano and Debra Street, "Antistatism in American Welfare State Development," in Julian Zelizer, *Taxing America: Wilbur D. Mills, Congress and the State, 1945–1975* (Cambridge: Cambridge University Press, 1999), p. 331.

7. We discuss Nixon's attempts at regulation and cost control at length in chapter 9.

8. Nixon Library, "White House Central File, Subject File Domestic Council: Box 5 (October 1973–December 1973)," quoted in Blumenthal and Morone, *Heart of Power*, p. 238.

9. Blumenthal and Morone, *Heart of Power*, p. 247.

10. The term *HMO* is often used indiscriminately to refer to any kind of managed care. However, today most Americans are not enrolled in prepaid plans but are instead enrolled in looser forms of managed care organizations (MCOs), such as preferred provider organizations (PPOs) or point of service plans (POSs). We will use HMOs as a general term for various forms of managed care.

11. Janet Adamy, "End of Life Provision Loses Favor." *Wall Street Journal*, August 13, 2009, http://online.wsj.com/article/SB125012322203627701.html (accessed August 25, 2009).

12. Kaiser Family Foundation, "Employer Health Benefits, 2008 Annual Survey," Exhibit 5.1, http://ehbs.kff.org/?page=charts&id=1&sn=4&p=1 (accessed August 12, 2009).

13. Ibid.

14. Wainess, "Ways and Means," p. 308.

15. Kaiser Family Foundation, "Employer Health Benefits, 2010 Annual Survey," Exhibit 4.4, http://ehbs.kff.or/?page=charts&id=1&sn=4&ch=1534 (accessed December 16, 2010).

16. Pete McCloskey, "Crises in Both Parties: The 'party of Lincoln' and Sen. Thurmond." *San Francisco Chronicle*, December 19, 2002, http://www.sfgate.com/cgi-bin/article.cgi?f=/c/a/2002/12/19/ED66198.DTL (accessed June 13, 2009).

17. Richard Nixon, "Special Message to Congress Proposing a National Health Strategy, February 18, 1971," in the *American Presidency Project*, ed. John T. Woolley and Gerhard Peters, http://www.presidency.ucsb.edu/ws/index.php?pid=3311&st=Nixon&st1=health (accessed June 14, 2009).

18. Blumenthal and Morone, *Heart of Power*, p. 236.

19. Memorandum from Stuart Altman to Casper Weinberger, prepared by Peter Fox, April 16, 1973.

20. Memorandum by Peter Fox to Melvin R. Laird, October 3, 1973.

21. US Department of Health and Human Services, Agency for Healthcare Research and Quality: Center for Financing, Access and Cost Trends, *Medical Expenditure Panel Survey-Insurance Component, 1998 and 2008*, http://www.meps.ahrq.gov/mepsweb/survey_comp/Insurance.jsp (accessed June 12, 2009).

22. Ibid.

23. Susan Jaffe, "Tax Debate," Health Affairs, Health Policy Brief, 2009, http://www.healthaffairs.org/healthpolicybriefs/brief.php?brief_id=7 (accessed June 14, 2009).

24. Prospective reimbursement means that providers receive a fixed amount according to the medical condition being treated as opposed to fee-for-service in which they are paid for each service and procedure.

25. Richard Nixon, "Special Message to Congress Proposing a Comprehensive Health Insurance Plan, February 6, 1974," in the *American Presidency Project*, ed. John T. Woolley and Gerhard Peters, http://www.presidency.ucsb.edu/ws/?pid=4337 (accessed June 15, 2009).

26. Stan Jones, telephone interview by the authors, August 19, 2009.

27. Ibid.

28. Ibid.

29. This conclusion drawn by the authors based on the contents of Wainess, "Ways and Means," pp. 318–21.

30. Stan Jones, telephone interview.

31. John Cushman Jr., "Russell B. Long, 84, Senator Who Influenced Tax Laws," *New York Times*, May 11, 2003, http://www.nytimes.com/2003/05/11/us/russell-b-long-84-senator-who-influenced-tax-laws.html?scp=1&sq=Russell long 84&st=nyt&pagewanted=1 (accessed June 15, 2009).

32. James Mongan, interview by the authors, May 29, 2009.

33. Ibid.

34. Stan Jones, telephone interview.

35. Steven Pearlstein, "Kennedy Saw Health Reform Fail in the '70s," *Washington Post*, August 28, 2009, http://www.washingtonpost.com/wp-dyn/content/article/2009/08/27/AR2009082703919.html (accessed June 16, 2009).

36. Editorial, New York Times, "Walkout on Health," *New York Times*, August

23, 1974, http://query.nytimes.com/mem/archive/pdf?res=FA0A11F73458147B93 C1AB1783D85F408785F9 (accessed June 16, 2009).

37. Stuart Auerbach, "Health Insurance Package is Unveiled by Wilbur Mills," *Washington Post*, August 15, 1974.

38. Wainess, "Ways and Means," p. 324.

39. Richard D. Lyons, "A Legislative Goal that Has No Foes Stalled by Differences in Approach," *New York Times*, August 27, 1974.

40. Ibid.

## Chapter 2: Clinton Chooses Wrong

1. Peter Gosselin, "Clinton Told Health Plan Will Carry Steep Price; Could Require Big Tax Hike," *Boston Globe*, January 24, 1993.

2. Haynes Johnson and David Broder, *The System: The American Way of Politics at the Breaking Point* (Boston: Little, Brown, 1996), p. 109.

3. Ibid.

4. Jacob Hacker, *The Road to Nowhere* (Princeton, NJ: Princeton University Press, 1997), p. 120.

5. Ibid., p. 122.

6. Judith Feder, interview by the authors, February 9, 2009.

7. Abigail Trafford, "Obama's Struggle with Health Care Reform Echoes Clinton's Failure in 1994," *Washington Post*, February 2, 2010, http://www.washingtonpost.com/wp-dyn/content/article/2010/02/01/AR2010020103200.html (accessed December 11, 2010).

8. Mary McGrory, "The Lessons of Pennsylvania," *Washington Post*, November 7, 1991.

9. US Department of Health and Human Services, Centers for Medicare and Medicaid Services, *National Health Expenditures Aggregate, Per Capita Amounts, percent distribution, and average Annual Percent Growth, by source of funds: Selected calendar years 1960–2008*, http://www.cms.gov/NationalHealthExpendData/downloads/tables.pdf (accessed March 10, 2009).

10. Ibid.

11. US Department of Commerce, Bureau of Economic Analysis, *Gross Domestic Product: Percent Change from Preceding Period*, http://www.bea.gov/national/#gdp (accessed March 10, 2009).

12. US Department of Labor, Bureau of Labor Statistics, *Employment Status of the Civilian Non-institutional Population 16 years and Over, 1970 to Date: Table A1*, http://www.bls.gov/web/empsit/cpseea1.pdf (accessed March 10, 2009).

13. Paul Fronstin, House of Representatives Committee on Ways and Means,

Subcommittee on Health, "Hearing: Health Insurance Coverage and the Uninsured," April 4, 2001, 107th Congress, 2nd sess., http://www.ebri.org/pdf/publications/testimony/T126.pdf (accessed March 10, 2009).

14. Employee Benefits Research Institute, *Sources of Health Insurance and Characteristics of the Uninsured: Analysis of the March 1992 Current Population Survey*, January 1993, http://www.ebri.org/pdf/briefspdf/0193ib.pdf (accessed March 10. 2009).

15. Accounting standards did not require firms to recognize the present cost of future health benefit obligations until 1992. When firms were told they had to recognize these mounting obligations on their current books, many decided to terminate the benefits, breaking their promises to retirees.

16. Milt Freudenheim, "A Health-Care Taboo is Broken," *New York Times*, May 8, 1989.

17. Ibid.

18. Ibid.

19. D. A. Pennebaker and Chris Hegedus, directors, *The War Room*, DVD, Universal City, CA: Universal Studios, 2004.

20. Theda Skocpol, "The Rise and Resounding Demise of the Clinton Health Security Plan," in *The Problem That Won't Go Away*, ed. Henry Aaron (Washington, DC: The Brookings Institution, 1996), p. 36.

21. Paul Fronstin, "Sources of Health Insurance and Characteristics of the Uninsured: Analysis of the March 2010 Current Population Survey," September 2010, http://www.ebri.org/pdf/briefspdf/EBRI_IB_09-2010_No347_Uninsured1.pdf (accessed December 20, 2010).

22. Lynn Etheredge, interview by the authors, February 9, 2009.

23. Jacob Hacker, *The Road to Nowhere* (Princeton, NJ: Princeton University Press, 1997), p. 63.

24. Ibid., p. 106.

25. Johnson and Broder, *The System*, p. 110.

26. Brown University Library, "Education for Everybody: Browns Innovation and Influence on Collegiate Education," http://www.brown.edu/Facilities/University_Library/exhibits/education/quest.html (accessed March 11, 2009).

27. Time Magazine, "Students: Peaceful Revolutionary," *Time Magazine*, July 4, 1969, http://www.time.com/time/magazine/article/0,9171,840189,00.html (accessed September 11, 2009).

28. Johnson and Broder, *The System*, p. 114.

29. Citation unknown.

30. Robert Pear, "Politically and Technically Complex, Medicare Defies a Sweeping Redesign," *New York Times*, March 18, 1999, http://www.nytimes.com/1999/03/18/us/politically-and-technically-complex-medicare-defies-a-sweeping-redesign.html?scp=5&sq=March+18 percent2C+1999&st=nyt (accessed September 11, 2009).

31. Robert Keith, Report for Congress: Government and Finance Division, "The Budget Reconciliation Process: The Senate's Byrd Rule," March 20, 2008, http://budget.house.gov/crs-reports/RL30862.pdf (accessed September 21, 2009).

32. This discussion is based on the account of Johnson and Broder, *The System*, pp. 420–23.

33. Ibid., p. 423.

34. Robert Reischauer, interview by the authors, May 19, 2009.

35. Ibid.

36. This discussion is from Johnson and Broder, *The System*, pp. 285–86.

37. Clay Chandler, "It's Reischauer's Hour; *CBO Chief*'s Report on Clinton's Health Care Plan Has the Hill Abuzz," *Washington Post*, February 11, 1994.

38. YouTube, "Harry and Louise on Clinton's health plan," http://www.youtube.com/watch?v=Dt31nhleeCg (accessed September 29, 2009).

39. Chip Kahn, interview by the authors, February 9, 2009.

40. Ibid.

41. Ibid.

42. Center for Public Integrity, "Well-Heeled: Inside the Lobbying for Health Care Reform," 1994, http://www.publicintegrity.org/assets/pdf/WELL-HEALED.pdf (accessed September 29, 2009).

43. The bill limited how much more companies could charge older people relative to younger people and did not allow differences in rates for a person's health status.

44. Bill Clinton, "Address to Congress on Health Care Reform," Washington, DC, September 22, 1993, http://millercenter.org/scripps/archive/speeches/detail/3926 (accessed October 9, 2009).

45. Alain Enthoven and Sara Singer, "A Single-Payer System in Jackson Hole Clothing," *Health Affairs* 1(1994): 81–95.

46. David Maraniss and Michael Weisskopf, *Tell Newt to Shut Up* (New York: Simon and Schuster, 1996), p. 33.

47. Ibid.

48. Jake Tapper, "Gingrich Admits to Affair During Clinton Impeachment," ABC News, March 9, 2007, http://abcnews.go.com/Politics/Story?id=2937633&page=1 (accessed, October 13, 2009).

49. In fact, Kristol had been urging the Party to oppose the Clinton plan before Clinton had a plan. In a well-known memo dated December 2, 1993, he wrote, "The Clinton proposal is also a serious *political* threat to the Republican Party." The memo stated, "It will revive the reputation of the party that spends and regulates, the Democrats, as the generous protector of middle-class interests. And it will at the same time strike a blow against Republican claims to defend the middle class by restraining government."

50. This discussion from Johnson and Broder, *The System*, p. 327.

51. Ibid.

52. Ibid., p. 448.

## Chapter 3: The Past Foreshadows the Present

1. Paul Starr, *The Social Transformation of American Medicine* (New York: Basic Books, 1984), p. 244.

2. Ibid., p. 249.

3. Ibid.

4. Ibid.

5. Ibid.

6. Ibid., p. 247.

7. Ibid., p. 254.

8. Ibid., p. 242.

9. Social Security Administration, Committee on Economic Security, "Unpublished 1935 Report on Health Insurance and Disability by the Committee on Economic Security," http://www.ssa.gov/history/reports/health.html (accessed March 7, 2010).

10. Starr, *Social Transformation*, p. 272.

11. Ibid.

12. Franklin Roosevelt, "State of the Union Address, January 7, 1943," in the *American Presidency Project*, ed. John T. Woolley and Gerhard Peters, http://www.presidency.ucsb.edu/ws/?pid=16386 (accessed March 10, 2010).

13. Harry Truman, "Special Message to Congress Recommending a Comprehensive Health Program, November 14, 1945," the Harry S. Truman Presidential Library and Museum, http://www.trumanlibrary.org/publicpapers/index.php?pid=483&st=&stl= (accessed March 8, 2010).

14. Robert Taft, Senate Committee on Education and Labor. "Hearings: National Health Program," April 2–16, 1946, 77th Congress, 2nd sess., part 1.

15. Ibid.

16. Harry Truman, "Special Message to the Congress recommending a Comprehensive Health Program, November 19, 1945," in the *American Presidency Project*, ed. John T. Woolley and Gerhard Peters, http://www.presidency.ucsb.edu/ws/index.php?pid=12288&st=Truman&stl= (accessed March 8, 2010).

17. David Blumenthal and James Morone, *The Heart of Power: Health and Politics in the Oval Office* (Berkeley: University of California Press, 2009), p. 7; Starr, *Social Transformation*, p. 283.

18. Richard Harris, *A Sacred Trust* (New York: New American Library, 1966), pp. 44–46.

19. Blumenthal and Morone, *Heart of Power*, p. 92.

20. Health Insurance Association of America, *Source Book of Health Insurance Data 1999/2000* (Washington, DC: Health Insurance Association of America, 2000), tables 2–10.

# PART 2: EXPANDING HEALTH COVERAGE PIECE BY PIECE

## Chapter 4: The Hill–Burton Program

1. American Hospital Association, "Uncompensated Hospital Care Cost Fact Sheet," http://www.aha.org/aha/content/2008/pdf/08-uncompensated-care.pdf (accessed December 12, 2010).

2. Stuart Auerbach, "Hospital Care for Poor Facing Benign Neglect," *Washington Post and Times–Herald*, July 14, 1972.

3. Ibid.

4. William Curran, "Medical Charity for the Poor: Hill–Burton and the Hospitals," *New England Journal of Medicine* 287, no. 10 (1972): 498–99.

5. United Press International, "Levels of Charity Care Set for U.S.-Financed Hospitals, *Washington Post and Times–Herald*, July 22, 1972.

6. Lewis Weeks and Howard Berman, *Shapers of American Health Care Policy: An Oral History* (Ann Arbor, MI: Health Administration Press, 1985), quoted in Harry Perlstadt, "The Development of the Hill–Burton Legislation: Interests, Issues and Compromises," *Journal of Health and Social Policy* 63, no. 3 (1995): 91–92.

7. Ibid., 89–90.

8. Roger Newman, "Major Acts of Congress: Hill–Burton Act of 1946," http://www.enotes.com/major-acts-congress/hill-burton-act (accessed January 29, 2010).

9. Ibid.

10. Ibid.

11. Ibid.

12. Ibid.

13. Paul Shaheen and Harry Perlstadt, "Class Action Suits and Social Change: The Organization and Impact of the Hill–Burton Cases," *Indiana Law Journal* 57 (1981–1982): 392.

14. Ibid., p. 393.

15. Ibid.

16. Ibid.

17. Ibid.

18. Ibid., p. 394.

19. Marilyn Rose, "Federal Regulation of Services to the Poor Under the Hill–Burton Act: Realities and Pitfalls," *Northwestern University Law Review* 70, no. 1 (1975): 173.

20. Ibid., p. 179.

21. James Blumstein, "Court Action, Agency Reaction: The Hill–Burton Act as a Case Study," *Iowa Law Review* 69, no. 1,227 (1984): 8.

22. Shaheen and Perlstadt, "Class Action Suits," p. 407.

23. Blumstein, "Court Action, Agency Reaction," p. 8.

24. Ibid., p. 10 (paraphrased).

25. Ibid., p. 12.

26. Nixon actually vetoed the renewal of Hill–Burton funding in 1970. However, the reason for his veto was that Hill–Burton had been so successful that the hospital industry was overbuilt and 20 percent of beds were vacant. At that time, the free care obligation was largely an unknown issue. Congress overrode the president's veto, but retrospective analysis reveals that Nixon's reason for the veto was probably correct.

## Chapter 5: The Three-Layer Cake

1. Theodore Marmor, *The Politics of Medicare*, 2nd ed. (Hawthorne, NY: Aldine de Gruyter, 2000), p. 36.

2. National Library of Medicine, "Profiles in Science, The Reports of the Surgeon General," http://profiles.nlm.nih.gov/NN/Views/Exhibit/narrative/smoking.html (accessed October 27, 2009).

3. James Sundquist, "Politics and Policy: The Eisenhower, Kennedy and Johnson Years," *Annals of the American Academy of Political and Social Science* 383, no. 1(1969): 173–75.

4. Richard Harris, *A Sacred Trust* (New York: New American Library, 1966), p. 161.

5. Ibid., p. 160.

6. US Department of Health and Human Services, *Chart Book of Basic Health Economics Data* (Washington, DC: Public Health Service, 1964).

7. Marmor, *Politics of Medicare*, p. 13.

8. Although, as we discussed, if there is no individual mandate some young and healthy people will drop out of the insurance pool, leaving more older and less healthy people remaining in the pool and causing rates to rise.

9. Kaiser Family Foundation, "Trends in Health Care Costs and Spending, September 2007," http://www.kff.org/insurance/upload/7692.pdf (accessed October 31, 2009).

10. Ibid.

11. Eugene Feingold, *Medicare: Policy and Politics* (San Francisco: Chandler, 1966), p. 10.

12. Harris, *Sacred Trust*, p. 80.

13. Feingold, *Medicare: Policy and Politics*, p. 10.

14. Ibid., p. 107.

15. Ibid., p. 113.

16. Marmor, *Politics of Medicare*, p. 44.

17. Feingold, *Medicare: Policy and Politics*, p. 124.

18. David Blumenthal and James Morone, *The Heart of Power: Health and Politics in the Oval Office* (Berkeley: University of California Press, 2009), p. 179.

19. Harris, *Sacred Trust*, p. 162.

20. Blumenthal and Morone, *Heart of Power*, pp. 179–80.

21. Ibid., p. 181.

22. Wilbur Mills, "Financing Health Care for the Aged," address before Downtown Little Rock Lions Club, quoted in Marmor, *Politics of Medicare*, p. 43.

23. Julian Zelizer, *Taxing America: Wilbur D. Mills, Congress and the State, 1945–1975* (Cambridge, Cambridge University Press, 1999), p. 135.

24. Barry Goldwater, "Washington News," *Journal of the American Medical Association* 189, no. 13 (1964): 17–18.

25. I am indebted to the entire description of the House–Senate conference to the work of Richard Harris in *Sacred Trust*, pp. 167–72.

26. Blumenthal and Morone, *Heart of Power*, p. 184.

27. Harris, *Sacred Trust*, p. 171.

28. Ibid., p. 172.

29. YouTube, "Daisy Girl Ad," http://www.youtube.com/watch?v=Tf-MedA PhYA (accessed November 17, 2009).

30. Jack Doyle, "LBJ's Atomic Ad," PopHistoryDig.com, http://www.pop historydig.com/?tag=us-senator-barry-goldwater (accessed November 17, 2009).

31. Mills, quoted in Harris, *Sacred Trust*, p. 170.

32. An alternative explanation is that Johnson engineered the entire process and gained Mills's support by quietly letting Mills take all the credit. Blumenthal and Morone proposed this theory, and no one can say for sure that they are incorrect. They cite Mills's oral history when he said of he and Johnson, "We planned that, yes. Oh yes." However, Mills's account may well have been self-serving, similar to his earlier denial in his Little Rock speech on September 28, 1964, that he never obstructed Medicare, which was patently false. Although LBJ was a master manipulator, such a cooperative plan seems inconsistent with Mills's repeated attempts to kill Medicare in 1964.

33. This was a phrase Mills used that was frequently cited by Ted Marmor in *Politics of Medicare* to describe Mills's actions.

34. Sheryl Stolberg, "Democrats Raise Alarms Over Health Bill Costs," *New York Times*, November 9, 2009, http://www.nytimes.com/2009/11/10/health/policy/10cost.html?_r=2&hp (accessed January 25, 2010).

35. Marmor, *Politics of Medicare*, p. 60.

36. Robert Cunningham III and Robert Cunningham Jr., *The Blues: A History of the Blue Cross and Blue Shield System* (Dekalb: Northern Illinois University Press, 1997), p. 140. This number comes from a letter from William Miller to Robert Ball dated November 6, 1963.

37. Walter McNerney, Senate Committee on Finance, "Testimony: Social Security Amendments of 1965," May 5, 1965, 89th Congress, 2nd sess.

38. Cunningham and Cunningham, *The Blues*, p. 154.

39. Ibid.

40. Marmor, *Politics of Medicare*, p. 98.

41. Ibid.

42. Ibid.

43. Ibid.

44. Ibid., p. 13.

45. US Census Bureau, "Poverty Status of People by Age, Race, and Hispanic Origin 1959–2009," http://www.census.gov/hhes/www/poverty/data/historical/people.html (accessed January 25, 2010).

46. Kaiser Family Foundation, "Medicaid/CHIP," http://www.kff.org/medicaid/index.cfm (accessed May 22, 2010).

47. Kaiser Family Foundation, "Medicaid Today," http://facts.kff.org/chart.aspx?ch=463 (accessed July 26, 2010).

48. Kaiser Family Foundation, "Medicaid/CHIP."

49. Paul Starr, *The Social Transformation of American Medicine* (New York: Basic Books, 1984), p. 373.

50. Marmor, *Politics of Medicare*, p. 58.

## Chapter 6: Ooops!

1. Eric Zorn, "Change of Subject: Ronald Reagan on Medicare circa 1961: Prescient Rhetoric or Familiar Alarmist Claptrap," Change of Subject (blog), *Chicago Tribune*, September 2, 2009, http://blogs.chicagotribune.com/news_columnists_ezorn/2009/09/ronald-reagan-on-medicare-circa-1961-prescient-rhetoric-or-familiar-alarmist-claptrap-.html (accessed December 7, 2009).

2. US Census Bureau, "Poverty Status of People by Age, Race, and Hispanic Origin 1959–2009," table 3, http://www.census.gov/hhes/www/poverty/data/historical/people.html (accessed January 25, 2010).

3. Richard Himelfarb, *Catastrophic Politics: The Rise and Fall of the Medicare Catastrophic Coverage Act of 1988* (University Park: Pennsylvania State University Press, 1988), pp. 16–17.

4. As stated in chapter 5, Medicare Part A covered ninety days of inpatient hospital days per year plus one lifetime extension of sixty days. After those days were used up, the patient was responsible for all charges. The commission's program would allow unlimited inpatient days and finance it through copayments, but individuals could buy insurance under Part B to cover the cost of the copayments.

5. Julie Rovner, "Reagan Sides with Bowen on Medicare Plan," *Congressional Quarterly*, February 14, 1988, p. 115.

6. Jonathan Oberlander, "Medicare's Coverage of Health Services," in *Renewing the Promise: Medicare and its Reform*, ed. David Blumenthal, Mark Schlesinger, and Pamela Brown, 26 (New York: Oxford University Press, 1988).

7. Jacqueline Calmes, "Reagan's Address Repeats Familiar Themes," *Congressional Quarterly*, February 8, 986, p. 261.

8. Robert Pear, "Political Medicine; Reagan, Apostle Of Less, Assures Expanded Health Care For Elderly," *New York Times*, February 15, 1987, http://www.nytimes.com/1987/02/15/weekinreview/political-medicine-reagan-apostle-less-assures-expanded-health-care-for-elderly.html?scp=5&sq=February 15, 1987 &st=nyt&pagewanted=1 (accessed December 14, 2009).

9. Theodore Marmor, *The Politics of Medicare*, 2nd ed. (Hawthorne, NY: Aldine de Gruyter, 2000), p. 13.

10. Theodore Marmor, "The Case for Universal Social Insurance," in *Policies for an Aging Society*, ed. Stuart Altman and David Shactman (Baltimore: Johns Hopkins University Press, 2002), p. 171.

11. Stuart Butler and Maya MacGuineas, "Rethinking Social Insurance," February 19, 2008, http://www.heritage.org/Research/Budget/wp021908.cfm (accessed December 14, 2009).

12. Beginning in 2003, the subsidy was income-related and reduced for those earning more than eighty thousand dollars.

13. Jonathan Oberlander, *The Political Life of Medicare* (Chicago: Chicago University Press, 2003), p. 69.

14. Ibid., p. 60.

15. Himelfarb, *Catastrophic Politics*, p. 21.

16. Ibid., p. 29.

17. Ibid.

18. Ibid., pp. 29–30.

19. Robert Pear, "Congress Seeks a Fair Way to Pay for Catastrophic Health Insurance," *New York Times*, June 7, 1987, http://www.nytimes.com/1987/06/07/weekinreview/congress-seeks-a-fair-way-to-pay-for-catasrophic-health-insurance

.html?scp=9&sq=June 7, 1987&st=nyt&pagewanted=1 (accessed December 14, 2009). From an interview with John Rother.

20. Ibid.

21. Congressional Budget Office, *The Medicare Catastrophic Coverage Act of 1988*, October 1988, http://www.cbo.gov/ftpdocs/84xx/doc8430/88doc14.pdf (accessed December 18, 2010).

22. Himelfarb, *Catastrophic Politics*, p. 40.

23. Ibid.

24. Stuart Butler, "On Catastrophic Health Care, Otis Bowen Undermines Reagan Policy," Heritage Foundation, November 25, 1986, http://www.heritage.org/Research/Reports/1986/11/On-Catastrophic-Health-Care-Otis-Bowen-Undermines-Reagan-Policy (accessed December 21, 2009).

25. Ibid.

26. The video can be viewed at http://www.youtube.com/watch?v=qre7Dz Etxyc (accessed December 21, 2009).

27. Stuart Altman, interview by David Shactman, December 22, 2009.

28. Himelfarb, *Catastrophic Politics*, p. 46.


## Chapter 7: Ted Kennedy and the Republican Congress

1. The report of Kennedy's meeting is from Elsa Walsh, "Kennedy's Hidden Campaign," *New Yorker*, March 31, 1997, http://archives.newyorker.com/?i=1997-03-31#folio=066, 69 (accessed March 3, 2010).

2. Ibid.

3. Nick Littlefield, interview by the authors, December 12, 2010.

4. Ibid.

5. Brian Atchinson and Daniel Fox, "The Politics of the Health Insurance Portability and Accountability Act," *Health Affairs* 16, no. 3 (1997): 148.

6. Ibid.

7. Ibid.

8. Robert Dreyfuss and Peter Stone, "Medikill," *Mother Jones*, January/ February 1996, http://motherjones.com/politics/1996/01/medikill (accessed December 2, 2010).

9. Ibid.

10. Robert Pear, "G.O.P. Plan Would Profit Insurer with Ties to Party," *New York Times*, April 14, 1996, http://www.nytimes.com/1996/04/14/us/gop-plan-would-profit-insurer-with-ties-to-party.html (accessed December 2, 2010).

11. Clay Chandler, "Favored Few Stand to Gain from Republican Tax Cuts," *Washington Post*, December 24, 1995.

12. Dreyfuss and Stone, "Medikill."

13. Kala Ladenheim, "Health Insurance in Transition: The Health Insurance Portability and Accountability Act of 1996," *Publius* 27, no. 2 (1997), http://www .jstor.org/stable/3330636 (accessed March 16, 2010).

14. Len Nichols and Linda Blumberg, "A Different Kind of New 'Federalism'? The Health Insurance Portability and Accountability Act of 1996," *Health Affairs* 17, no. 3 (1998): 25–42.

15. Ibid.

16. Ibid.

17. Ladenheim, "Health Insurance in Transition."

18. Jerry Gray, "Through Senate Alchemy, Tobacco Is Turned Into Gold for Children's Health," *New York Times*, August 11, 1997, http://www.nytimes.com/1997/ 08/11/us/through-senate-alchemy-tobacco-is-turned-into-gold-for-children-s -health.html?pagewanted=3 (accessed December 18, 2010).

19. Robert Bennefield, "Current Population Reports: Health Insurance Coverage: 1996," pp. 60–199, http://www.census.gov/prod/3/97pubs/P60-199.PDF, (accessed December 5, 2010).

20. Ibid.

21. Michael Doonan, "American Federalism and Contemporary Health Policy," PhD diss., Brandeis University, 2002, 67.

22. Ibid., p. 72.

23. Ibid., p. 71.

24. American Conservative Union, "Congressional Ratings 2009," http:// www.conservative.org/ratings/ratingsarchive/2009/Senatepercent20Ratings.htm #UT (accessed December 5, 2010).

25. Senator Orrin Hatch, statement, *Congressional record*, May 21, 1997, 105th Congress, 1st sess., S4782.

26. Senator Ted Kennedy, statement, *Congressional record*, May 21, 1997, 105th Congress, 1st sess., S4815.

27. Gray, "Senate Alchemy."

28. Paul Fronstin, "Sources of Health Insurance and Characteristics of the Uninsured: Analysis of the March 2010 Current Population Survey," September 2010, http://www.ebri.org/pdf/briefspdf/EBRI_IB_09-2010_No347_Uninsured1 .pdf (accessed December 20, 2010), p. 5.

29. Ibid.

30. Congressional Budget Office, *The State Children's Health Insurance Program*, 8, http://www.cbo.gov/ftpdocs/80xx/doc8092/05-10-SCHIP.pdf, (accessed December 6, 2010).

31. Fronstin, "Sources of Health," p. 27.

32. US Department of Health and Human Services, Centers for Medicare and

Medicaid Services, *Overview of National CHIP Policy: CHIP Ever Enrolled Year Graph*, http://www.cms.gov/NationalCHIPPolicy/downloads/CHIPEverEnrolledYear Graph.pdf (accessed December 6, 2010).

33. Congressional Budget Office, *State Children's Health*, p. 11.

34. Robert Pear, "Obama Signs Children's Health Insurance Bill," *New York Times*, February 4, 2009, http://www.nytimes.com/2009/02/05/us/politics/05 health.html?_r=1&hp (accessed December 6, 2010).

35. Congressional Budget Office, *Cost Estimate. H.R. 2: Children's Health Insurance Reauthorization Act of 2009*, 6, http://www.cbo.gov/ftpdocs/99xx/doc9985/hr2 paygo.pdf (accessed December 6, 2010).

36. Ibid., p. 1.

37. Congressional Budget Office, Fact Sheet for CBO's March 2010 Baseline: CHIP, http://www.cbo.gov/ftpdocs/115xx/doc11521/CHIP.pdf (accessed December 7, 2010).

38. Walsh, "Kennedy's Hidden Campaign," p. 81.

## Chapter 8: The Unlikely Saga

1. Robert Cunningham, "The Wheels of Policy Grind Slowly: Top Story of 1999 is Medicare Commission's Decision to Punt," *Medicine and Health Perspectives* 54, no. 1 (2000).

2. Thomas Oliver, Philip Lee, and Helene Lipton, "A Political History of Medicare and Prescription Drug Coverage," *Millbank Quarterly* 82, no. 2 (2004): 319.

3. David Broder and Amy Goldstein, "AARP Decision Followed a Long GOP Courtship," *Washington Post*, November 20, 2003.

4. Henry Aaron and Robert Reischauer, "The Medicare Reform Debate: What Is the Next Step?" *Health Affairs* 14, no. 4 (1995). A thorough analysis of the premium support concept was undertaken by the Congressional Budget Office and can be found at http://www.cbo.gov/ftpdocs/76xx/doc7697/12-08-Medicare.pdf.

5. Bradley Strunk and Paul Ginsburg, "Tracking Health Care Costs: Trends Slow in First Half of 2003," *Center for Studying Health System Change: Data Bulletin* no. 26 (2003): 1.

6. Ibid.

7. Jonathan Oberlander, "Through the Looking Glass: The Politics of the Medicare Prescription Drug, Improvement, and Modernization Act," *Journal of Health Politics, Policy and Law* 32, no. 2 (2007): 198.

8. Oliver et al., "Political History of Medicare," p. 309. The amount was never exactly specified but a range of $5,500 to $7,000 was discussed.

9. Michael Heaney, "Brokering Health Policy: Coalitions, Parties, and Interest Group Influences," *Journal of Health Politics, Policy and Law* 31 (2006): 920.

10. The CMS summary can be found at http://www4.cms.gov/MMAUpdate/downloads/PL108-173summary.pdf; and the Kaiser summary at http://www.kff.org/medicare/med011604pkg.cfm.

11. Congressional Budget Office, *The Long-Term Budget Outlook* (Washington, DC: Government Printing Office, 2005), p. 26.

12. Robert Pear and Walt Bogdanich, "Some Successful Models Ignored As Congress Works on Drug Bill, *New York Times*, September 4, 2003, accessed May 21, 2010, http://www.nytimes.com/2003/09/04/business/some-successful-models-ignored-as-congress-works-on-drug-bill.html?src=pm.

13. Peter Orszag, Congressional Budget Office, Senate Committee on Finance. "Testimony: The Medicare Advantage Program: Enrollment and Budgetary Effects," April 11, 2007, 110th Congress, 2nd sess., http://cbo.gov/ftpdocs/79xx/doc7994/04-11-MedicareAdvantage.pdf (accessed May 21, 2010,).

14. Ibid.

15. Dee Mahan, "Falling Short: Medicare Prescription Drug Plans Offer Meager Savings," Families USA Special Report, December 2005, http://www.familiesusa.org/assets/pdfs/PDP-vs-VA-prices-special-report.pdf (accessed April 25, 2010). The study was conducted in two states.

16. Bill Thomas, interview by the authors, May 12, 2010.

17. John Iglehart, "The New Prescription-Drug Benefit—A Pure Power Play," *New England Journal of Medicine* 350, no. 8 (2004): 826–33.

18. This story is from R. Jeffrey Smith, "GOP's Pressing Question on Medicare Vote: Did Some Go Too Far to Change a No to a Yes?" *Washington Post*, December 23, 2003.

19. Amy Goldstein, "Foster: White House Had Role in Withholding Medicare Data; HHS Actuary Feels Bush Aide Put Hold on Medicare Data," *Washington Post*, March 19, 2004.

20. Ibid.

21. Sheryl Stolberg and Robert Pear, "Mysterious Fax Adds to Intrigue Over the Medicare Bill's Cost," *New York Times*, March 18, 2004.

22. Robert Pear, "Inquiry Confirms Top Medicare Official Threatened Actuary Over Cost of Drug Benefits," *New York Times*, July 7, 2004, http://query.nytimes.com/gst/fullpage.html?res=9B02E0D9143BF934A35754C0A9629C8B63 (accessed May 21, 2010).

23. Ibid.

24. Ibid.

25. Robert Pear, "Medicare Official Testifies on Cost Figures," *New York Times*, March 25, 2004, http://www.nytimes.com/2004/03/25/us/medicare-official-testifies-on-cost-figures.html (accessed May 21, 2010).

26. Robert Pear, "Bush's Aides Put Higher Price Tag on Medicare Law," *New York Times*, January 30, 2004.

27. Ibid.

28. Editorial, "The Drug Benefit: A Report Card," *New York Times,* June 5, 2006, http://query.nytimes.com/gst/fullpage.html?res=9E04E7DE1431F936A35755C0A 9609C8B63&scp=2&sq=New percent20York percent20Times percent20Editorial, percent20 percentE2 percent80 percent9CThe percent20Drug percent20Benefit: percent20A percent20Report percent20Card&st=cse (accessed May 21, 2010).

29. Robert Pear, "Federal Costs Dropping Under New Medicare Drug Plan," *New York Times,* February 3, 2006, http://www.nytimes.com/2004/03/25/us/ medicare-official-testifies-on-cost-figures.html?pagewanted=all (accessed May 21, 2010).

30. Ibid.

31. Ibid.

32. Ibid.

33. Authors' calculations based on data from the Center for Medicare and Medicaid Services, "2009 Annual Report of the Boards of Trustees of the Federal Hospital Insurance and Federal Supplementary Medical Insurance Trust Funds," http://www.cms.gov/ReportsTrustFunds/downloads/tr2009.pdf (accessed April 27, 2010).

34. The Trustee's projections can only be approximately compared to those of the CBO.

35. John Rother, interview by the authors, April 15, 2010.

36. Bill Thomas, interview by the authors, May 12, 2010.

37. Barbara S. Klees, Christian Wolfe, and Catherine Curtis, US Department of Health and Human Services, Office of the Actuary, Centers for Medicare and Medicaid Services, "Brief Summaries of Medicare and Medicaid: Title XVIII and Title XIX of the Social Security Act," November 1, 2009, http://www.cms.gov/MedicareProgramRates Stats/Downloads/MedicareMedicaidSummaries2009.pdf (accessed April 27, 2010).

# PART 3: WHY CAN'T AMERICANS AFFORD THEIR HEALTH CARE?

## Chapter 9: Controlling Health Costs

1. US Department of Health and Human Services, Office of the Actuary, *National Health Expenditure Projections 2009–2019,* January 2010, https://www.cms .gov/NationalHealthExpendData/downloads/proj2009.pdf (accessed July 3, 2010).

2. Organization for Economic Co-operation and Development (OECD), *OECD Health Data 2006,* October 10, 2006, http://www.oecd.org/health/healthdata (accessed July 3, 2010).

3. Stuart Altman, US Department of Health, Education, and Welfare, *Present and Future Supply of Registered Nurses* (Washington, DC: Government Printing Office, 1971).

4. Economic Stabilization Program, *Economic Stabilization Program: Quarterly Reports, August 15, 1971–January 10, 1973*, vol. 1 (Washington, DC: Government Printing Office, 1973).

5. Medicare excluded some costs in the calculation that would not be incurred by the Medicare population such as certain costs associated with newborns.

6. US Department of Health and Human Services, Centers for Medicare and Medicaid Services, *Historical National Health Expenditures Data*, http://www.cms.gov/NationalHealthExpendData/02_NationalHealthAccountsHistorical.asp#TopOf Page (accessed December 22, 2010).

7. Economic Stabilization Program, *Economic Stabilization Program: Quarterly Reports, January 11, 1973–December 31, 1973*, vol. 2 (Washington, DC: Government Printing Office, 1973).

8. Rick Mayes, "The Origins, Development, and Passage of Medicare's Revolutionary Prospective Payment System," *Journal of The History of Medicine and Allied Sciences* (2006): 12.

9. Wilbur Cohen and Robert Ball, "Social Security Amendments of 1965: Summary and Legislative History," *Social Security Bulletin* 28, no. 9 (1965).

10. House of Representatives, Committee on Ways and Means, "Summary of Major Provisions of P.L. 89–97, the Social Security Amendments of 1965," September 1965, 89th Congress, 1st sess., part F, 20–21; House of Representatives, Committee on Ways and Means, Subcommittee on Oversight, "Hearing: Administration of Medicare Cost-Saving Experiments," May 14–17, 1976, 94th Congress, 2nd sess.

11. Ibid.

12. Jonathan Oberlander, "Medicare: The End of Consensus," Paper presented at the Annual Meeting of the American Political Science Association, Boston, Massachusetts, 1998.

13. Robert Ball, "Social Security Amendments of 1972: Summary and Legislative History," *Social Security Bulletin* 36, no. 3 (1972).

14. This was a term used by Theodore Marmor, *The Politics of Medicare*, 2nd ed. (Hawthorne, NY: Aldine de Gruyter, 2000), pp. 96–99.

15. Robert Ball, in personal conversation with Stuart Altman.

16. Glenn Markus, Congressional Research Service, Education and Public Welfare Division, *How Medicare Pays for Doctors' Services* (Washington, DC: Government Printing Office, 1972).

17. Paul Starr, *The Social Transformation of American Medicine* (New York: Basic Books, 1984), p. 244.

18. House of Representatives, Committee on Ways and Means, "Third Annual

Report of the Health Insurance Benefits Advisory Council of the Medicare Program," January 27, 1972, 92nd Congress, 2nd sess., 1–14.

19. Rick Mayes and Robert Berenson, *Medicare Prospective Payment and the Shaping of US Health Care* (Baltimore: Johns Hopkins University Press, 2006), p. 20.

20. Rick Mayes, interview by Stuart Altman, July 22, 2002. This interview was conducted for the article by Rick Mayes, "Causal Chains and Cost Shifting: How Medicare's Rescue Inadvertently Triggered the Managed-Care Revolution," *Journal of Policy History* 16, no. 2 (2002): 144–74.

21. Rosemary Stevens, *In Sickness and in Wealth: American Hospitals in the Twentieth Century* (Baltimore: Johns Hopkins University Press, 1989).

22. Frank Sloan, "Rate Regulation as a Strategy for Hospital Cost Control: Evidence from the Last Decade," *Milbank Memorial Quarterly* 61, no. 2 (1983): 195–221.

23. Ibid.

24. Frank Sloan, "State Regulatory Strategies," Presentation, Health Industry Forum Breakfast Series, Waltham, MA, October 2008.

25. Milton Roemer, "Bed Supply and Hospital Utilization: A Natural Experiment," *Hospitals* 35 (1961): 36–42.

26. Drew Altman, "Creating a National Health Planning System," in *Federal Health Programs*, ed. Stuart Altman and Harvey Sapoksly (Lexington: Lexington Books, 1981), p. 122.

27. American Health Planning Association, *Final Report on 1978 Survey of Health Planning Agencies* (Washington, DC: Government Printing Office, 1979).

28. Anthony Robbins, "Who Should Make Public Policy for Health?" *American Journal of Public Health* 66, no. 5 (1976): 431; Bruce Vladeck, "Interest-Group Representation and the HSAs; Health Planning and Political Theory," *American Journal of Public Health* 67, no. 1 (1977): 23–29.

29. For detailed analysis of trends in the rate of growth in hospital spending, see Medicare Board of Trustees Reports, 1970–1985. Annual reports can be found online at http://www.ssa.gov/history/reports/trust/trustyears.html.

30. Senate Committee on Human Resources, Subcommittee of Health and Scientific Research, *The Hospital Cost Containment Act of 1977: An Analysis of the Administration's Proposal*, 1977, 95th Congress, 1st sess. The estimates included pass-throughs for increases in wages, admissions, and some exceptional expenses.

31. Ibid.

32. Marsha Gold and Karyen Chu, "Effects of Selected Cost-Containment Efforts: 1971–1993," *Health Care Financing Review* 14, no. 3 (1993): 183–225.

33. Congressional Budget Office, *Hospital Cost Containment Model: A Technical Analysis* (Washington, DC: Government Printing Office, 1981).

34. David Blumenthal and James Morone, *The Heart of Power: Health and Politics in the Oval Office* (Berkeley: University of California Press, 2009), pp. 267–68.

35. Ibid., p. 271.

36. Alain Enthoven, "Consumer Choice Health Plan: A National Health Insurance Proposal Based on Regulated Competition in the Private Sector," *New England Journal of Medicine* 298, no. 12, Part 1, (1978): 650–58; Alain Enthoven, "Consumer Choice Health Plan: A National Health Insurance Proposal Based on Regulated Competition in the Private Sector," *New England Journal of Medicine* 298, no. 13, Part 2 (1978): 709–20.

37. Leslie Stahl, "Jimmy Carter: My Presidency was a Success," *CBS News*, September 19, 2010, http://www.cbsnews.com/stories/2010/09/16/60minutes/main 6872344.shtml (accessed October 10, 2010).

38. Robert VanGiezen and Albert Schwenk. Bureau of Labor Statistics, "Historical Data: Labor Force Statistics from the Current Population Survey," *Compensation and Working Conditions* (2001): 20.

39. David Smith, *Paying For Medicare: The Politics of Reform* (New York: Aldine De Gruyter, 1992), p. 63. See chapter 9, endnote 13.

40. Ibid., p. 29.

41. Ibid., p. 30.

42. Thomas Oliver, "Health Care Market Reform in Congress: The Uncertain Path from Proposal to Policy," *Political Science Quarterly* 106, no. 3 (1991): 453–77.

43. Mayes and Berenson, *Medicare Prospective Payment*, pp. 37–38.

44. Robert Fetter, John Thompson, Ronald Mills, and Donald Riedel, "The Application of Diagnostic Specific Cost Profiles to Cost and Reimbursement Control in Hospitals," *Journal of Medical Systems* 1, no. 2 (1977): 137–49; Robert Fetter, Youngsoo Shin, Jean Freeman, Richard Averill, and John Thompson, "Case Mix Definition by Diagnosis-Related Groups," *Medical Care* 18, no. 2 (1980): 1–53.

45. Richard Schweicker, "Executive Summary: The Report to Congress on Hospital Prospective Payment for Medicare," *Health Care Financial Management* 37, no. 3 (1983): 67–69.

46. Tim Brady, Barbie Robinson, and Tricia Davis, Office of Inspector General, Office of Evaluation and Inspections, *Medicare Hospital Prospective Payment System: How DRG Rates Are Calculated and Updated* (Washington, DC: Government Printing Office, 2001).

47. James Morone and Andrew Dunham, "The Waning of Professional Dominance: DRGs and the Hospitals," *Health Affairs* 3, no. 73 (1984): 73–87.

48. Smith, *Paying for Medicare*, p. 42.

49. Uwe Reinhardt, "Future Trends in the Economics of Medical Care," *American Journal of Cardiology* 56, no. 5 (1985): 50c–59c.

50. Schweicker, "Executive Summary."

51. US Department of Health, Education, and Welfare, "Medical Technology: The Culprit Behind Health Care Costs?" in *Proceedings of the 1977 Sun Valley Forum on*

*National Health*, ed. Stuart Altman and Robert Blendon (Washington, DC: US Government Printing Office, 1979).

52. Smith, *Paying for Medicare*, p. 49.

53. Ibid.

54. Association of American Medical Colleges, "Medicare Indirect Medical Education (IME) Payment," http://www.aamc.org/advocacy/library/gme/gme 0002.htm (accessed July 8, 2010).

55. Ibid.

56. Mayes and Berenson, *Prospective Payment*, p. 44.

57. This information is from the authors' private discussion with Richard Knapp, a former senior member of the AAMC staff who participated in these discussions.

58. Congressional Budget Office, *The Indirect Teaching Adjustment for Medicare's Prospective Payment System: Issues and Options* (Washington, DC: Government Printing Office, 1985), p. 22.

59. Congressional Budget Office, *Setting Medicare's Indirect Teaching Adjustment for Hospitals* (Washington, DC: Government Printing Office, 1989).

60. Gail Wilensky and Joseph Newhouse, MedPac, *Report to Congress: Rethinking Medicare's Payment Policies for Graduate Medical Education and Teaching Hospitals* (Washington, DC: Government Printing Office, 1999).

61. Stuart Altman, ProPac, Senate Committee on Finance, Subcommittee on Health, "Testimony: Prospective Payment Assessment Commission," July 29,1985, 99th Congress, 2nd sess.

62. Smith, *Paying for Medicare*, pp. 40, 61.

63. ProPac, *Prospective Payment Assessment Commission: Annual Report, March 1, 1991* (Washington, DC: Prospective Payment Assessment Commission 1991), p. 16.

64. See the Omnibus Budget Reconciliation Act of 1990, HR 5835, 101st Congress, 2nd sess. Available online (organized by congressional session) at http://thomas.loc.gov/home/thomas.php.

65. Centers for Medicare and Medicaid Services, "Fact Sheet: Sole Community Hospital," http://www.cms.gov/MLNProducts/downloads/solecommhospfct sht 508-09.pdf (accessed July 8, 2010).

66. Robert Pokras, Lola Kozak, Eileen McCarthy, and Edmund Graves, "Trends in Hospital Utilization: United States, 1965–86," *Vital Health Statistics* 13, no. 101 (1989); Patricia Adams, Kathleen Heyman, and Jackline Vickerie; "Summary Health Statistics for the US Population: National Health Interview Survey, 2008," *Vital Health Statistics* 10, no. 243 (2009).

67. Smith, *Paying for Medicare*, p. 136.

68. Centers for Medicare and Medicaid Services, Office of Information Services, *Data from the Medicare Data Extract System, Table 61a* (Washington, DC: Government Printing Office, 2009).

69. Smith, *Paying for Medicare*, p. 141.

70. Ibid., p. 153.

71. See the Consolidated Omnibus Budget Reconciliation Act of 1985, HR 3128, 99th Congress, 2nd sess. Available online (organized by congressional session) at http://thomas.loc.gov/home/thomas.php.

72. William Hsiao, Peter Braun, Douweand Ynteme, and Edmund Becker, "Estimating Physicians' Work for a Resource Based Relative Value Scale," *New England Journal of Medicine* 319, no. 13 (1988): 835–41.

73. John Goodson, "Unintended Consequences of Resource Based Relative Value Scale Reimbursement," *Journal of the American Medical Associtaion* 298 (2007): 2308–10.

74. William Hsiao, Peter Braun, Daniel Dunn, Edmund Becker, and Thomas Ketcham, "Results and Policy Implications of the Resource Based Relative Value Study," *New England Journal of Medicine* 319, no. 13 (1988): 881–88.

75. William Hsiao, Peter Braun, Nancy Kelly, and Edmund Becker, "Results, Potential Effects, and Implementation Issues of the Resource Based Relative Value Scale," *Journal of the American Medical Association* 260, no. 16 (1988): 2429–38.

76. Catherine Hoffman, "Medicaid Payment for Nonphysician Practitioners: An Access Issue," *Health Affairs* 13, no. 4 (1994): 140–52.

77. Smith, *Paying for Medicare*, p. 204.

78. Ibid., pp. 207–208.

79. National Health Statistics Group, "National Health Care Expenditures Data," table 12, http://www.cms.gov/NationalHealthExpendData/downloads/tables.pdf (accessed July 10, 2010).

80. Edward Salsberg and Gaetano Forte, "Trends in the Physician Workforce, 1980–2000," *Health Affairs* 21, no. 5 (2002): 166.

81. Stuart Altman and Marc Rodman, "Halfway Competitive Markets and Ineffective Regulation: The American Health Care System," *Journal of Health Politics, Policy and Law* 13, no. 2 (1988): 323–39.

## Chapter 10: The Last Twenty Years

1. US Department of Health and Human Services, Centers for Medicare and Medicaid Services, Office of the Actuary, National Health Statistics Group, "National Health Care Expenditures Data," (Washington, DC: Government Printing Office, 2010), table 1.

2. Henry Aaron and Paul Ginsburg, "Is Health Spending Excessive? If So, What Can We Do About It?," *Health Affairs* 28, no. 5 (2009): 1262.

3. Kaiser Family Foundation, "Employer Health Benefits, 2009 Annual

Survey," September 2009, http://ehbs.kff.org/pdf/2009/7936.pdf.ion (accessed July 8, 2010).

4. Centers for Disease Control and Prevention, National Center for Health Statistics, *Health, United States, 2006 with Chartbook on Trends in the Health of Americans* (Hyattsville, MD: Center for Disease Control and Prevention, 2006).

5. Kaiser Family Foundation, "Employer Health Benefits, 2009."

6. US General Accounting Office, *Federal Employees' Health Plans: Premium Growth and OPM's Role in Negotiating Benefits* (Washington, DC: Government Printing Office, 2002).

7. David Hilzenrath, "Costly Savings: Downside of the New Health Care," *Washington Post*, August 7, 1995.

8. James Robinson, "The End of Managed Care," *Journal of the American Medical Association* 285, no. 20 (2001): 2622–28.

9. This core belief of Sidney Garfield was told to Stuart Altman by one of the early pioneers of Kaiser Permanente, Scott Fleming. Fleming and Altman worked together in the Department of Health, Education, and Welfare in the early '70s.

10. Stuart Guterman, "The Balanced Budget Act of 1997: Will Hospitals Take a Hit on Their PPS Margins?" *Health Affairs* 17, no. 1 (1998): 159–66.

11. Cathy Cowan, Helen Lazenby, Anne Martin, Patricia McDonnell, Arthur Sensenig, Cynthia Smith, Lekha Whittle, Mark Zezza, Carolyn Donham, and Madie Stewart, "National Health Expenditures, 1999." *Health Care Financing Review* 22, no. 4 (2001): 77–110.

12. US Congress, House, *Annual Report of the Boards of Trustees of the Federal Hospital Insurance and Federal Supplementary Medical Insurance Trust Funds*, 104th Congress, 1st sess, (Washington, DC: Government Printing Office, 1995).

13. Clinton Brass, Government Organization and Management, Congressional Research Service, *Shutdown of the Federal Government: Causes, Processes, and Effects* (Washington, DC: Government Printing Office, 2010).

14. Balanced Budget Act of 1997, H.R. 2015, 105th Congress, 1st sess. (1997).

15. Gail Wilensky, Medicare Payment Advisory Commission, House Committee on Commerce. Subcommittee on Health and Environment, "Testimony: The Balanced Budget Act of 1997: A Current Look at its Impact on Patients," July 19, 2000, 106th Congress, 2nd sess.

16. US Department of Health and Human Services, Centers for Medicare and Medicaid Serivces, Office of the Medicare Actuary, *1998 Annual Report of the Boards of Trustees of the Federal Hospital Insurance and Federal Supplementary Medical Insurance Trust Funds* (Washington, DC: Government Printing Office, 1998).

17. US Department of Health and Human Services, "National Health Expenditures Data."

18. Aaron and Ginsburg, "Is Health Spending Excessive?," p. 1262.

19. Vivian Wu, "Hospital Cost Shifting Revisited: New Evidence from the Balanced Budget Act of 1997," *International Journal of Health Care Finance and Economics* 10, no. 1 (2010): 61–83.

20. US General Accounting Office, *Non-profit, For-profit, and Government Hospitals: Uncompensated Care and Other Community Benefits* (Washington, DC: Government Printing Office, 2005).

21. Almanac of Hospital Financial and Operating Indicators, *Financial Indicators: Profitability Ratios*, 2010 ed., http://www.ingenix.com/content/attachments/ALM.pdf (accessed December 22, 2010).

22. Kaiser Family Foundation, "Employer Health Benefits, 2007 Annual Survey," http://www.kff.org/insurance/7672/index.cfm (accessed, July 10, 2010).

23. Linda Blumberg and Lisa Clemans-Cope, "High-Deductible Health Plans with Health Savings Accounts: Emerging Evidence and Outstanding Issues," Urban Institute, http://www.urban.org/UploadedPDF/411833_health_saving_account.pdf (accessed July 8, 2010).

24. Christopher Tompkins, Stuart Altman, and Ephrat Eilat, "The Precarious Pricing System for Hospital Service," *Health Affairs* 25, no. 1 (2006): 45–56.

25. Reza Fazel, Harlan Krumholz, Yongfei Wang, Joseph Ross, Jersey Chen, Henry Ting, Nilay Shah, Khurman Nasir, Andrew Einstein, and Brahmajee Nallamathu, "Exposure to Low-Dose Ionizing Radiation from Medical Imaging Procedures," *New England Journal of Medicine* 361, no. 9 (2009): 849–57.

26. National Institute for Health and Clinical Effectiveness, "Incorporating Health Economics in Guidelines and Assessing Resource Impact," *Guideline Development Methods*, http://www.nice.org.uk/search/guidancesearchresults.jsp?keywords=Incorporating+health+economics+in+guidelines&searchSite=on&searchType=All&newSearch=1 (accessed July 8, 2010,).

27. National Institute for Health and Clinical Effectiveness, "Measuring Effectiveness and Cost Effectiveness: The QALY," April 20, 2010, http://www.nice.org.uk/newsroom/features/measuringeffectivenessandcosteffectivenesstheqaly.jsp (accessed December 9, 20010).

28. Organization for Economic Co-operation and Development (OECD), *Health at a Glance 2009—OECD Indicators* (Paris: Organisation for Economic Co-operation and Development; 2009).

29. Ibid.

30. Ibid.

31. Ibid.

32. Ibid.

33. Chris Peterson and Rachel Barton, Congressional Research Service, *US Health Care Spending: A Comparison with other Countries* (Washington, DC: Government Printing Office, 2007).

34. Ibid.

35. Ibid.

36. Sherry Glied, "Single-Payer as a Financing Mechanism," *Journal of Health Politics, Policy and Law* 34 no. 4 (2009): 593–615.

## PART 4: SUCCESS AT LAST!

### Chapter 11: Obama Develops His Plan

1. Organizing for America, "Full Text of Senator Barack Obama's Announcement for President," February 10, 2007, http://www.barackobama.com/2007/02/10/remarks_of_senator_barack_obam_11.php (accessed October 6, 2010).

2. Adam Negaunee and Jeff Zeleny, "In Mostly Sedate Debate, Democrats Show More Unity Than Strife," *New York Times*, April 27, 2007, http://query.nytimes.com/gst/fullpage.html?res=9400E7DD123EF934A15757C0A9619C8B63&scp=1&sq=In+mostly+sedate+debate&st=nyt (accessed October 6, 2010).

3. Robert Toner, "Obama Calls for Wider and Less Costly Health Care Coverage," *New York Times*, May 30, 2007, http://www.nytimes.com/2007/05/30/us/politics/30obama.html?_r=1&scp=1&sq=Obama+calls+for+wider+and+less+costly+health&st=nyt (accessed October 6, 2010).

4. The White House, Office of the Press Secretary, "Remarks by the President to a Joint Session of Congress, Washington, DC, September 9, 2009," http://www.whitehouse.gov/the_press_office/remarks-by-the-president-to-a-joint-session-of-congress-on-health-care/ (accessed October 8, 2010).

5. It is effectively 138 percent for many people because some previous components of income are now disregarded.

### Chapter 12: Early Players and Done Deals

1. Robert Pear, "Health Care Industry in Talks to Shape Policy," *New York Times*, February 19, 2009.

2. Ibid.

3. John Bresnahan and Carrie Budoff Brown, "Is a Top Dem Stirring Daschle Trouble?" *Politico*, February 2, 2009, http://www.politico.com/news/stories/0209/18271.html (accessed October 8, 2010).

4. Center for Responsive Politics, "Senator Max Baucus 2003–2008," http://www.opensecrets.org/politicians/industries.php?type=C&cid=N00004643&newMem=N&recs=20&cycle=2008 (accessed June 3, 2011).

5. Tom Hamburger, "Obama Gives Powerful Drug Lobby a Seat at the Healthcare Table," *Los Angeles Times*, August 4, 2009, http://www.latimes.com/features/health/la -na-healthcare-pharma4-2009aug04,0,4078424,full.story (accessed December 22, 2010).

6. Ibid.

7. David Kirkpatrick, "White House Affirms Deal on Drug Costs," *New York Times*, August 6, 2009.

8. John Boehner, "Letter to Billy Tauzin," August 17, 2009, http://www .kaiserhealthnews.org/Stories/2009/August/17/~/media/Images/KHN percent20 Features/2009/Aug/17/Boehnerletter.ashx (accessed October 11, 2010).

9. "The Arena: Profile: Karen Ignagni," *Politico*, http://www.politico.com/ arena/bio/karen_ignagni.html (accessed October 11, 2010).

10. Ibid.

11. Jason Rosenbaum, "Best Protector of Profits at the Expense of Our Health," *Huffington Post*, March 10, 2009, http://www.huffingtonpost.com/jason-rosenbaum/ best-protector-of-profits_b_173628.html (accessed October 11, 2010).

12. Washington Post, "Who Runs Government: Profile: Karen Ignagni," *Washington Post*, http://www.whorunsgov.com/Profiles/Karen_Ignagni (accessed October 11, 2010).

13. Liz Fowler, interview by the authors, May 12, 2010.

14. Ibid.

15. Karen Ignagni, interview by the authors, May 12, 2010.

16. Ibid.

17. Glenn Thrush, "Pelosi Slams Insurers as Immoral Villains," *Politico*, July 30, 2009, http://www.politico.com/blogs/glennthrush/0709/Pelosi_slams_insurers _as_immoral_villains.html (accessed October 11, 2010).

18. The figures in the paragraph were reported by Jeffrey Young, "Snowe, Democrats Unite on Crucial Healthcare Deal," *The Hill*, October 1, 2009, accessed October 12, 2010, http://thehill.com/homenews/senate/61299-snowe-democrats -unite-on-crucial-healthcare-deal.

19. Ezra Klein, "Pricewaterhouse Coopers Backs Away from AHIP," *Washington Post*, October 13, 2009, http://voices.washingtonpost.com/ezra-klein/2009/10/ pricewaterhousecoopers_backs_a.html (accessed October 12, 2010).

20. Liz Fowler, interview by the authors, May 12, 2010.

21. America's Health Insurance Plans, "AHIP Statement on Health Reform Legislation," March 18, 2010, http://www.ahip.org/content/pressrelease.aspx?docid =29767 (accessed December 1, 2010).

22. Peter Stone, "Health Insurers Funded Chamber Attack Ads," *National Journal Under the Influence*, January 12, 2010, http://undertheinfluence.national journal.com/2010/01/health-insurers-funded-chambers.php (accessed October 11, 2010).

23. Jonathan Cohn, "The Operator: Why is the Most Powerful Health Care Lobbyist Playing Nice?" *New Republic*, July 1, 2009, http://www.tnr.com/article/health-care/the-operator?page=0,3 (accessed December 1, 2010).

24. Stuart Altman, presentation at the Health Industry Forum, Brandeis University, "American Hospital Association Survey Data 1980–2007." The percent of uncompensated care does not include losses on Medicare, Medicaid, and SCHIP.

25. John Holahan and Bowen Garrett, *The Cost of Uncompensated Care with and without Health Reform, March 2010*, The Urban Institute, http://www.urban.org/publications/412045.html (accessed November 12, 2010).

26. Katie Connolly, "No Harry and Louise: Why Health-Care Reform Might Be Different Now," *Newsweek*, March 14, 2009, http://www.newsweek.com/2009/03/13/no-harry-and-louise.html# (accessed December 11, 2010).

27. Ibid.

28. Chip Kahn, interview by the authors, May 19, 2009.

29. "Modern Healthcare Announces 100 Most Powerful People in Healthcare," *Modern Healthcare*, August 27, 2007, http://www.modernhealthcare.com/assets/pdf/CH25102828.PDF (accessed November 13, 2010).

30. Catholic News Agency, "Catholic Health Association Summit in Denver Attracts Praise from Obama," June 5, 2010, http://www.catholicnewsagency.com/news/catholic-health-association-summit-in-denver-attracts-praise-from-obama/ (accessed November 13, 2010).

31. United States Conference of Catholic Bishops, "Pulpit Announcement and Prayer Petition," March 16, 2010, http://usccb.org/healthcare/ (accessed December 23, 2010).

32. Sister Carol Keehan, interview by the authors, November 8, 2010.

33. Chip Kahn, interview by the authors, May 12, 2010.

34. Carol Glatz, "Jesuit Journal Praises U.S. Health Reform Law as Needed, Long-Awaited," Catholic News Service, June 3, 2010, accessed November 10, 2010, http://www.catholicnews.com/data/stories/cns/1002303.htm.

35. David Kirkpatrick, "Hospital Lobbyists Say Baucus Has Not Yet Lived Up to Their Deal," Prescriptions: The Business of Health Care Blog, *New York Times*, October 7, 2009, http://prescriptions.blogs.nytimes.com/2009/10/07/hospial-lobbyists-say-baucus-has-not-yet-lived-up-to-their-deal/ (accessed December 23, 2010).

36. Karen Ignagni, interview by the authors, May 12, 2010.

37. Glenn Hackbarth, Medicare Payment Advisory Commission, House Committee on Ways and Means, Subcommittee on Health, "Hearing: Report to Congress: Medicare Payment Policy," March 17, 2009, 111th Congress, 1st sess., http://www.medpac.gov/documents/Mar09_March%20report%20testimony_WM%20FINAL.pdf (accessed December 23, 2010).

38. Amy Sorrel and Emily Berry, "Obama Tells AMA 'I need your help,'" AMEDNews.com, June 15, 2009, http://www.ama-assn.org/amednews/2009/06/15/prsc0615.htm (accessed October 25, 2010).

39. Alexander Bolton, "Reid Offers Doctors a Deal," *The Hill*, October 20, 2009, http://thehill.com/homenews/senate/63811-reid-offers-docs-a-deal (accessed October 27, 2010).

40. Ibid.

## Chapter 13: Baucus, Grassley, and the Gang of Six

1. Parts of the following discussion are taken from Liz Halloran, Audie Cornish, Peter Overby, and Julie Rovner, "What the Gang of Six Wants From Health Care Bill," National Public Radio, September 9, 2009, http://www.npr.org/templates/story/story.php?storyId=112222617 (accessed November 1, 2010).

2. Bob Cusack, "Liberal Talk Show Hosts Attack Baucus Plan," *The Hill*'s Healthcare Blog, September 21, 2009, http://thehill.com/blogs/blog-briefing-room/news/59587-liberal-talk-show-hosts-attack-baucus-plan (accessed November 1, 2010).

3. Republican National Committee, "Congressman Kevin Brady (R-TX) Delivers Weekly Republican Address," October 17, 2009, http://www.gop.com/index.php/news/comments/media_advisorycongressman_kevin_brady_r-tx_delivers_weekly_republican_addre (accessed November 1, 2010).

## Chapter 14: The Summer of Death Panels

1. Fox News, "Health Care Town Halls Turn Violent in Tampa and St. Louis," Fox News.com, August 7, 2009, http://www.foxnews.com/politics/2009/08/07/health-care-town-halls-turn-violent-tampa-st-louis/ (accessed November 9, 2010).

2. Kathy Kiely and Mimi Hall, "End-of-Life Counseling Had Bipartisan Support," *USA Today*, August 18, 2009, http://www.usatoday.com/news/health/2009-08-17-deathpanel_N.htm (accessed November 9, 2010).

3. Sam Stein, "Grassley Endorses 'Death Panel' Rumor: 'You Have Every Right to Fear,'" *Huffington Post*, August 12, 2009, http://www.huffingtonpost.com/2009/08/12/grassley-endorses-death-p_n_257677.html (accessed November 9, 2010).

4. Robert Pear and David Herzenhorn, "Democrats Push Health Care Plan While Issuing Assurances on Medicare," *New York Times*, July 28, 2009, http://www

.nytimes.com/2009/07/29/health/policy/29health.html (accessed November 9, 2010).

5. Harold Sox and Sheldon Greenfield, "Comparative Effectiveness Research: A Report from the Institute of Medicine," *Annals of Internal Medicine* 151. no. 3 (2009): 203–5.

6. The text quoted here is available online at http://www.gpo.gov/fdsys/pkg/PLAW-111publ148/pdf/PLAW-111publ148.pdf.

7. Health Affairs, "Comparative Effectiveness Research," *Health Affairs*, October 5, 2010, http://www.healthaffairs.org/healthpolicybriefs/brief.php?brief_id=28 (accessed November 10, 2010).

8. Alicia Mundy, "Drug Makers Fight Stimulus Provision," *Wall Street Journal*, February 10, 2009.

## Chapter 15: The Speaker Carries the Day

1. American Civil Liberties Union, "Public Funding for Abortion," July 21, 2004, http://www.aclu.org/reproductive-freedom/public-funding-abortion (accessed August 9, 2010).

2. David Kirkpatrick and Robert Pear, "For Abortion Foes, a Victory in Health Care Vote," *New York Times*, November 9, 2009.

3. Thomas Langhorne, "Ellsworth Angers Abortion Foes," *Evansville Courier and Press*, November 6, 2009, http://www.courierpress.com/news/2009/nov/06/ellsworth-angers-abortion-foes/ (accessed November 5, 2010).

4. Julian Pecquet, "Defeated Ellsworth Was One Election Target of Abortion Opponents," *The Hill*, November 2, 2010, http://thehill.com/blogs/healthwatch/politics-elections/127143-defeated-ellsworth-was-target-of-abortion-opponents-ire (accessed November 5, 2010).

5. Tom Daschle, *Getting It Done: How Obama and Congress Finally Broke the Stalemate to Make Way for Health Care Reform* (New York: St. Martin's, 2010) Kindle edition pp. 3,957–93.

6. Patricia Murphy, "Nancy Pelosi: Abortion Debate not Over; Afghanistan Vote Harder than Health care," The Capitolist (blog), *Politics Daily*, November 16, 2009, http://www.politicsdaily.com/2009/11/16/nancy-pelosi-abortion-debate-not-over-afghanistan-vote-harder/ (accessed November 5, 2010).

7. Sheryl Stolberg, "Obama Presses Senate to Pass its Health Bill," *New York Times*, November 9, 2009.

## Chapter 16: The Senate and the Christmas Eve Health Bill

1. Carol Morello and Ashley Halsey III, "Massive Storm Sets December Record, Cripples Transit," *Washington Post*, December 20, 2009.

2. Helen Halpin and Peter Harbage, "The Origin and Demise of the Public Option," *Health Affairs* 29, no. 6 (2010): 1118.

3. Clay Chandler, "Letter to Honorable Harry Reid," December 19, 2009, http://cbo.gov/ftpdocs/108xx/doc10868/12-19-Reid_Letter_Managers _Correction_Noted.pdf (accessed October 5, 2010).

4. Ibid., p. 1.

5. Currently, if you are in a 33 percent tax bracket and you deduct an expense from income, it would reduce your taxes by 33 percent of the amount of the deduction. Obama's proposal would reduce the amount of the deduction to 28 percent for those in the highest income brackets.

6. Richard Wolf, "Lawmakers Target Health Insurance Tax Break," *USA Today*, June 11, 2009, http://www.usatoday.com/news/health/2009-06-10-health cost_N.htm (accessed November 5, 2010). The data cited in the articles are figures provided by the Office of Management and Budget.

7. This description of events from Paul Kane, "To Sway Nelson, A Hard-Won Compromise on Abortion Issue," *Washington Post*, December 20, 2009, http://www .washingtonpost.com/wp-dyn/content/article/2009/12/19/AR2009121902383 .html (accessed August 17, 2010).

8. Robert Pear and David Herszenhorn, "Senate Clears Final Hurdle to Vote on Health Care Bill, *New York Times*, December 24, 2009.

9. Shailagh Murray, "Senators ready to Vote Again; With 60 Backers, Measure May Pass on Christmas Eve," *Washington Post*, December 22, 2009.

10. Dana Millbank, "An Ugly Finale for Health Reform," *Washington Post*, December 21, 2009, http://www.washingtonpost.com/wp-dyn/content/article/2009/ 12/20/AR2009122002872.html (accessed August 18, 2010).

11. This and balance of paragraph from Rachel Maddow, "OMG—Republican Senators Pray to Kill Healthcare," broadcast Dec. 17, 2009. The full contents of this broadcast can be accessed at http://www.youtube.com/watch?v=RHXXPeN84yY.

12. Description of Whitehouse speech from Millbank, "Ugly Finale."

13. Description from Mark Leibovich, "Despite Fragile Health, Byrd is Present for Votes," *New York Times*, December 24, 2009, http://query.nytimes.com/gst/ fullpage.html?res=9903E7D8113CF937A15751C1A96F9C8B63&scp=1&sq =december+24+2009+despite+fragile+health&st=nyt (accessed August 18, 2010).

14. Millbank, "Ugly Finale."

15. The full contents of President Obama's speech can be heard at http://www .youtube.com/watch?v=GALYnnAQFKA.

## Chapter 17: Success at Last

1. Sheryl Stolberg, Jeff Zeleny, and Carl Hulse, "Health Vote Caps a Journey-back from the Brink," *New York Times*, March 20, 2010.

2. Staff Writers, *Washington Post, Landmark: The Inside Story of America's New Health-Care Law and What It Means for Us All* (New York: Public Affairs, 2010), pp. 49–50.

3. Huma Khan, "Lawmakers Blast Anthem Blue Cross Executives for Insurance Rate Hikes," *ABC News*, February 24, 2010, http://abcnews.go.com/WN/Politics/anthem-blue-cross-owner-wellpoint-fire-lawmakers-insurance/story?id=9931601 (accessed August 25, 2010).

4. Office of the Press Secretary, "Remarks by the President on Health Reform," March 3, 2010, http://www.whitehouse.gov/the-press-office/remarks-president-health-care-reform (accessed August 25, 2010).

5. Seattle Times News Service, "Senate's Rule Referee out of Obscurity, into Spotlight," *Seattle Times*, http://seattletimes.nwsource.com/html/nationworld/2011372817_rulesguy18.html (accessed September 12, 2010).

6. Ibid.

7. Dan Amira, "New Yorker Alan Frumin, Senate Parliamentarian, Back in the Hot Seat Once More," *New York Magazine*, http://nymag.com/daily/intel/2010/01/new_yorker_alan_frumin_senate.html (accessed September 14, 2010).

8. Ibid.

9. A little known oddity was an impediment. CBO had to score the reconciliation bill under current law, and the Senate health reform bill was not yet current law. Without the Senate bill, the reconciliation bill would have increased the deficit and, hence, could not be allowed under the Byrd Rule.

10. Jeff Zeleny, "Millions Spent to Sway Democrats on Health Care," *New York Times*, March 14, 2010.

11. Ibid.

12. David Herzenhorn, "Obama Delays Trip as Report Aids Final Push on Health Care," *New York Times*, March 17, 2010.

13. James Martin, "60 Women's Religious Orders Support Health Care Bill," In All Things: Our Group Blog, *America Magazine*, March 17, 2010, http://www.america magazine.org/blog/entry.cfm?blog_id=2&entry_id=17992010 (accessed September 14, 2010).

14. Statement of Sister Carol Keehan, "The Time is Now for Health Reform," *Catholic Health World*, 26 no. 5 (2010), http://www.chausa.org/The_time_is_now_for_health_reform.aspx (accessed September 14, 2010).

15. Stephanie Condon, "Bart Stupak Received Threatening Messages for Health Care Vote," *CBS News Political Hotsheet*, March 24, 2010, http://www.cbsnews.com/8301-503544_162-20001091-503544.html (accessed September 15, 2010).

16. Ibid.

17. Robert Pear and David Herszenhorn, "Obama Hails Vote on Health Care as Answering 'the Call of History,'" *New York Times*, March 21, 2010.

18. Ibid.

19. The full text video of Obama's speech can be found at http://www .youtube.com/watch?v=GALYnnAQFKA (accessed September 17, 2010).

20. Sheryl Stolberg and Robert Pear, "Obama Signs Health Care Overhaul Bill with a Flourish," *New York Times*, March 23, 2010.

21. Ibid.

22. These estimates are from Chuck Marr, "Changes in Medicare Tax on High-Income People Represent Sound Additions to Health Reform," March 4, 2010, http:// www.cbpp.org/cms/index.cfm?fa=view&id=3102 (accessed August 13, 2010).

23. Ibid.

24. The data for the balance of this summary (through page 139) is from the Democratic Policy Committee, "The Health Care and Education Reconciliation Act: Section-by-Section Analysis," http://dpc.senate.gov/healthreformbill/health bill63.pdf (accessed September 17, 2010).

## Chapter 18: How He Did It

1. Kavita Patel and John McDonough, "From Massachusetts to 1600 Pennsylvania Avenue: Aboard the Health Reform Express," *Health Affairs* 29, no. 6 (2010): 1106–11.

2. The full text and audio of Obama's speech given on September 9, 2009 before a joint session of Congress can be found at http://www.pbs.org/newshour/ updates/politics/july-dec09/speechtext_09-09.html (accessed July 23, 2010).

3. The full text of Obama's 2010 State of the Union address can be found online at http://www.whitehouse.gov/the-press-office/remarks-president-state -union-address.

## Chapter 19: The Future Is Cost Control

1. Cathy Schoen, Jennifer Nicholson, and Sheila Rustgi, *Paying the Price: How Health Insurance Premiums Are Eating Up Middle Class Incomes, State Health Insurance Premium Trends and the Potential of National Health Reform* (New York: The Commonwealth Fund, 2009).

2. US Department of Labor, Bureau of Labor Statistics, *Occupational Outlook Handbook*, 2010-2011 ed. (Washington, DC: Government Printing Office, 2010).

3. Association of American Medical Colleges, "Policy Brief: Physician Shortages to Worsen without Increases in Residency Training," June 2010, https://www.aamc.org/download/153160/data/physician_shortages_to_worsen_without_increases_in_residency_tr.pdf (accessed December 23, 2010).

4. Partnership for Solutions, *Chronic Conditions: Making the Case for Ongoing Care* (Baltimore: Johns Hopkins University, 2002).

5. Robert Graham Center, *The Patient Centered Medical Home: History, Seven Core Features, Evidence and Transformational Change* (Washington, DC: Robert Graham Center, 2007), p. 2.

6. Ibid., p. 5.

7. Barbara Starfield, Leiyu Shi, and James Macinko, "Contribution of Primary Care to Health Systems and Health," *Milbank Quarterly* 83, no. 3 (2005): 457–502.

8. US Department of Health and Human Services, Centers for Medicare and Medicaid Services, Office of Legislation, "Medicare 'Accountable Care Organizations' Shared Savings Program—New Section 1899 of Title XVIII," https://www.cms.gov/OfficeofLegislation/Downloads/AccountableCareOrganization.pdf (accessed December 22, 2010).

9. Kelly Devers and Robert Berenson, "Can Accountable Care Organizations Improve the Value of Health Care by Solving the Cost and Quality Quandaries?" *Robert Wood Johnson Foundation and Urban Institute*, 2009 http://www.urban.org/publications/411975.html (accessed May 16, 2011).

10. Peter Orszag, Congressional Budget Office, Senate Committee on Finance, "Testimony: The Medicare Advantage Program: Enrollment and Budgetary Effects," April 11, 2007, 110th Congress, 2nd sess, http://cbo.gov/ftpdocs/79xx/doc7994/04-11-MedicareAdvantage.pdf (accessed May 21, 2010).

11. James Capretta, "The Independent Payment Advisory Board and Health Care Price Controls," *Kaiser Health News*, May 6, 2010, http://www.kaiserhealthnews.org/Columns/2010/May/050610Capretta.aspx (accessed December 22, 2010).

## Epilogue

1. Andrea Sisko, Christopher Truffer, Sean Keehan, John Poisal, Joseph Lizonitz, M. Clemens, and Andrew Madison, "National Health Spending Projections: The Estimated Impact of Reform Through 2019," *Health Affairs* 29 no. 10 (2010): 1933–41.

# GLOSSARY

**ACCOUNTABLE CARE ORGANIZATION (ACO):** An integrated group of health care providers who assume responsibility for the quality and cost of patients, and who coordinate care across providers.

**ADVERSE SELECTION:** A situation in which patients who have greater than average expected health care costs select an insurer or health plan.

**AGENCY FOR HEALTHCARE RESEARCH AND QUALITY (AHRQ):** A government agency responsible for helping to improve the quality, safety, efficiency, and effectiveness of American health care.

**AMERICAN ASSOCIATION OF HEALTH PLANS (AAHP):** An organization that represented large private health insurance companies and integrated health systems. AAHP merged with the Health Insurance Association of America (HIAA) in 2000 to become America's Health Insurance Plans (AHIP).

**AMERICAN ASSOCIATION OF MEDICAL COLLEGES (AAMC):** An organization representing academic medical centers including medical schools, teaching hospitals, and health systems.

**AMERICAN ASSOCIATION OF RETIRED PERSONS (AARP):** A membership and advocacy organization for individuals fifty years of age and over. The organization formally changed its name to AARP.

**AMERICAN FEDERATION OF LABOR AND CONGRESS OF INDUSTRIAL ORGANIZATIONS (AFL-CIO):** A federation of national and international labor unions with over twelve million members. The federation was formed in 1955 by the merger of the AFL with the CIO.

**AMERICAN HOSPITAL ASSOCIATION (AHA):** The largest member organization representing American hospitals. The AHA provides extensive educational services to member hospitals.

**AMERICAN MEDICAL ASSOCIATION (AMA):** The largest organization representing American physicians. The AMA provides extensive educational services to member physicians.

**AMERICA'S HEALTH INSURANCE PLANS (AHIP):** The largest organization representing American health insurance companies and health plans. AHIP was created by the merger of the American Association of Health Plans and the Health Insurance Association of America in the year 2000. AHIP was also an acronym for a Nixon administration proposal called the "Assisted Health Insurance Plan." It was a comprehensive plan to replace Medicaid but was never enacted.

**ASSIGNMENT:** A financial arrangement in which a doctor agrees to be paid in full directly by Medicare for approved medical services.

**BALANCE BILLING:** A financial arrangement in which a patient agrees to pay a doctor some amount above what the doctor collects from an insurer.

**BENEFIT PACKAGE:** The collection of services an insurer contractually agrees to provide to a customer that it insures. A minimum benefit package (often required by state or federal regulations) prescribes the minimum collection of services that an insurer must provide.

**BLUE CROSS PLANS:** Hospital insurance plans that were originally developed by hospitals, but are now private, independent health insurance plans. They are often combined with Blue Shield plans that provide insurance for physician services.

**BLUE DOG:** A name referring to Democratic members of Congress from the South whose political philosophy is often conservative.

**BLUE SHIELD PLANS:** Insurance plans for physician services that were originally developed by physicians, but are now private, independent health insurance plans. They are often combined with Blue Cross plans that provide insurance for hospital services.

**BUNDLED PAYMENT:** A payment methodology in which the unit of payment is for the entire package of services associated with a distinct medical event. This contrasts with fee-for-service in which the unit of payment is for each separate service provided to a patient.

**BYRD RULE:** A budget rule named after the late senator Robert Byrd. Under the Byrd Rule, a senator can raise a point of order if a bill being considered under the budget reconciliation process (see **RECONCILIATION**) were to contain any provision that is not directly germane to the budget (either increases or decreases revenues). If the point of order were to be sustained, the provision would be stricken unless the Senate could muster three-fifths (currently sixty votes) to waive the rule.

**CADILLAC TAX:** A tax levied on an expensive health plan. The tax is levied on a health plan, the cost of which exceeds a threshold amount, in order to discourage such complete health insurance coverage that beneficiaries will not be cost conscious.

**CAPITATION:** A payment methodology in which a provider (or a health plan) receives a predetermined amount of money to take care of all of a person's health needs for a fixed period of time (usually one year). In theory, the prospective payment amount is an incentive to keep the patient healthy and provide services in the most efficient manner so that the provider's cost does not exceed the advance payment.

**CASE MIX:** The various types (mix) of patients treated by a hospital or medical plan. Patients can be defined by certain attributes such as age, sex, severity of illness, and so on.

**CATASTROPHIC INSURANCE:** An insurance policy that insures against very large (catastrophic) costs, but in which the insured usually pays out-of-pocket for all costs that are below the catastrophic threshold. This is in contrast to "first-dollar" insurance in which the policy covers all costs. In theory, catastrophic insurance makes insured people more cost conscious because they are paying with their own money for services below the threshold.

**CATHOLIC HEALTH ASSOCIATION (CHA):** An organization that represents Catholic hospitals, health systems, and nursing homes.

**CENTERS FOR MEDICARE AND MEDICAID SERVICES (CMS):** The federal agency that administers the Medicare, Medicaid, and Children's Health Insurance programs.

**CERTIFICATE OF NEED (CON):** A certificate issued by a state government or planning agency permitting a hospital to make a capital investment in constructing a building, providing a service, or purchasing an expensive piece of equipment.

**CHAIRMAN'S MARK:** The recommendation (usually in the form of a bill) by a committee chairperson that is brought to the floor for markup.

**CHILDREN'S HEALTH INSURANCE PROGRAM:** A federal/state program to provide health insurance to children (and in some cases parents of children) who qualify by being below an income threshold.

**CLAW-BACK:** A federal requirement that states pay back to the federal government funds that it had been spending for a program when that program is taken over and paid for by the federal government.

CLOTURE: A vote to end debate in the Senate. Cloture votes are used to end the threat that a bill cannot be brought to a vote because of continuous debate (i.e., a filibuster). Cloture requires a three-fifths vote (currently sixty members) of the Senate.

CODING: A process of classifying medical diagnoses in accordance with an international system. Codes can be translated into Medicare or insurance payments by assigning a dollar amount to each code.

COINSURANCE: The portion of a total medical bill that the insured person must pay out-of-pocket. For example, Medicare Part B requires beneficiaries to pay 20 percent of most doctor bills.

COMMUNITY RATE: An insurance term meaning that everyone within a designated geographical area pays the same premium regardless of how much medical care they are expected to use based upon such characteristics as age, sex, health status, and so on.

COMPARATIVE EFFECTIVENESS RESEARCH (CER): Research that compares the efficacy of different kinds of treatments to provide information on what constitutes the best medical practice. The research could compare two drugs, drugs versus surgery, different surgical techniques, and so on.

COMPREHENSIVE HEALTH INSURANCE PLAN (CHIP): President Richard Nixon's universal health insurance plan that he proposed in 1974.

CONFERENCE COMMITTEE: See HOUSE–SENATE CONFERENCE COMMITTEE.

CONGRESSIONAL BUDGET OFFICE (CBO): A congressionally appointed, nonpartisan agency that is required to determine the budgetary implications of any bill before it can be voted upon.

CONSUMER OPERATED AND ORIENTED PLAN (CO-OP): A nonprofit insurance plan controlled by the patients it insures. The Obama health plan requires each state to include such a plan in its insurance exchange.

COPAYMENT: A predetermined dollar payment that an insured person must pay each time they receive a medical service. For example, a visit to a doctor, regardless of the reason, often obligates the insured to pay a small, predetermined amount—usually about twenty dollars.

COST/CHARGE RATIO: In hospital billing, the cost of a billed service divided by the retail listed price of that service. Often hospital statistics are reported in terms of price, and analysts who wish to determine the cost of a service multiply the price by an estimated cost/charge ratio.

**COST EFFECTIVENESS ANALYSIS:** Research that compares the cost of a treatment regimen with the expected benefit. The most frequently used methodology employs "quality-adjusted life years" as a component of the benefit. That measure includes both the additional length of life and the quality of life expected from a treatment regimen. The benefit is monetized by adding a dollar value for each quality-adjusted life year.

**COST PER ADMISSION:** The cost of an inpatient admission to the hospital. Medicare originally calculated the average cost per admission as all the expenses (costs) incurred by a hospital divided by the number of admissions. Medicare now uses the DRG methodology to calculate this measure.

**COST PER CASE:** See **COST PER ADMISSION**.

**COST PER DIEM:** The cost to stay in the hospital as an inpatient for a day. The average cost per diem is calculated as hospital total cost/total number of hospital inpatient days for a given period of time.

**COST SHARING:** The amount insured individuals must pay toward each service covered by his or her insurance plan. Cost sharing generally takes the form of copayments, coinsurance, and/or deductibles.

**DEATH PANEL:** An erroneous description of some aspects of the Obama health plan. A death panel was supposedly a government or government-sponsored group that would decide if a public program, such as Medicare, would pay for a potentially life-saving course of treatment. The claim had no basis in fact.

**DEATH SPIRAL:** A situation that occurs when an insurer is subject to adverse selection and enrolls a higher proportion of sicker people than its competitors. In such cases the insurer has to raise its prices, but higher prices cause its healthiest people to drop out, and then it has to raise prices even more, and so on.

**DEDUCTIBLE:** An amount insured people must pay within any billing period (usually one year) before insurance begins to cover their expenses. For example, people enrolled in the Medicare Prescription Drug program must pay the first $250 in any benefit year.

**DEFINED BENEFIT:** A package of benefits that is guaranteed to an eligible recipient. For example, Medicare provides every beneficiary a defined set of benefits.

**DEFINED CONTRIBUTION:** In health care, an amount contributed or given to a recipient (sometimes periodically) that the recipient can use to purchase insurance (similar to a voucher).There is no guarantee that the amount will be adequate to purchase the desired package of benefits. Also the amount an insurance policy will reimburse a patient for a given medical procedure.

DEPARTMENT OF HEALTH AND HUMAN SERVICES (DHHS): The US government's principal agency responsible for protecting the health of all Americans and providing essential human services, particularly to those in need.

DIAGNOSIS RELATED GROUP (DRG): A system used to classify hospital patients into groups according to their medical diagnoses. In the United States, the Medicare program uses the DRG system to pay most hospitals.

DIAGNOSIS RELATED GROUP CREEP (DRG CREEP): A situation in which hospitals classify patients into higher-paying DRGs in order to increase revenue (also called upcoding or code creep).

DUAL ELIGIBLE: A person who qualifies for both Medicare and Medicaid.

EARLY PERIODIC SCREENING, DIAGNOSIS, AND TREATMENT (EPSDT): A screening and prevention program for all children under twenty-one years of age who are enrolled in Medicaid. The program requires screening and subsequent treatment for a variety of conditions, even if those treatments are not required under a particular state's Medicaid program.

EMERGENCY MEDICAL TREATMENT AND ACTIVE LABOR ACT (EMTALA): A federal law that requires hospitals and ambulance services to provide care to anyone needing emergency treatment, regardless of citizenship or ability to pay. The law only applies to hospitals and ambulance services that participate in the Medicare program, but that is virtually all of them.

EMPLOYER MANDATE: A law requiring employers to provide health insurance to their employees. Obligations under the law may vary according to types of coverage and employer attributes such as firm size, level of employee compensation, and so on.

EXPERIENCE RATE: An insurance term meaning that insurers set the premium rates of insured persons or groups according to past spending patterns or certain attributes such as age, health status, gender, past health history, and so on.

FEDERAL EMPLOYEES HEALTH BENEFITS PROGRAM (FEHBP): An insurance program for federal employees that permits them to choose among a number of competing private health insurance plans.

**FEDERATION OF AMERICAN HOSPITALS (FAH):** An organization that represents for-profit hospitals.

**FEE-FOR-SERVICE:** A payment methodology in which providers are paid for each service that they render. This contrasts with payment for an entire hospital admission or episode of care.

**FILIBUSTER:** A Senate procedure in which a member may delay a proceeding by speaking endlessly and not yielding the floor. Ending a filibuster requires a cloture vote. See **CLOTURE.**

**FIRST-DOLLAR COVERAGE:** An insurance policy that has no deductible, copayment, or coinsurance. The policy provides coverage beginning with the "first-dollar" charged.

**FISCAL INTERMEDIARY:** In health insurance, an organization that helps to administer a health insurance policy or plan for the company or government entity that provides the insurance.

**FORMULARY:** In health insurance, the list of drugs that are covered by an insurance policy. It also is used to designate certain drugs which are given a preferred payment amount within a class of drugs considered to have similar medical attributes.

**GLOBAL BUDGET:** In health care, the total amount paid to provide medical coverage for an entire population in a geographic area, such as a city, state, or country.

**GUARANTEED ISSUE:** A policy that requires insurance companies to issue insurance to all applicants, regardless of their age, gender, health status, and so on. Under guaranteed issue, premium increases among enrollees with different risk profiles are limited by government regulation or company policy.

**HEALTH AND HUMAN SERVICES (HHS):** See **DEPARTMENT OF HEALTH AND HUMAN SERVICES.**

**HEALTH CARE FINANCING ADMINISTRATION:** The federal agency that administered the Medicare and Medicaid programs. The agency's name was changed to the Centers for Medicare and Medicaid Services (CMS) in 2001.

**HEALTH, EDUCATION, AND WELFARE (HEW):** A federal cabinet office that is now the Department of Health and Human Services. See **DEPARTMENT OF HEALTH AND HUMAN SERVICES.**

**HEALTH INSURANCE ASSOCIATION OF AMERICA (HIAA):** An organization that represented insurance companies. It merged with the American Association of Health Plans (AAHP) in 2000 to become America's Health Insurance Plans (AHIP).

**HEALTH INSURANCE PURCHASING COOPERATIVE (HIPC):** An organization that acts as an intermediary to assists individuals or groups to purchase insurance. Under the Clinton health plan, all insurance would be purchased through such quasi-governmental entities.

**HEALTH MAINTENANCE ORGANIZATION (HMO):** An organization that provides health insurance and/or health care with a commitment to manage the care of its enrollees. In some cases, an HMO owns its hospitals and clinics. To varying degrees, HMOs integrate the financing and delivery of health care. An HMO requires enrollees to choose care from a limited panel of doctors that could be independent or salaried. Some HMOs operate on a capitated basis. See CAPITATION.

**HEALTH SAVINGS ACCOUNT (HSA):** An account belonging to an individual that is funded by "before tax" earnings. It is paired with a high deductible health plan and is used to pay for medical expenses up to the amount of the deductible.

**HEALTH SYSTEMS AGENCY (HSA):** A federal organization that carried out health planning functions during the '70s.

**HIGH-DEDUCTIBLE HEALTH PLAN:** A health plan with a deductible that is generally higher than two thousand dollars. Such a plan is often paired with a health savings account (HSA).

**HILL–BURTON PROGRAM:** A federal program that distributed funds to the states for the construction of hospitals and other health care facilities. The program required participating hospitals to provide a "reasonable amount" of free care to the poor.

**HOUSE–SENATE CONFERENCE:** A meeting or series of meetings among designated members of both houses of Congress to reconcile different versions of a bill that was passed by the House and the Senate.

**HYDE AMENDMENT:** An amendment named after Henry Hyde (R-IL) that bans the use of most federal funds for abortions, except in cases of rape, incest, or danger to the life of the mother. The amendment is in the form of a rider that has been attached to annual appropriation bills every year since 1976.

**INCOME-RELATED PREMIUMS:** Health insurance premiums that vary with an insured person's income. For example, in Medicare Part B, higher income enrollees are charged higher premiums.

**JOB LOCK:** A situation in which employees feel that they cannot leave or change their places of employment because replacing their employer-provided health coverage may be difficult or unaffordable.

**LENGTH OF STAY:** The number of days a person spends in the hospital for an episode of care.

**MANAGED CARE:** An arrangement in which an insurer can act as an intermediary to regulate (or manage) some aspects of the doctor–patient relationship. For example, the insurer may limit the choice of doctor or influence the doctor's treatment by establishing practice guidelines, reviewing the doctor's utilization of services, or providing monetary incentives and disincentives. The primary goal of managed care is to ensure the best practice in the most appropriate setting.

**MANAGED COMPETITION:** A system proposed as part of the Clinton health plan in which managed care companies would compete against each other, but the competition would be structured (managed) by intermediaries called health insurance purchasing cooperatives.

**MANAGER'S AMENDMENT:** An amendment or group of amendments added to a piece of legislation by the majority leader before the legislation is brought to the floor of the chamber.

**MEDICAID:** The government program that provides health insurance to low-income citizens. The program is jointly financed by the federal government and the states and is administered and structured by the states within federal guidelines.

**MEDICAL LOSS RATIO:** The proportion of insurance premiums that an insurance company spends on direct medical care (as opposed to marketing, administration, etc.).

**MEDICAL PAYMENT ASSESSMENT COMMISSION (MEDPAC):** An independent agency created by Congress to provide advice about issues pertaining to the Medicare program.

**MEDICARE:** The federal government program that provides health insurance to people sixty-five years of age or over and to the disabled.

**MEDICARE ADVANTAGE (MA):** A program that allows private health insurance plans to offer Medicare benefits. Medicare Advantage plans are paid by Medicare but compete with the traditional Medicare program. The authorization for MA plans is included in Part C of the Medicare program.

**MEDICARE + CHOICE:** A program in which private health insurance plans offered Medicare benefits and competed with the traditional Medicare program. Medicare + Choice was succeeded by the Medicare Advantage program in 1997.

**MEDICARE PART A:** The part of the Medicare program that insures all inpatient hospital care and limited amounts of other care following an inpatient stay (such as inpatient rehabilitation or home health care). Part A is a universal insurance program funded by payroll tax deductions.

**MEDICARE PART B:** The part of the Medicare program that insures outpatient and doctor care, as well as some other medical services. Part B is an optional program partially funded by premiums and cost sharing, but heavily subsidized from federal general revenues.

**MEDICARE PART C:** See **MEDICARE ADVANTAGE.**

**MEDICARE PART D:** A provision in the Medicare program that authorizes stand-alone drug plans for people who are enrolled in the traditional Medicare program.

**MEDICARE PRESCRIPTION DRUG, IMPROVEMENT, AND MODERNIZATION ACT (MEDICARE MODERNIZATION ACT OR MMA):** The legislation enacted in 2003 that provides for prescription drug coverage under the Medicare program.

**MEDICARE WITHHOLDING TAX:** A payroll tax deduction that funds Medicare Part A.

**MORAL HAZARD:** The tendency of people to demand more products or services because they are not required to pay the full costs. For example, health insurance that shields people from paying the full cost of health services may encourage the extra use of medical services that are of marginal value.

**NATIONAL FEDERATION OF INDEPENDENT BUSINESS (NFIB):** An association representing small business.

**NATIONAL INSTITUTES OF HEALTH (NIH):** In health care, a number of federally funded institutes that support and conduct medical research. NIH is part of the Department of Health and Human Services (DHHS).

**NEAR-ELDERLY:** People between the ages of fifty-five and sixty-five.

**OFFICE OF MANAGEMENT AND BUDGET (OMB):** An executive branch agency that oversees the financial operations of government and government agencies.

**OFFICES OF THE ACTUARY:** In health care, a component of the Medicare program that provides Medicare and various parts of the government with statistical analysis related to medical spending and utilization.

**OPEN ENROLLMENT PERIOD:** In insurance, a time period in which anyone can apply for insurance coverage.

**OUTLIER:** A patient who requires an unusually long and/or costly hospital stay.

**PARLIAMENTARIAN:** The person who judges whether the rules and procedures of Congress are being properly followed.

**PATIENT-CENTERED OUTCOME RESEARCH INSTITUTE (PCORI):** In the Obama health plan, a federally appointed board to oversee comparative effectiveness research.

**PHARMACEUTICAL RESEARCH AND MANUFACTURERS OF AMERICA (PHRMA):** An organization representing pharmaceutical research and biotechnology companies.

**POINT OF SERVICE PLAN (POS):** A health insurance plan that permits enrollees to choose health providers outside of their networks for no additional charge.

**PREEXISTING CONDITION:** A medical condition that exists before a person enrolls in an insurance plan.

**PREFERRED PROVIDER ORGANIZATION (PPO):** A health insurance plan with a limited number of network providers. An enrollee can seek care from network providers or choose out-of-network providers for an additional charge.

**PREPAID GROUP PRACTICE:** A group of providers that is paid prospectively. See **PROSPECTIVE PAYMENT**.

**PROSPECTIVE PAYMENT:** A payment rate that is set in advance for a service or a complete set of services. The Medicare Prospective Payment System sets rates in advance according to a patient's diagnosis.

**PROSPECTIVE PAYMENT ASSESSMENT COMMISSION (PROPAC):** An independent agency created by Congress to provide advice pertaining to the Medicare prospective payment system. ProPAC was merged with PPRC to form MedPAC in 1997.

**PROSPECTIVE PAYMENT REVIEW COMMISSION (PPRC):** An independent agency created by Congress to provide advice pertaining to payment of doctors under the Medicare program.

**PROSPECTIVE PAYMENT SYSTEM (PPS):** A system for setting the rates for services before they are performed. The Medicare program pays for most services prospectively utilizing DRGs. See DIAGNOSIS RELATED GROUPS.

PUBLIC OPTION: In the debate over the Obama health plan, a publicly-run health insurance plan that would compete with private insurers in state or federal insurance exchanges.

QUALITY-ADJUSTED LIFE YEAR (QALY): A methodology for monetizing the value of an added period of life by considering both the added living time and the quality of life experienced during the added living time.

RATING BAND: The difference in premium rates that an insurer charges because of certain attributes of the insured. For example, if an insurer charged a sixty-year-old person three times as much as a twenty-year-old person, it would represent a rating band of three-to-one. Rating-band differences are regulated by some states and by the Obama health plan.

RECONCILIATION: A procedure in the US Senate that limits the debate on bills pertaining only to the budget so that the bills cannot be filibustered and, hence, can be enacted by a simple majority vote.

RESOURCE-BASED RELATIVE VALUE SCALE (RBRVS): A system that rates the relative values of physician services according to a number of attributes such as years of education required, practice expenses, risk to the patient, and so on. The relative values are used by the Medicare program and some health plans to pay doctors for their services.

RETROSPECTIVE PAYMENT: Payment, or the determination of payment amount, for services that have already been performed.

RISK ADJUSTMENT: In health insurance, a process of adjusting an insurer's premium payments according to the risk profile of the patient or group of patients. For example, the insurer might receive a higher premium for an older person. The adjustment would be paid from a fund administered by a third party and would not come from the insured person.

ROE V. WADE: The 1973 Supreme Court decision that legalized most abortions in the United States.

SINGLE-PAYER: A health insurance system in which one single entity (the government) sets payment rates and pays for all health services excluding patient cost-sharing.

SOCIAL INSURANCE: Insurance that covers everyone in a population, is paid for by tax revenues, and generally provides everyone the same package of benefits.

**SOCIAL SECURITY TRUST FUND:** The fund that collects money from payroll withholding taxes and disburses funds to Social Security recipients.

**SOCIAL SECURITY WITHHOLDING TAX:** The payroll tax deduction that funds Social Security benefits.

**SOLE COMMUNITY HOSPITAL:** A hospital that meets certain requirements for serving an area with few other hospital services. The Medicare program pays such hospitals mainly according to cost rather than by DRGs.

**STATE CHILDREN'S HEALTH INSURANCE PROGRAM (SCHIP):** See CHILDREN'S HEALTH INSURANCE PROGRAM.

**SUSTAINABLE GROWTH RATE (SGR):** A designated growth target that limits the total payment Medicare can pay doctors based on the growth in GDP and medical inflation.

**TAX EQUITY AND FISCAL RESPONSIBILITY ACT OF 1982 (TEFRA):** A law enacted by Congress that limited allowable hospital costs for payment under the Medicare and Medicaid programs.

**THIRD PARTY ADMINISTRATOR:** An organization that acts as a fiscal agent to process payments and perform administrative tasks for employers that self-insure the health policies of employees.

**THIRD PARTY REIMBURSEMENT:** In health care, a payment for medical services that are rendered by someone other than the patient; usually an insurer or government.

**UNCOMPENSATED CARE:** The sum of free care and bad debt expenses incurred by hospitals.

**UNIVERSAL ACCESS:** A system in which everyone has access to buy or receive health insurance, but may not be insured because of affordability, personal choice, and so on.

**UNIVERSAL COVERAGE:** A system in which all people have health insurance.

**UPCODING:** See **DIAGNOSIS RELATED GROUP CREEP.**

**UTILIZATION REVIEW:** The practice by health insurance plans of reviewing doctors' records in order to analyze their performances in using the proper amount and type of resources and procedures.

**WAIVER:** In health policy, permission for a state to circumvent certain federal requirements. A waiver is generally given in response to a state application to implement its own set of policies.

**ZERO-PREMIUM PLAN:** A health insurance plan that does not charge the enrollee any premium because it is receiving sufficient payment from the government for its service obligations.

# BIBLIOGRAPHY

Aaron, Henry, and Paul Ginsburg. "Is Health Spending Excessive? If So, What Can We Do About It?" *Health Affairs* 28, no. 5 (2009): 1260–75.

Aaron, Henry, and Robert Reischauer. "The Medicare Reform Debate: What is the Next Step?" *Health Affairs* 14, no. 4 (1995): 8–30.

Adams, Patricia, Kathleen Heyman, and Jackline Vickerie. "Summary Health Statistics for the US Population: National Health Interview Survey, 2008." *Vital Health Statistics* 10, no. 243 (2009).

Almanac of Hospital Financial and Operating Indicators. *Financial Indicators: Profitability Ratios*, 2010 edition. http://www.ingenix.com/content/attachments/ALM.pdf.

Altman, Drew. "Creating a National Health Planning System." *Federal Health Programs*. Edited by Stuart Altman and Harvey Sapoksly. Lexington, MA: Lexington Books, 1981.

Altman, Stuart. US Department of Health, Education, and Welfare. *Present and Future Supply of Registered Nurses*. Washington, DC: Government Printing Office, 1971.

———. Presentation at the Health Industry Forum, Brandeis University. "American Hospital Association Survey Data 1980–2007."

Altman, Stuart, and Marc Rodman. "Halfway Competitive Markets and Ineffective Regulation: The American Health Care System." *Journal of Health Politics, Policy and Law* 13, no. 2 (1988): 323–39.

Association of American Medical Colleges. "Medicare Indirect Medical Education (IME) Payment." https://www.aamc.org/download/86186/data/moranime.pdf.

———. "Policy Brief: Physician Shortages to Worsen without Increases in Residency Training." June 2010. https://www.aamc.org/download/153160/data/physician_shortages_to_worsen_without_increases_in_residency_tr.pdf.

American Health Planning Association. *Final Report on 1978 Survey of Health Planning Agencies*. Washington, DC: Government Printing Office, 1979.

American Hospital Association. "Uncompensated Hospital Care Cost Fact Sheet." http://www.aha.org/aha/content/2008/pdf/08-uncompensated-care.pdf.

Amira, Dan. "New Yorker Alan Frumin, Senate Parliamentarian, Back in the Hot Seat Once More." *New Yorker Magazine*, January 20, 2010. http://nymag .com/daily/intel/2010/01/new_yorker_alan_frumin_senate.html.

Atchinson, Brian, and Daniel Fox. "The Politics of the Health Insurance Portability and Accountability Act." *Health Affairs* 16, no. 3 (1997): 146–50.

Ball, Robert. "Social Security Amendments of 1972: Summary and Legislative History." *Social Security Bulletin* 36, no. 3 (1972).

Bennefield, Robert. "Current Population Reports: Health Insurance Coverage: 1996." http://www.census.gov/prod/3/97pubs/P60-199.pdf.

Blumberg, Linda, and Lisa Clemans-Cope. "High-Deductible Health Plans with Health Savings Accounts: Emerging Evidence and Outstanding Issues." Urban Institute, http://www.urban.org/UploadedPDF/411833_health_saving_account.pdf.

Blumenthal, David, and James Morone. *The Heart of Power: Health and Politics in the Oval Office.* Berkeley: University of California Press, 2009.

Blumstein, James. "Court Action, Agency Reaction: The Hill–Burton Act as a Case Study." *Iowa Law Review* 69, no. 1,227 (1984).

Brady, Tim, Barbie Robinson, and Tricia Davis. Office of Inspector General. Office of Evaluation and Inspections. *Medicare Hospital Prospective Payment System: How DRG Rates Are Calculated and Updated.* Washington, DC: Government Printing Office, 2001.

Brass, Clinton. Government Organization and Management, Congressional Research Service. *Shutdown of the Federal Government: Causes, Processes, and Effects.* Washington, DC: Government Printing Office, 2010.

Center for Public Integrity. "Well-Heeled: Inside the Lobbying for Health Care Reform." 1994. http://www.publicintegrity.org/assets/pdf/WELL-HEALED .pdf.

Cohen, Wilbur, and Robert Ball. "Social Security Amendments of 1965: Summary and Legislative History." *Social Security Bulletin* 28, no. 9 (1965).

Congressional Budget Office. *Cost Estimate. H.R. 2: Children's Health Insurance Reauthorization Act of 2009.* http://www.cbo.gov/ftpdocs/99xx/doc9985/hr2paygo.pdf.

———. *Fact Sheet for CBO's March 2010 Baseline: CHIP.* http://www.cbo.gov/ftpdocs/ 115xx/doc11521/CHIP.pdf.

———. *Hospital Cost Containment Model: A Technical Analysis.* Washington, DC: Government Printing Office, 1981.

———. *The Indirect Teaching Adjustment for Medicare's Prospective Payment System: Issues and Options.* Washington, DC: Government Printing Office, 1985.

———. *The Long-Term Budget Outlook.* Washington, DC: Government Printing Office, 2005.

————. *The Medicare Catastrophic Coverage Act of 1988.* October 1988. http://www.cbo.gov/ftpdocs/84xx/doc8430/88doc14.pdf.

————. *Setting Medicare's Indirect Teaching Adjustment for Hospitals.* Washington, DC: Government Printing Office, 1989.

————. *The State Children's Health Insurance Program.* http://www.cbo.gov/ftp docs/80xx/doc8092/05-10-SCHIP.pdf.

Cowan, Cathy, Helen Lazenby, Anne Martin, Patricia McDonnell, Arthur Sensenig, Cynthia Smith, Lekha Whittle, et al. "National Health Expenditures, 1999." *Health Care Financing Review* 22, no. 4 (2001): 77–110.

Cunningham, Robert. "The Wheels of Policy Grind Slowly: Top Story of 1999 is Medicare Commission's Decision to Punt." *Medicine and Health Perspectives* 54, no. 1 (2000): supplement 1–4.

Cunningham, Robert, III, and Robert Cunningham Jr. *The Blues: A History of the Blue Cross and Blue Shield System.* DeKalb: Northern Illinois University Press, 1997.

Curran, William. "Medical Charity for the Poor: Hill–Burton and the Hospitals." *New England Journal of Medicine* 287, no. 10 (1972): 498–99.

Daschle, Tom. *Getting It Done: How Obama and Congress Finally Broke the Stalemate to Make Way for Health Care Reform.* New York: St. Martin's, 2010.

Davis, Karen, Stuart Guterman, Sara Collins, Kristol Stemilds, Shiela Rustgi, and Rachel Nuzum. *Starting on the Path to a High Performance Health System: Analysis of Payment and System Reform Provisions in the Patient Protection and Affordability Care Act of 2010.* New York: The Commonwealth Fund, 2010.

Debt Reduction Task Force. "Restoring America's Future: Reviving the Economy, Cutting Spending and Debt, and Creating a Simple, Pro-Growth Tax System," November 2010. http://www.bipartisanpolicy.org/sites/default/files/BPC %20FINAL%20REPORT%20FOR%20PRINTER%2002%2028%2011.pdf.

Democratic Policy Committee. "The Health Care and Education Reconciliation Act: Section-by-Section Analysis." http://dpc.senate.gov/healthreformbill/healthbill63.pdf.

Devers, Kelly, and Robert Berenson. "Can Accountable Care Organizations Improve the Value of Health Care by Solving The Cost and Quality Quandaries?" Robert Wood Johnson Foundation and Urban Institute, 2009. http://www.urban.org/publications/411975.html.

Doonan, Michael. "American Federalism and Contemporary Health Policy." PhD diss., Brandeis University, 2002.

Economic Stabilization Program. *Economic Stabilization Program: Quarterly Reports, August 15, 1971–January 10, 1973,* vol. 1. Washington, DC: Government Printing Office, 1973.

————. *Quarterly Reports, January 11, 1973–December 31, 1973,* vol. 2. Washington, DC: Government Printing Office, 1973.

Employee Benefits Research Institute. *Sources of Health Insurance and Characteristics of the Uninsured: Analysis of the March 1992 Current Population Survey,* January 1993. http://www.ebri.org/pdf/briefspdf/0193ib.pdf.

Enthoven, Alain. "Consumer Choice Health Plan: A National Health Insurance Proposal Based on Regulated Competition in the Private Sector." *New England Journal of Medicine* 298, no. 12, Part 1 (1978): 650–58.

———. "Consumer Choice Health Plan: A National Health Insurance Proposal Based on Regulated Competition in the Private Sector," *New England Journal of Medicine* 298, no. 13, Part 2 (1978): 709–20.

Enthoven, Alain, and Sara Singer. "A Single-Payer System in Jackson Hole Clothing." *Health Affairs* 1(1994): 81–95.

Fazel, Reza, Harlan Krumholz, Yongfei Wang, Joseph Ross, Jersey Chen, Henry Ting, Nilay Shah, et al. "Exposure to low-dose ionizing radiation from medical imaging procedures." *New England Journal of Medicine* 361, no. 9 (2009): 849–57.

Feingold, Eugene. *Medicare: Policy and Politics.* San Francisco: Chandler, 1966.

Fetter, Robert, John Thompson, Ronald Mills, and Donald Riedel. "The Application of Diagnostic Specific Cost Profiles to Cost and Reimbursement Control in Hospitals." *Journal of Medical Systems* 1, no. 2 (1977): 137–49.

Fetter, Robert, Youngsoo Shin, Jean Freeman, Richard Averill, and John Thompson. "Case Mix Definition by Diagnosis-Related Groups." *Medical Care* 18, no. 2 (1980): 1–53.

———. "Sources of Health Insurance and Characteristics of the Uninsured: Analysis of the March 2010 Current Population Survey." September 2010. http://www.ebri.org/pdf/briefspdf/EBRI_IB_09-2010_No347_Uninsured1 .pdf.

Glied, Sherry. "Single-Payer as a Financing Mechanism." *Journal of Health Politics, Policy and Law* 34 no. 4 (2009): 593–615.

Gold, Marsha, and Karyen Chu. "Effects of Selected Cost-Containment Efforts: 1971–1993." *Health Care Financing Review* 14, no. 3 (1993): 183–225.

Goldwater, Barry. "Washington News." *Journal of the American Medical Association* 189, no. 13 (1964): 17–18.

Goodson, John. "Unintended Consequences of Resource Based Relative Value Scale Reimbursement." *Journal of the American Medical Association* 298 (2007): 2308–10.

Guterman, Stuart. "The Balanced Budget Act of 1997: Will Hospitals Take a Hit on Their PPS Margins?" *Health Affairs* 17, no. 1 (1998): 159–66.

Hacker, Jacob. *The Road to Nowhere.* Princeton, NJ: Princeton University Press, 1997.

Halpin, Helen and Peter Harbage,. "The Origin and Demise of the Public Option." *Health Affairs* 29, no. 6 (2010): 1117–24.

Harris, Richard. *A Sacred Trust.* New York: New American Library, 1966.

Health Insurance Association of America. *Source Book of Health Insurance Data 1999/2000.* Washington, DC: Health Insurance Association of America, 2000.

Heaney, Michael. "Brokering Health Policy: Coalitions, Parties, and Interest Group Influences." *Journal of Health Politics, Policy and Law* 31 (2006): 887–954.

Himelfarb, Richard. *Catastrophic Politics: The Rise and Fall of the Medicare Catastrophic Coverage Act of 1988.* University Park: Pennsylvania State University Press, 1988.

Hoffman, Catherine."Medicaid Payment for Nonphysician Practitioners: An Access Issue." *Health Affairs* 13, no. 4 (1994): 140–52.

Holahan, John, and Bowen Garrett. *The Cost of Uncompensated Care With and Without Health Reform, March 2020.* The Urban Institute. http://www.urban.org/publications/412045.html.

Hsiao, William, Peter Braun, Daniel Dunn, Edmund Becker, Margaret DeNicola, and Thomas Ketcham. "Results and Policy Implications of the Resource Based Relative-Value Study." *New England Journal of Medicine* 319, no. 13 (1988): 881–88.

Hsiao, William, Peter Braun, Douweand Yntema, and Edmund Becker. "Estimating Physicians' Work for a Resource Based Relative Value Scale." *New England Journal of Medicine* 319, no. 13 (1988): 835–41.

Hsiao, William, Peter Braun, Nancy Kelly, and Edmund Becker. "Results, Potential Effects, and Implementation Issues of the Resource Based Relative Value Scale." *Journal of the American Medical Association* 260, no. 16 (1988): 2429–38.

Iglehart, John. "The New Prescription-Drug Benefit—A Pure Power Play." *New England Journal of Medicine* 350, no. 8 (2004): 826–33.

Johnson, Haynes, and David Broder. *The System.* Boston: Little, Brown, 1996.

Kaiser Family Foundation. Health Research & Educational Trust. "Employer Health Benefits 2009 Annual Survey." http://ehbs.kff.org/pdf/2009/7936.pdf.

———. "Trends in Health Care Costs and Spending, September 2007." http://www.kff.org/insurance/upload/7692.pdf.

Keehan, Sister Carol. "The Time Is Now for Health Reform." *Catholic Health World* 26, no. 5 (2010). http://www.chausa.org/The_time_is_now_for_health_reform.aspx.

Keith, Robert. Report for Congress: Government and Finance Division. "The Budget Reconciliation Process: The Senate's Byrd Rule." March 20, 2008. http://democrats.budget.house.gov/crs-reports/RL30862.pdf.

Klees, Barbara, Christian Wolfe, and Catherine Curtis. US Department of Health and Human Services. Office of the Actuary. Centers for Medicare and Medicaid Services. "Brief Summaries of Medicare and Medicaid: Title XVIII and Title XIX of the Social Security Act," November 1, 2009. http://www.cms .gov/Medicare ProgramRatesStats/Downloads/MedicareMedicaidSummaries 2009.pdf.

Ladenheim, Kala. "Health Insurance in Transition: The Health Insurance Portability and Accountability Act of 1996." *Publius* 27, no. 2 (1997). http://www.jstor.org/stable/3330636.

Mahan, Dee. "Falling Short: Medicare Prescription Drug Plans Offer Meager Sav-
    ings." Families USA Special Report, December 2005. http://www.familiesusa
    .org/assets/pdfs/PDP-vs-VA-prices-special-report.pdf.
Maraniss, David, and Michael Weisskopf. *Tell Newt to Shut Up.* New York: Simon and
    Schuster, 1996.
Markus, Glenn. Congressional Research Service. Education and Public Welfare
    Division. *How Medicare Pays for Doctors' Services.* Washington, DC: Government
    Printing Office, 1972.
Marmor, Theodore. "The Case for Universal Social Insurance." *Policies for an Aging
    Society.* Edited by Stuart Altman and David Shactman. Baltimore: Johns Hopkins
    University Press, 2002.
————. *The Politics of Medicare.* 2nd ed. Hawthorne, NY: Aldine de Gruyter, 2000.
Mayes, Rick. "The Origins, Development, and Passage of Medicare's Revolutionary
    Prospective Payment System." *Journal of The History of Medicine and Allied Sci-
    ences* (2006): 12.
Mayes, Rick, and Robert Berenson. *Medicare Prospective Payment and the Shaping of U.S.
    Health Care.* Baltimore: Johns Hopkins University Press, 2006.
Mills, Wilbur. "Financing Health Care for the Aged." Address before Downtown
    Little Rock Lions Club. Quoted in Theodore Marmor, *The Politics of Medicare.*
    2nd ed. Hawthorne, NY: Aldine de Gruyter, 2000.
Modern Healthcare. "Modern Healthcare Announces 100 Most Powerful People in
    Healthcare." August 27, 2007. http://www.modernhealthcare.com/assets/pdf/
    CH25102828.pdf.
Morone, James, and Andrew Dunham. "The Waning of Professional Dominance:
    DRGs and the Hospitals." *Health Affairs* 3, no. 73 (1984): 73–87.
Murray, Shailagh. "Senators Ready to Vote Again; With 60 Backers, Measure May
    Pass on Christmas Eve." *Washington Post,* December 22, 2009.
National Institute for Health and Clinical Effectiveness. "Incorporating health eco-
    nomics in guidelines and assessing resource impact." *Guideline Development
    Methods.* http://www.nice.org.uk/niceMedia/pdf/GDM_Chapter8_0305.pdf.
Nichols, Len, and Linda Blumberg. "A Different Kind of New 'Federalism'? The
    Health Insurance Portability and Accountability Act of 1996." *Health Affairs* 17,
    no. 3 (1998): 25–42.
Nixon, Richard. "Special Message to Congress Proposing a Comprehensive Health
    Insurance Plan, February 6, 1974." *American Presidency Project.* Edited by John T.
    Woolley and Gerhard Peters. http://www.presidency.ucsb.edu/ws/?pid=4337.
————. "Special Message to Congress Proposing a National Health Strategy," Feb-
    ruary 18, 1971. *American Presidency Project.* Edited by John T. Woolley and Ger-
    hard Peters. http://www.presidency.ucsb.edu/ws/index.php?pid=3311&st
    =Nixon&st1=health.

Nixon Library. "White House Central File, Subject File Domestic Council: Box 5 (October 1973–December 1973)." Quoted in David Blumenthal and James Morone, *Heart of Power: Health and Politics in the Oval Office.* Berkeley: University of California Press, 2009.

Oberlander, Jonathan. "Medicare's Coverage of Health Services." In *Renewing the Promise: Medicare and its Reform.* Edited by David Blumenthal, Mark Schlesinger, and Pamela Brown. New York: Oxford University Press, 1988.

———. "Medicare: The End of Consensus." Paper presented at the annual meeting of the American Political Science Association, Boston, Massachusetts, 1998.

———. *The Political Life of Medicare.* Chicago: Chicago University Press, 2003.

———. "Through the Looking Glass: The Politics of the Medicare Prescription Drug, Improvement, and Modernization Act." *Journal of Health Politics, Policy and Law* 32, no. 2 (2007): 187–219.

Oliver, Thomas. "Health Care Market Reform in Congress: The Uncertain Path from Proposal to Policy." *Political Science Quarterly* 106, no. 3 (1991): 453–77.

Oliver, Thomas, Philip Lee, and Helene Lipton. "A Political History of Medicare and Prescription Drug Coverage." *Millbank Quarterly* 82, no. 2 (2004): 283–354.

Organization for Economic Co-operation and Development (OECD). *Health at a Glance 2009—OECD Indicators.* Paris: Organisation for Economic Co-Operation and Development, 2009.

Organizing for America. "Full Text of Senator Barack Obama's Announcement for President." February 10, 2007. http://www.barackobama.com/2007/02/10/remarks_of_senator_barack_obam_11.php.

Patel, Kavita, and John McDonough. "From Massachusetts to 1600 Pennsylvania Avenue: Aboard The Health Reform Express." *Health Affairs* 29, no. 6 (2010): 1106–11.

Partnership for Solutions. *Chronic Conditions: Making the Case for Ongoing Care.* Baltimore, MD: Johns Hopkins University, 2002.

Pennebaker, D. A., and Chris Hegedus, directors. *The War Room.* DVD. Universal City, CA: Universal Studios, 2004.

Peterson, Chris, and Rachel Barton. Congressional Research Service. *US Health Care Spending: A Comparison with other Countries.* Washington, DC: Government Printing Office, 2007.

Pokras, Robert, Lola Kozak, Eileen McCarthy, and Edmund Graves. "Trends in Hospital Utilization: United States, 1965–86." *Vital Health Statistics* 13, no. 101 (1989).

ProPac. *Prospective Payment Assessment Commission: Annual Report, March 1, 1991.* Washington, DC: Prospective Payment Assessment Commission, 1991.

Quadagno, Jill, and Debra Street. "Antistatism in American Welfare State Development." In Julian Zelizer, *Taxing America: Wilbur D. Mills, Congress, and the State, 1945–1975.* Cambridge: Cambridge University Press, 1999.

Reinhardt, Uwe. "Future Trends in the Economics of Medical Care." *American Journal of Cardiology* 56, no. 5 (1985): 50c–59c.

Robbins, Anthony. "Who Should Make Public Policy for Health?" *American Journal of Public Health* 66, no. 5 (1976): 431.

Robert Graham Center. *The Patient Centered Medical Home: History, Seven Core Features, Evidence and Transformational Change.* Washington, DC: Robert Graham Center, 2007.

Robinson, James. "The End of Managed Care." *Journal of the American Medical Association* 285, no. 20, (2001): 2622–28.

Roemer, Milton. "Bed Supply and Hospital Utilization: A Natural Experiment." *Hospitals* 35 (1961): 36–42.

Roosevelt, Franklin. "State of the Union Address, January 7, 1943." *American Presidency Project.* Edited by John T. Woolley and Gerhard Peters. http://www.presidency.ucsb.edu/ws/?pid=16386.

Rose, Marilyn. "Federal Regulation of Services to the Poor under the Hill–Burton Act: Realities and Pitfalls." *Northwestern University Law Review* 70, no. 1 (1975): 168–201.

Salsberg, Edward, and Gaetano Forte. "Trends in the Physician Workforce, 1980–2000." *Health Affairs* 21, no. 5 (2002): 165–73.

Schoen, Cathy, Jennifer Nicholson, and Sheila Rusgi. *Paying the Price: How Health Insurance Premiums Are Eating Up Middle Class Incomes, State Health Insurance Premium Trends, and the Potential of National Health Reform.* New York: The Commonwealth Fund, 2009.

Schweicker, Richard. "Executive Summary: The Report to Congress on Hospital Prospective Payment for Medicare." *Health Care Financial Management* 37, no. 3 (1983): 67–69.

Shaheen, Paul, and Harry Perlstadt. "Class Action Suits and Social Change: The Organization and Impact of the Hill–Burton Cases." *Indiana Law Journal* 57 (1981–1982): 385–423.

Sisko, Andrea, Christopher Truffer, Sean Keehan, John Poisal, Joseph Lizonitz, M. Clemens, and Andrew Madison. "National Health Spending Projections: The Estimated Impact of Reform Through 2019." *Health Affairs* 29 no. 10 (2010): 1933–41.

Skocpol, Theda. "The Rise and Resounding Demise of the Clinton Health Security Plan." In *The Problem That Won't Go Away.* Edited by Henry Aaron. Washington, DC: The Brookings Institution, 1996.

Sloan, Frank. "Rate Regulation as a Strategy for Hospital Cost Control: Evidence from the Last Decade." *Milbank Memorial Quarterly* 61, no. 2 (1983): 195–221.

———. "State Regulatory Strategies." Presentation, Health Industry Forum Breakfast Series, Waltham, MA, October 2008.

Smith, David. *Paying For Medicare: The Politics of Reform.* New York: Aldine De Gruyter, 1992.

Social Security Administration. Committee on Economic Security. "Unpublished 1935 Report on Health Insurance and Disability by the Committee on Economic Security." http://www.ssa.gov/history/reports/health.html.

Sox, Harold, and Sheldon Greenfield. "Comparative Effectiveness Research: A Report from the Institute of Medicine." *Annals of Internal Medicine* 151, no. 3 (2009): 203–5.

Staff Writers, *Washington Post. Landmark: The Inside Story of America's New Health-Care Law and What It Means for Us All.* New York: PublicAffairs, 2010.

Stahl, Leslie. "Jimmy Carter: My Presidency was a Success." CBS News, September 19, 2010. http://www.cbsnews.com/stories/2010/09/16/60minutes/main6872344.shtml.

Starfield, Barbar, Leiyu Shi, and James Macinko. "Contribution of Primary Care to Health Systems and Health." *Milbank Quarterly* 83, no. 3 (2005): 457–502.

Starr, Paul. *The Social Transformation of American Medicine.* New York: Basic Books, 1984.

Stevens, Rosemary. *In Sickness and in Wealth: American Hospitals in the Twentieth Century.* Baltimore: Johns Hopkins University Press, 1989.

Stone, Peter. "Health Insurers Funded Chamber Attack Ads." *National Journal Under the Influence,* January 12, 2010. http://undertheinfluence.nationaljournal.com/2010/01/health-insurers-funded-chambers.php.

Strunk, Bradley, and Paul Ginsburg. "Tracking Health Care Costs: Trends Slow in First Half of 2003." *Center for Studying Health System Change: Data Bulletin* no. 26 (2003): 1–2.

Sundquist, James. "Politics and Policy: The Eisenhower, Kennedy and Johnson Years." *Annals of the American Academy of Political and Social Science* 383, no. 1 (1969): 173–75.

Time Magazine. "Students: Peaceful Revolutionary." *Time Magazine,* July 4, 1969. http://www.time.com/time/magazine/article/0,9171,840189,00.html.

Tompkins, Christopher, Stuart Altman, and Ephrat Eilat. "The Precarious Pricing System for Hospital Service." *Health Affairs* 25, no. 1 (2006): 45–56.

Truffer, Christopher, Sean Keehan, Sheila Smith, Jonathan Cyclus, Andrea Sisko, John Poisal, Josephy Lizonitz, et al. "Health Spending Projections Through 2019: The Recession's Impact Continues." *Health Affairs* 29 no. 3 (2010): 522–29.

Truman, Harry. "Special Message to Congress Recommending a Comprehensive Health Program, November 14, 1945." The Harry S. Truman Presidential Library and Museum. http://www.trumanlibrary.org/publicpapers/index.php?pid=483&st=&st1=.

———. "Special Message to the Congress recommending a Comprehensive Health

Program, November 19, 1945." *American Presidency Project.* Edited by John T. Woolley and Gerhard Peters. http://www.presidency.ucsb.edu/ws/index.php ?pid=12288&st=Truman&st1=.

US Census Bureau. "Poverty Status of People by Age, Race, and Hispanic Origin 1959–2009." Historical Poverty Tables. http://www.census.gov/hhes/www/ poverty/data/historical/people.html.

United States Conference of Catholic Bishops. "Pulpit Announcement and Prayer Petition." March 16, 2010. http://flrl.org/PDFs_and_Docs/Health%20Care %20Reform%20—%20USCCB%201-7-2010%20Pulpit%20Announcement .pdf.

US Department of Health, Education, and Welfare. "Medical technology: The Culprit Behind Health Care Costs?" In *Proceedings of the 1977 Sun Valley Forum on National Health*, edited by Stuart Altman and Robert Blendon. Washington, DC: Government Printing Office, 1979.

US Department of Health and Human Services. Agency for Healthcare Research and Quality: Center for Financing, Access and Cost Trends. *Medical Expenditure Panel Survey-Insurance Component: 1998 and 2008.* http://www.meps.ahrq.gov/ mepsweb/survey_comp/Insurance.jsp.

———. Centers for Disease Control and Prevention. National Center for Health Statistics. *Health, United States, 2006 with Chartbook on Trends in the Health of Americans.* Hyattsville, MD: Centers for Disease Control and Prevention, 2006.

———. Centers for Medicare and Medicaid Services. "2009 Annual Report of the Boards of Trustees of the federal Hospital Insurance and Federal Supplementary Medical Insurance Trust Funds." http://www.cms.gov/ReportsTrust Funds/downloads/tr2009.pdf.

———. Centers for Medicare and Medicaid Services. *National Health Expenditures Aggregate, Per Capita Amounts, Percent Distribution, and Average Annual Percent Growth, by Source of Funds: Selected Calendar Years 1960–2008.* http://www.cms.gov/ NationalHealthExpendData/downloads/tables.pdf.

———. Centers for Medicare and Medicaid Services. "Fact Sheet: Sole Community Hospital." http://www.cms.gov/MLNProducts/downloads/solecommhospfct sht508-09.pdf.

———. Centers for Medicare and Medicaid Services. Office of the Actuary, National Health Statistics Group. "National Health Care Expenditures Data." http://www.cms.gov/NationalHealthExpendData/downloads/tables.pdf.

———. Centers for Medicare and Medicaid Services. Office of Legislation. "Medicare 'Accountable Care Organizations' Shared Savings Program—New Section 1899 of Title XVIII." https://www.cms.gov/OfficeofLegislation/ Downloads/AccountableCareOrganization.pdf.

———. Centers for Medicare and Medicaid Services. *Overview of National CHIP*

*Policy: CHIP Ever Enrolled Year Graph.* http://www.cms.gov/NationalCHIP
Policy/downloads/CHIPEverEnrolledYearGraph.pdf.

———. Centers for Medicare and Medicaid Services, Office of the Medicare
Actuary. *1998 Annual Report of the Boards of Trustees of the Federal Hospital Insurance
and Federal Supplementary Medical Insurance Trust Funds.* Washington, DC: Government Printing Office, 1998.

———. Office of Information Services. *Data from the Medicare Data Extract System,
Table 61a.* Washington, DC: Government Printing Office, 2009.

———. Office of The Actuary. *National Health Expenditure Projections 2009–2019,* January 2010. https://www.cms.gov/NationalHealthExpendData/downloads/
proj2009.pdf.

———. *Chart Book of Basic Health Economics Data.* Washington, DC: Public Health
Service, 1964.

US Department of Labor. Bureau of Labor Statistics. *Employment Status of the Civilian
Non-institutional Population 16 years and Over, 1970 to Date: Table A1.* ftp://ftp
.bls.gov/pub/special.requests/lf/aat2.txt.

———. *Occupational Outlook Handbook,* 2010–2011 ed. Washington, DC: Government
Printing Office, 2010.

US General Accounting Office. *Federal Employees' Health Plans: Premium Growth and
OPM's Role in Negotiating Benefits.* Washington, DC: Government Printing Office,
2002.

———. *Non-profit, For-profit, and Government Hospitals: Uncompensated Care and Other
Community Benefits.* Washington, DC: Government Printing Office, 2005.

VanGiezen, Robert, and Albert Schwenk. Bureau of Labor Statistics. "Historical
Data: Labor Force Statistics from the Current Population Survey." *Compensation
and Working Conditions* (2001). http://www.bls.gov/opub/cwc/archive/fall
2001art3.pdf.

Vladeck, Bruce. "Interest-Group Representation and the HSAs; Health Planning
and Political Theory." *American Journal of Public Health* 67, no. 1 (1977): 23–29.

Wainess, Flint. "The Ways and Means of National Health Care Reform, 1974 and
Beyond." *Journal of Health Politics, Policy and Law* 24, no. 2 (1999): 305–33.

Walsh, Elsa. "Kennedy's Hidden Campaign." *New Yorker,* March 31, 1997.
http://archives.newyorker.com/?i=1997-03-31#folio=066.

Weeks, Lewis, and Howard Berman. *Shapers of American Health Care Policy: An Oral
History.* Ann Arbor, MI: Health Administration Press, 1985. Quoted in Harry
Perlstadt, "The Development of the Hill–Burton Legislation: Interests, Issues
and Compromises," *Journal of Health and Social Policy* 63, no. 3 (1995): 91–92.

Wilensky, Gail, and Joseph Newhouse. MedPac. *Report to Congress: Rethinking
Medicare's Payment Policies for Graduate Medical Education and Teaching Hospitals.*
Washington, DC: Government Printing Office, 1999.

Wu, Vivian. "Hospital Cost Shifting Revisited: New Evidence from the Balanced Budget Act of 1997." *International Journal of Health Care Finance and Economics* 10, no. 1 (2010): 61–83.

Zelizer, Julian. *Taxing America: Wilbur D. Mills, Congress, and the State, 1945–1975*. Cambridge: Cambridge University Press, 2000.

# INDEX

Aaron, Henry, 178

Abbott Laboratories, 259

abortion issue, 21, 269–70, 287–91, 309, 310, 313, 322–23

accountable care organizations [ACOs], 340–41, 381

Adams, Jim, 27

Adler, John, 320

Administrative Procedures Act, 119

adverse selection, 84, 86, 164, 186, 196, 381

Advisory Commission on Social Security, 151

Advisory Committee on Economic Security, 99

Affordable Care Act. *See* Patient Protection and Affordable Care Act (2010)

Agency for Healthcare Research and Quality [AHRQ], 283, 381

Aiken, George, 105

Alger, Bruce, 133–34

Altman, Florence, 11, 12, 159–60, 225

Altman, Stuart, 7, 9, 177, 206, 217, 229

"Altman's Law," 44, 60, 96, 98, 106

and Clinton's administration, 11, 14, 17–18, 62, 63–64, 74, 75, 81, 94, 95, 163, 177, 179, 230, 231

and Medicare, 11–12, 81, 177, 179, 208, 210, 221, 223, 225

and Nixon's administration, 14, 17, 27, 30, 34–35, 44–47, 51, 52, 53, 61, 96, 169–70, 204–205

and Hill–Burton Program, 111–12, 117, 120

and national health planning, 204, 206–208, 210–12

and Obama's administration, 12–13, 17–18, 22, 96, 245, 249, 252

and Reagan's administration, 159–60, 221, 223, 225

and Ted Kennedy, 18, 57, 58, 60

American Academy of Pediatrics, 85, 340

American Association for Labor Legislation [AALL], 97–99, 105

American Association of Health Plans [AAHP], 260–61, 381

*See also* America's Health Insurance Plans

American Association of Medical Colleges [AAMC], 220, 381

American Association of Retired Persons [AARP], 21, 78, 156, 157, 160, 177, 184, 191–92, 197, 301, 381

American Bar Association, 103

American College of Surgeons [ACS], 227

American Federation of Labor and Congress of Industrial Organiza-

tions [AFL-CIO], 28, 56, 97, 164,
  260, 381
American Health Planning Association,
  212
American Hospital Association [AHA],
  103, 112–13, 119–20, 143, 207, 213,
  257, 265–67, 268, 301, 381
American Medical Association [AMA],
  36, 104, 226, 254, 381–82
  alternative health care proposals from,
    44, 59, 97, 101, 128, 139, 140
  fears of regulation and price-controls
    on doctors, 20, 29, 98, 127, 128,
    224, 226, 227, 228
  and Medicare, 139, 142, 144, 149,
    271–72
    and Medicare Part D, 193
    siding with the tobacco industry,
      122–23, 133, 134, 333
  and Obama's health plan, 254, 257,
    267, 271–73, 301
  opposing all efforts to enact national
    health insurance, 20, 44, 56, 98,
    100, 101, 103, 128, 271, 333
  lobbying programs, 104, 106, 122,
    139, 140
America's Health Insurance Plans
  [AHIP], 254, 257, 260–64, 382
America's Healthy Future Act, 8
Anderson, Clinton, 135, 136
Angle, Sharron, 320
Anthem Blue Cross, premium hikes by,
  316
assignment, 225, 382
Assisted Health Insurance Program
  [AHIP], 54, 382

balance billing, 142, 225, 382
Balanced Budget Act of 1997 [BBA],
  176, 178, 180, 228, 234, 304

Balanced Budget Reform Act of 1999,
  234
Ball, Robert, 208
Baucus, Max, 256
  and Medicare drug benefit, 177, 181,
    184, 186–87, 195, 256
  and Obama's health plan, 263,
    274–77, 286, 300, 327
  negotiations with health care
    groups, 257, 258, 259, 261–62,
    265, 306–307
Beck, Glenn, 324
Begala, Paul, 68
benefit package, 47, 50, 54, 59, 94, 147,
  155, 170, 179, 341, 382
  Federal Employees Health Benefits
    Program, 47, 175, 301, 386
  limiting scope of, 40, 43, 52, 73, 127,
    138
  Medicaid benefits package, 172, 173,
    174, 175
Bennett, Bob, 93
Bentsen, Lloyd, 156
Berman, Richard, 205
Biden, Joe, 76, 325, 336
Bierring, Walter, 100
Bingaman, Jeff and the Gang of Six,
  275
Bismarck, Otto von, 140
Bjorkland, Cybele, 195
block grants for states, 172
Blue Cross/Blue Shield plans, 124–25,
  143–44, 164, 175, 205, 208–209,
  218, 285, 316, 382
Blue Dogs. *See* Democrats
Blue Shield plans. *See* Blue Cross/Blue
  Shield plans
Blumenauer, Earl, 281
Blumstein, James, 118, 119
Boccieri, John, 321

Boehner, John, 259, 282, 325

*Boston Globe* (newspaper), 314

Boustany, Charles, 281

Bowen, Otis, 150–52, 161

Boxer, Barbara, 309

Bradley, Bill, 247

Brady, Kevin, 277

Breaux, John, 177, 178, 179, 184, 195

Broder, David, 62

Brown, Scott, 259, 313–14, 316, 337

Brownback, Sam, 21, 312

Brown University, 74

*Brown v. Board of Education*, 132

Budget Improvement and Protection Act of 2000, 234

budget neutrality
  Clinton's health plan, 71, 74, 75, 79, 80, 81, 90, 95
  Obama's health plan, 250, 251, 253, 272, 302
  Reagan's health plan, 152, 156, 157, 159, 220

budget reconciliation, 77–78, 227, 316–26, 335, 382

bundled payment, 20, 21, 304, 382

Bunning, Jim, 313

Burke, Sheila, 93

Burton, Harold, 112, 113

Bush, George H. W., 68, 161

Bush, George W., 46, 70, 76, 77–78, 150, 176, 261, 278, 333
  and Medicare Part D, 157, 177–99, 330
  use of budget reconciliation rules, 316, 317, 335

businesses and health care, 20, 66–67, 98, 279
  and Medicare Part D, 190, 193
  and Obama's health plan, 263
  *See also* employer mandate; managed competition; pharmaceutical companies; private insurance

Business Roundtable, 193

Butler, Lewis, 36, 41

Butler, Stuart, 158

Butterfield, Alexander, 58

Byrd, Robert, 76–79, 92, 136, 292, 294, 295, 311–12, 313, 317, 335

Byrd Rule and budget reconciliation, 77–78, 318–19, 382–83

Byrnes, John, 133, 139, 141

Byrnes bill, 139–40, 142

Cadillac tax, 21, 276, 286–87, 307–308, 313, 383
  final Obama health care law postpones, 319, 328, 341

Califano, Joseph, 72, 214

Campaign America, 167

Cao, Anh, 291

capitation, 37–39, 73, 76, 98, 105, 231, 304, 339, 340, 341, 383
  *See also* prepaid group practices

Capretta, James, 342

Caro, Robert, 131

Carter, Jimmy, 72
  cost controls rather than universal coverage, 163, 213–15, 229

Carville, James, 68

case mix, 217, 383

Casey, Bill, 65

Castor, Kathy, 278

catastrophic insurance, 51, 85, 87, 214–15, 236, 237, 383
  Long's plan for, 44, 47, 57, 147, 214
  and Medicare Part D, 182
  Nixon's plan for, 43, 54, 56, 59, 147
  Reagan's Medicare Catastrophic insurance, 149–61, 178, 180, 189, 330, 332

Catholic Health Association [CHA], 103, 269–70, 321, 383

Catholic nuns coalition, 321, 322

CBS (TV network), 301, 323

Cellar, Edward, 105

Centers for Medicare and Medicaid Services [CMS], 148, 186, 197, 383

Certificates of Need [CON], 54, 211–12, 229, 383

Chafee, John, 92, 253

chairman's mark, 177, 276, 383

Chamber of Commerce, 20, 48, 247, 254, 264, 320

Cheney, Richard "Dick," 91, 183, 204–205

children and health insurance. *See* State Children's Health Insurance Program

Children's Defense Fund, 173

Christmas Eve vote on Obama's health care reform, 8, 292–313

Civil Rights Act (1960), 132

Civil Rights Act (1964), 7, 41, 77, 140

*La Civilta Cattolica* (journal), 270

Clark, Louise, 84, 85

claw-back, 188, 383–84

Cleaver, Emanuel, 324

Clinton, Bill, 8, 11, 14, 17, 40, 162, 163, 180, 314, 336

    efforts to control health care costs, 157, 230–35

    and national health insurance, 62–96, 178, 260, 268

        reasons for failure of plan, 94–96, 330–33, 336

    and uninsured children, 171, 173–74

Clinton, Hillary, 62, 63, 74, 83, 85, 171, 173

    on Obama's health plan, 245, 246, 249

cloture, 77, 194, 294, 311, 384

Coakley, Martha, 314–15

COBRA health coverage for the unemployed, 317

Coburn, Tom, 294, 311, 318, 319–20

coding, 222, 384

Cohen, Wilbur, 32, 139, 140

coinsurance, 43, 50, 56, 146–47, 148, 384

Committee of 100 for National Health Insurance, 28–29

community rate, 40, 86, 124–25, 384

community service obligation, 114, 116

comparative effectiveness research [CER], 87, 238–39, 281–84, 384

comparative rate, 384

competition among insurance plans. *See* insurance exchanges; managed care; managed competition

competitive managed care, 166–67

Comprehensive Health Insurance Plan [CHIP], 47, 52, 53–61, 384

Congressional Budget Office [CBO], 79, 318, 384

    analysis of Hospital Cost Containment Act, 213

    on costs of Clinton's health plan, 75, 79–80, 81, 90

    on costs of Medicare Part D, 196, 197

    on government negotiating prices with drug companies, 188

    on Medicare Advantage plans, 187

    on Obama's health plan, 251, 263, 286, 290, 298, 302, 321–22, 322, 327

    projecting a surplus over the next decade in 2001, 180

    on the SCHIP Program, 176

*Congressional Quarterly*, 132

Connally, John, 204

Conrad, Kent, 274–75, 276, 318

Constantine, Jay, 57

"Consumer Choice Health Plan," 72

Consumer Operated and Oriented Plan [CO-OP], 301, 384

"Contract with America, The" (of the Republican Party), 93, 162, 233

*Cook Political Report* (newsletter), 314

*Cook v. Ochsner Foundation Hospital,* 116–17

Cooper, Jim, 72

copayment, 30, 47, 50, 56, 148, 151, 155–56, 174, 182, 186, 234, 307, 328, 384

"Cornhusker kickback," 309–310, 329

cost/charge ratio, 384

cost effectiveness analysis, 238–39, 284, 385

Cost of Living Council, 204, 205–207, 216

cost per admission (cost per case), 206–207, 208, 385

cost per diem, 147, 205–206, 207–209, 385

cost per QALY. *See* quality-adjusted life year

cost sharing, 43, 47, 50–51, 54, 56, 59, 172, 175, 189–90, 339, 385

cost shifting, 69, 235

costs of health care, 66–67, 124, 234–35
    and CBO. *See* Congressional Budget Office
    concerns about, 144–45, 190–91, 203–204, 263–64
    efforts to control costs, 203–229
        "bending the cost curve," 12–13, 20–21, 252, 304, 334
        cost control in Obama's health plan, 220
        cost control under Carter, 213–15, 229

cost control under Nixon, 204–208
cost control under Reagan, 215–29, 345
during the 1990s, 230–35
rate regulation/health planning, 208–215, 345
methods suggested to reduce costs
    accountable care organizations [ACOs], 340–41
    changing health care delivery and finance, 338–42
    comparative effectiveness research, 238
    Diagnosis Related Group system, 207–208, 217–24, 386
    eliminating tax deduction for health insurance, 236–37
    government regulation of prices/supply of services, 237
    managed care, 237–38
    patient-centered medical home [PCMH], 340
    primary care and prevention, 338–39
    regulatory measures, 341–42
    using high deductibles to limit use of health care, 237
reasons for higher costs, 69, 235–40, 241, 334
statistics on
    comparison of US with other countries, 67, 203, 239, 240–41
    geographical differences in US, 222–24, 226
    for Medicare Part D, 195–97
    between 1948 and 1958, 107
    percentages of people and amount spent on health care, 125
    as share of US economy, 18, 235–41

systems for paying, 68–70. *See also* play-or-pay systems; single-payer systems; tax incentive plans

Council of Economic Advisors, 52, 204

Council on Medical Education, 100

Crane, Dan, 91

Crane, Philip, 160

Cutler, David, 63, 245

Danforth, John, 92

Daschle, Tom, 17, 172, 184, 194, 255–57, 274

David, Geoff, 281

Dean, Howard, 277

death panels, 87, 239, 277, 324, 335, 385
  summer of the death panels, 278–84

"death spiral," 86, 183, 385
  *See also* adverse selection

deductibles, 43, 47, 50, 56, 146, 148, 155–56, 160, 182, 185–86, 307, 385
  high-deductible health plans, 165–66, 237, 341, 388

deemer clause, 169

deficits, US budget, 18, 323, 331, 335
  and banking crisis of 2008, 19, 278
  in Carter administration, 215
  Medicare Part D adding to, 191, 192
  Obama's health care not adding to, 19, 21, 246, 251, 253, 277, 302, 308
    CBO saying would reduce, 321, 327
    concerns that it would add to, 293, 302, 324
  in Reagan administration, 150, 155, 219, 220

defined benefit, 94, 178, 385

defined contribution, 178, 385–86

DeMint, Jim, 21, 312, 318

Democrats, 20–21, 95, 106, 153–54, 191, 246, 272

Blue Dogs (conservative Democrats), 21, 95, 266, 285, 286, 321–22, 382

pro-life Democrats, 269, 288, 322

rejecting Nixon's health plan, 44, 55, 301

southern Democrats, 31, 32, 59, 100–101, 104, 115, 122, 127–28, 129–30, 131, 133, 134, 330

DeParle, Nancy-Ann, 257

Department of Health and Human Services [DHHS], 17, 256–57, 288, 386

Diagnosis Related Group system [DRG], 207–208, 217–25, 386
  Diagnosis Related Group creep, 221–22, 386

Dingell, John, 92, 95, 105

Dingell, John, Jr., 113

Dobson, James, 312

Dole, Robert "Bob," 92–93, 165, 167, 253

Dole–Packwood proposal, 92–93, 165

Domestic Council on Health, 34

Domestic Policy Council, 46, 155

donut hole, 20, 185–86, 197, 259
  final Obama health care law closes donut hole, 328
  reasons for, 182–83

Dove, Robert, 318

Doyle, Mike, 289

Doyle Dane Bernbach (advertising firm), 137

drug benefit under Medicare. *See* Medicare, Medicare Part D

dual eligibles, 142, 188, 196, 386

Dunlop, John, 206

Durenberger, David, 92, 217

Early Periodic Screening, Diagnosis, and Treatment [EPSDT], 172, 386

Economic Stabilization Act of 1970, 204

Edelman, Marian Wright, 173

Edwards, John, 245, 246, 249, 299

efficiency-versus-cost and managed care, 37–38

Ehrlichman, John, 31, 39, 46

Eichenholz, Joseph, 205, 207

Eisenhower, Dwight D., 123, 127

Eldercare bill, 139–40

   as an expansion of Kerr–Mills bill, 139

elderly

   near-elderly, 300, 301, 390

   poverty rate reduction, 150

   reaction to Medicare Catastrophic Health Bill, 159–61

   and the social contract, 153

   *See also* Medicaid; Medicare

Electronic Data Systems, 32

eligibility and a public option, 297

Ellsworth, Brad, 289–90

Ellwood, Paul, 35–37, 39, 71–72

Emanuel, Rahm, 140–41, 259, 273, 309, 310, 315, 316, 336, 337

Emergency Medical Treatment and Active Labor Act of 1986 [EMTALA], 121, 264–65, 386

Employee Retirement Income Security Act of 1974 [ERISA], 169–70

employer mandate, 22, 48–49, 247, 386

   and Obama's health plan, 20, 250–51, 253, 275, 276, 329

   and play-or-pay systems, 69–70

   small businesses worries about, 20, 279

   use of in pre-Obama plans, 42–44, 53, 56, 58–59, 75, 79, 83, 89, 94, 163, 214–15

   *See also* benefit package; businesses and health care

employer-provided insurance and Obama's health plan, 247–48, 250–51, 253, 338

end-of-life counseling, 281–82

end-of-life treatments, costs in last year of life, 38

end-stage renal disease, coverage for, 148, 210, 343

Engel, Lew, 312

Enthoven, Alain, 72, 90, 214

Enzi, Mike and the Gang of Six, 275

Etheredge, Lynn, 72

Ethics and Public Policy Center, 342

Ewing, Oscar, 105

experience rate, 125–26, 386

Families USA, 254–55

Feder, Judy, 62–63, 74, 192

Federal Employees Health Benefits Program [FEHBP], 47, 175, 301, 386–87

Federal Hospital Council, 113, 115

federal matching assistance program [FMAP], 175

Federation of American Hospitals [FAH], 265, 267–69, 387

fee-for-service, 22, 35–37, 39–40, 98, 105, 178, 186, 303, 339–40, 387

Feingold, Russ, 294

Felt, Mark, 46

Fetter, Robert, 207–208, 217

filibuster, 76, 77, 177, 194, 198

   and Obama's health plan, 293–95, 296, 301, 308–309, 311, 316, 325, 326, 330, 335, 387

Finch, Robert, 36, 41, 42

first-dollar coverage, 52, 182, 307, 387

"first-dollar insurance," 50, 52

fiscal intermediary, 30, 49, 56, 142, 144, 233, 387

Fleming, Scott, 111–12
Flick, Jeffrey, 195
Focus on the Family group, 312
Foley, Tom, 95
Food and Drug Administration, 238
Forand bill, 127, 130
Ford, Gerald, 58–59
    and National Health Planning and
        Resource Development Act
        (1975), 211–12
Ford Motors, 230
formulary, 188, 387
Foster, Rick, 195, 197
Fowler, Liz, 262, 264
Fox, Fannie "Tidal Basin Bombshell,"
    17, 60
Fox, Peter, 46, 47
Foxx, Virginia, 325
Frank, Barney, 324
free care. See uncompensated care
"free riders," 49, 87
Frist, Bill, 184
Frumin, Alan, 317–20
Fullerton, Bill, 28, 32, 33, 59

Gang of Six and Obama's health plan,
    274–77
gap insurance. See Medigap insurance;
    supplemental insurance
Garfield, Sidney, 232
Gawande, Atul, 72
Geisinger Medical System, 39
Geithner, Tim, 257
George, Francis Cardinal, 270
George, Walter, 101
Gibbons, Sam, 78, 84
G.I. Bill (1944), 7
Gingrich, Newt, 21, 90–91, 93, 162, 167,
    170, 173, 176, 233, 258, 268, 276,
    304

global budget, 29, 39, 70, 80, 81–82, 90,
    94, 99, 106, 213, 228, 334, 387
Goddard, Ben, 84, 85
Goddard Claussen (advertising firm),
    84, 85
Golden Rule Insurance Company,
    166–67
Goldman, Lee, 32
Goldman Sachs, 46
Goldwater, Barry, 135, 137, 330
Gompers, Samuel, 97
Goolsbee, Austan, 245
GOPAC, 167
Gordon, Bart, 322
Gore, Al, 62, 134–35, 136, 301
government regulation of prices or
    supply of services, 237
government shutdowns, 233
government subsidies. See subsidies for
    insurance
Gradison, Bill, 82–84, 155, 156
Graham, Lindsey, 194
Grassley, Chuck, 181, 184, 186–87, 256,
    274–77, 282, 307, 308
Green, William, 59
Greenspan Commission (1982), 150
Gregg, Judd, 317
Group Health of Puget Sound, 37
guaranteed issue, 86, 387
Gundersen Lutheran Health system,
    281

Haldeman, Bob, 46, 58
HarperCollins, 91
Harry and Louise commercials, 82–85,
    88, 89, 93, 137, 267–69, 333
Hart, Peter, 177
Harvard School of Public Health, 226
Hastert, Dennis, 184
Hatch, Orrin, 172–73, 174, 311

Hatch–Kennedy bill. *See* State Children's Health Insurance Program

Health, Education, and Welfare, Department of [HEW], 34, 36, 41, 45, 105, 178, 204, 211–12, 217–18, 387
  and efforts to give uninsured poor legal right to receive medical care, 111–12, 116–19, 120
  Health Civil Rights Branch, 116–17
  on Nixon's universal health care, 21
  and patient "case-mix" indexes for hospitals, 217
  *See also* Department of Health and Human Services

health alliances. *See* health insurance purchasing cooperatives

Health and Human Services. *See* Department of Health and Human Services

Health Care Financing Administration [HCFA], 260, 387

Health Care for America group, 260

health care in US. *See* national health care in the US; rural areas, health care in; urban areas, health care in

Health Care Task Force, 171

Health Insurance Association of America [HIAA], 82, 83–85, 255, 260, 261, 268, 388
  *See also* American Association of Health Plans

Health Insurance Company of Greater New York [HIP], 261

Health Insurance Portability and Access Act (1996) [HIPAA], 163–68, 248

health insurance purchasing cooperatives [HIPC], 73, 75, 79, 388

Health Maintenance Act of 1973, 40, 42, 111, 231, 339

Health Maintenance Organizations [HMOs], 13, 29, 175, 231–33, 235, 339, 388
  backlash against, 13, 195, 232–33, 234
  Nixon bringing HMOs to Americans, 35–42, 43, 54, 71–72
  *See also* managed care; prepaid group practices

Health Policy Group, 62

Health Policy Task Force, 63–64

Health Reform Dialogue Group, 255, 271

health savings accounts [HSAs], 166, 183–84, 388

Health Security Act (failed Clinton bill), 178

"Health Security Plan." *See* Kennedy–Griffiths bill

health system agencies [HSAs], 212, 388

Heritage Foundation, 158

Herlock, Sidney, 122

high-deductible health plans, 165–66, 237, 341, 388

Hill, Lister, 105, 112, 113, 115

Hill–Burton Program, 104, 111–21, 128, 150, 343, 388
  use of to gain free care for uninsured poor, 111–12, 116–19, 120

Holtz-Eaton, Douglas, 196

Hospital Cost Containment Act of 1977, 213

hospitals
  construction of, 113, 114–15, 120, 150, 211–12
  efforts to control costs
    changing from per diem to per admission basis, 206–207
    concerns about outliers, 219–20
    Cost of Living Council's efforts, 205–207
    Diagnosis Related Group creep, 221–22

efforts in the 1970s, 209–215
Medicare Prospective Payment
    System, 217–25
need for teaching adjustments,
    220–21
TEFRA changing costs to average
    cost per case, 216
use of "case-mix" indexes, 217
use of Diagnosis Related Group
    system, 217–21
high costs of, 124, 235
    and per diem basis, 205–206, 209
    using DRG to increase profits, 222
and Medicare
    and Medicare Part D, 193
    shifting costs from Medicare to
        privately insured patients, 235
    splitting hospital and physician
        care in, 139–40, 144–45
and Obama's health plan, 264–71
providing free care for the poor. See
    Emergency Medical Treatment
    and Active Labor Act of 1986;
    Hill–Burton Program; uncom-
    pensated care
racial issues facing until into the
    1960s, 130
sole community hospitals, 223
statistics on
    comparison of average discharge
        rate in US and other coun-
        tries, 239–40
    decline in numbers of from 1980
        to 2000, 235
House–Senate Conference Committee,
    134, 293, 315, 388
Hsiao, William, 226
Humphrey, Hubert, 105, 136
Hyde Amendment, 288, 388

Iacocca, Lee, 65, 67
Ignagni, Karen, 260–64
income-related premiums, 148, 150,
    153, 156–57, 189–90, 388–89
Independent Payment Advisory Board
    [IPAB], 266–67, 271, 273, 341–42
individual mandate, 49–50
    in Obama's health plan, 249–50, 253,
        262–63, 308, 329
    weakening of, 263, 267, 270–71,
        276–77
Institute of Medicine, 11–12, 283, 286
insurance companies. See private
    insurance
insurance exchanges, 75, 249–51, 253
interest groups,
    and Medicare Part D, 191–93
    opposition to Clinton health plan, 19,
        20, 191
        Harry and Louise commercials,
            82–85, 88, 89, 94
    opposition to Obama health plan,
        19–21, 191
    working with stakeholders and spe-
        cial interests, 333
    See also businesses and health care;
        pharmaceutical companies; pri-
        vate insurance
Internal Revenue Service
    ruling that employer contributions
        for health not counted as wages,
        101, 107
    Tax Equity and Fiscal Responsibility
        Act of 1982, 216–17, 393

Jackson Hole Group, 71–72, 89
Javits, Jacob, 105, 131, 135
Jefferson, William, 78, 291
Jeffords, Jim, 181
job lock, 163, 164, 389

Johnson, Doug, 290
Johnson, Harry, 84
Johnson, Haynes, 62
Johnson, Jack, 292
Johnson, Lyndon, 76, 116, 127, 137, 331
  and passage of Medicare, 28, 31, 33,
    131–37, 330
Jones, Stan, 27, 32, 55, 56, 57

Kahn, Chip, 82–84, 255, 261, 267–69,
  270, 302, 316
Kaiser, Edward, 39
Kaiser Family Foundation, 185
Kaiser Permanente, 36, 37, 40, 111, 232,
  261
Kasich, John, 80
Kassebaum, Nancy, 163, 165
Keehan, Carol, 269–70, 321
Kennedy, Edward "Ted," 8, 28–30, 80,
  162–63, 313
  brain tumor diagnosis, 18, 254, 274
  and death of Mary Jo Kopechne, 45, 61
  health care reform efforts
    bills introduced by Kennedy, 28–
      29, 30, 32, 33, 43–44, 47, 55–
      56, 57–60, 163–68, 171–76
    and HMOs, 40
    with Jimmy Carter, 214–15
    and Medicare Part D, 177, 181,
      194, 195, 198
    and Obama's health plan, 254–55
    and State Children' Health Insur-
      ance Program, 171–76
  as possible presidential opponent of
    Nixon, 32, 34, 42
Kennedy, John F., 28, 122, 128, 130–31
Kennedy–Griffiths bill, 28–29, 43–44, 47
Kennedy–Kassebaum bill. See Health
  Insurance Portability and Access
  Act (1996)

Kennedy–Mills bill, 30, 32, 33, 55–56,
  59, 60
Kerrey, Bob, 179, 191
Kerr–Mills bill, 127–28, 132, 139, 141
  See also Eldercare bill; Medicaid
Kerry, John, 7–9, 171, 310
Keynes, John Maynard, 48
"Kids First" proposal of Hillary
  Clinton, 171
Kildee, Dale, 321
King–Anderson bill, 122–23, 130–34
  See also Medicare
Kirk, Paul, 55
Kitzhaber, John, 203
Knowles, John, 36
Kopechne, Mary Jo, 45, 61
Kristol, William, 92
Kucinich, Dennis, 321, 322

Ladenheim, Kala, 170
Laird, Melvin, 59
Landrieu, Mary, 296, 301, 310, 311
Leahy, Patrick, 310
length of stay, 223, 240, 389
Levin, Carl, 310
Lewis, John, 324
Lieberman, Joe, 300–301, 310
lifetime limits on coverage, 246, 253
Lincoln, Blanche, 296
Long, Russell, 44, 56–57, 134, 136, 137,
  208, 214
Long–Ribicoff bill, 57, 59
Lott, Trent, 172, 173, 174, 194, 318
*Lugo v. Simon*, 118

Madian, Bob, 41
Magazine, George, 260
Magaziner, Ira, 62, 83, 331
  and managed competition, 63, 74–76,
    79, 80, 81–82, 88

malpractice reform, 272, 273

managed care, 37–39, 89, 166, 231–33, 237–38, 341, 389

   backlash against, 232–33, 234–35. *See also* Preferred Provider Organizations

   IPAB as "government driven" managed care, 342

   percentage of Americans enrolled in, 38

managed competition in Clinton's health plan, 62–96, 333, 334, 389

   managed competition within a budget, 81–82, 90, 334

manager's amendment, 295–96, 301, 302, 308–312, 327, 389

Markey, Betsy, 322

Marmor, Theodore, 146

Massachusetts health plan, 81, 249–50, 253, 334

Matalin, Mary, 68

Maxwell, Elliott, 74

Mayo Clinic, 39

McCain, John, 161

McCarren–Ferguson Act of 1945, 169

McCarthy, Joe, 33, 105

McCloskey, Pete, 41

McConnell, Mitch, 276, 310–11, 320

McDonough, John, 171, 334

McGovern, George, 32, 45

McGrory, Mary, 65

McNerney, Walter J., 143–44

means testing, 129, 154, 181

Medicaid, 7, 14, 36, 107, 112, 139–40, 141, 142, 145–46, 163, 173, 288, 343, 389

   *Cook v. Ochsner Foundation Hospital* and denial of service, 117–18

   costs of, 36, 39, 67, 144–45, 150, 250

      hospitals transferring costs to non-Medicaid patients, 235, 297

   subsidies varying by state, 52

   Medicaid benefits package, 148, 172, 173, 174, 175

   in Obama's health plan, 246, 250–51, 253, 255, 279, 287, 293, 296, 309–310, 329, 333, 339

   passage of, 7, 14, 33, 36, 107, 140, 145, 204, 325, 343

      starting as the Kerr–Mills bill, 141

   replacements for

      Assisted Health Insurance Program, 54, 382

      combining catastrophic insurance with, 57

      efforts to change to block grants, 172

      National Health Insurance Partners Program, 42–43

"medical home," 340

medical loss ratio, 263, 341–42, 389

Medical Payment Assessment Commission [MedPAC], 389

medical savings accounts [MSAs], 165–67

Medicare, 7, 12, 13–14, 28, 36, 107, 389

   benefits of, 146–48

   and Blue Cross, 143–44, 208–209

   costs of, 233–34

      changing per diem to per admission basis, 206–207

      costing more than originally planned for, 31, 39, 67, 144–45

      Diagnosis Related Group system, 208, 217–21

      hospitals transferring costs to non-Medicare patients, 235

      limiting growth in physicians' fees, 209

      setting target growth rates, 342

   efforts to control costs and slow growth, 230–35, 303–304

Reagan's efforts, 215–29
use of rate regulation and health
 planning in the '70s, 208–215
and end-of-life counseling, 281–82
legacy of, 140–46
Medicare Advantage [MA], 185,
 186–88, 190, 193, 197, 262, 280,
 286, 304–305, 328, 389
Medicare Part A, 139–40, 141, 144,
 146–47, 148, 154, 390
Medicare Part B, 139–40, 141, 144,
 147, 148, 151, 152, 154, 156–57,
 160, 189–90, 390
Medicare Part C. *See* Medicare,
 Medicare Advantage
Medicare Part D, 148, 157, 177–99,
 282, 390
 details of the plan, 185–91
 donut hole, 20, 182–83, 185–86,
  197, 259
 government prohibited from negotiating prices, 20, 187–88, 246,
  258
Medicare + Choice program, 180,
 181, 185, 304, 390. *See also*
 Medicare, Medicare Advantage
Medicare withholding tax, 157, 179,
 306, 313, 327, 390
and Obama's health plan, 302–305,
 306, 327
 allowing near-elderly to join,
  296–300
passage of, 76, 126–40
 Forand bill, 127
 Kerr–Mills bill as a way to head
  Medicare off, 127–28
 King–Anderson bill, 122–23,
  130–35, 138–39
 splitting hospital and physician
  care in, 139–40, 144–45

"three-layer cake strategy," 59,
 139–40
Wilbur Mills as an impediment to,
 122–23, 127–28, 130–37
physicians' fees
 AMA opposing reduction in reimbursement, 228, 271–72
 Medicare Physician Payment bill,
  227–28
 and Physician Payment Reform,
  224–26
 and the Sustainable Growth Rate
  formula, 228, 271–72
popularity of, 12, 145
reorienting toward the private sector
 after 2002, 181, 183
as a single-payer plan (Medicare for
 all), 68, 69, 154, 171, 246,
 298–99, 300
and Sustainable Growth Rate, 228,
 271–72, 273, 393
*See also* Medicare Catastrophic
 Health Bill (1989)
Medicare Catastrophic Health Bill
 (1989), 149–61, 180, 189, 330, 332
including prescription drugs, 178
repealed in 1989, 149, 161
Medicare Modernization Act [MMA].
 *See* Medicare, Medicare Part D
Medicare Payment Advisory Committee, 234
Medicare Physician Payment bill,
 227–28
Medicare Prescription Drug, Improve-
 ment, and Modernization Act
 [MMA]. *See* Medicare, Medicare
 Part D
Medicare Prospective Payment System.
 *See* prospective payment system
 [PPS]

Medicare Trust Funds, 190, 306

*Medicine and Health Perspectives*
(newsletter), 177

Medigap insurance, 148, 154

Merck & Co., Inc., 259

Messina, Jim, 259, 316

Michel, Bob, 91

Mikulski, Barbara, 292

Milbank, Dana, 312

"millionaire's tax," 306, 313

Mills, Wilbur, 28, 30–33, 55, 331–32
and Medicare, 141
obstructing, 122–23, 127–28,
130–37
supporting, 138
"three-layer cake strategy," 17, 59,
139–46
scandal involving, 17, 60, 61

Mitchell, George, 77, 80, 95

Mongan, James, 57

Moorhead, Carlos, 92

moral hazard, 52, 87, 236, 390

Morgan, Jim, 209

Morris, Dick, 162

Morton, Judge, 118, 119

"Mother's Day Massacre," 207, 208

Moynahan, Daniel Patrick, 92, 95

Murray, James, 102, 104, 105, 113, 114

Murray, Patricia, 309

Murray–Humphrey–Dingell–Celler
bill, 105

National Abortion Rights Action
League, 310, 323

National Bipartisan Commission on the
Future of Medicare, 11, 14, 177,
178–80

National Committee to Preserve Social
Security and Medicare, 159

National Federation of Independent
Business [NFIB], 20, 48, 56, 254,
390

National Governors Association, 57

National Grange, 104

National Health Board, 81, 90

national health care in the US
American Association for Labor Legislation plan, 97–99
Carter's catastrophic insurance plan,
214–15
changing health care delivery and
finance, 338–42
Clinton's efforts to establish, 62–96,
157, 171, 178, 230–35, 260, 268,
330–33
cost figures
average discharge rate compar-
isons, 239–40
costs compared to other countries,
203, 239, 240–41
costs growing faster than GDP,
344–45
geographical differences in costs in
US, 222–23, 226
growth of per capita costs in the
1980s, 230
as a percentage of federal budget,
344
as a share of US economy, 18
slowing of increases between 1997
and 2000, 234
efforts to control costs
Carter's controlling costs rather
than expanding coverage,
213–15
changing health care delivery and
finance, 338–42
during the 1990s, 230–35
Nixon's nationwide wage and price
controls, 204–208

Reagan's use of DRGs and procompetition, 215–29
use of rate regulation and health
planning in the '70s, 208–215
Eisenhower not pursuing, 123–26
Employee Retirement Income Secu-
rity Act of 1974, 169–70
Forand bill, 127, 130
Franklin Roosevelt's efforts to estab-
lish, 99–102
health insurance as interstate com-
merce, 169
Health Insurance Portability and
Access Act (1996), 163–68
Hill–Burton Program, 111–21
impact of on businesses, consumers,
and government, 66
Kerr–Mills bill, 127–28, 132
King–Anderson bill, 130–34, 138–39.
See also Medicare
Medicare Part D, 177–99
Murray–Humphrey–Dingell–Celler
bill, 105
Nixon's efforts to establish, 27–61
Obama's efforts to establish, 17–22,
245–77, 285–329. See also Patient
Protection and Affordable Care
Act (2010)
economic constraints, 19
learning strategy for passage from
history, 330–37
public reaction to (summer of the
death panels), 278–84
obstacles to reform
during Clinton's administration,
19, 20, 90–94
during Obama's administration,
19–22, 86
only industrialized country not providing universal coverage, 344

polls
Americans fear of federal government compared to private
insurance, 13
Americans preferring independent
choice of health care options,
39
Americans wanting universal
health care, 11, 335
Reagan's Medicare Catastrophic
insurance, 149–61
State Children's Health Insurance
Program, 171–76
Wagner–Murray–Dingell bill,
102–105, 113
See also Medicaid; Medicare; rural
areas, health care in; urban areas,
health care in
national health care systems in other
countries, 13
comparison of average discharge
rates, 239–40
costs compared to US, 67, 203, 239,
240–41
industrialized countries providing
universal coverage, 344
relying on public regulation, 39
successful techniques to regulated
spending and use, 237
United Kingdom use of cost effectiveness analysis, 238–40
National Health Insurance Partners
Program, 42–46
National Health Law Program [Nhelp],
116, 117
National Health Planning and
Resource Development Act,
211–12
National Health Service (United
Kingdom), 238–39

National Institute for Clinical Effectiveness (United Kingdom) [NICE], 238

National Institutes of Health [NIH], 283, 390

National Legal Program on Health Problems. *See* National Health Law Program

National Organization of Women, 310

National Right to Life Committee, 290

NBC (TV network), 223

near-elderly, 300, 301, 390

Nebraska and the "Cornhusker kickback," 309–310

Nelson, Ben, 301, 309–310, 311, 322

Neugebauer, Randy, 323

New Jersey Hospital Association, 218

Newsom, Callie Mae, 118, 119

*Newsom v. Vanderbilt*, 118

*Newsweek* (magazine), 267, 268

*New York Times* (newspaper), 58, 60, 72, 75, 135, 245, 260

Nixon, Richard, 8, 14, 90, 105, 163, 180, 344

    bringing HMOs to Americans, 27–42, 339

    Comprehensive Health Insurance Plan, 47, 53–61

    efforts to control healthcare costs through wage and price controls, 204–208

    interest in providing national health insurance, 120, 127, 178, 330

    and the National Health Insurance Partners Program, 42–46, 253, 301

Obama, Barack, 14, 272

    lessons learned from earlier presidents

        build on current system and minimize change, 330–37

        learning from Clinton's health care mistakes, 75–76, 78, 274

    and national health insurance, 17–22, 244–77, 285–329. *See also* Patient Protection and Affordable Care Act (2010)

    financing of, 302–308

    personal efforts to finalize, 320–21

    public reaction to (summer of the death panels), 278–84

    signing bill into law, 326

    reauthorizing SCHIP, 176

"Obamacare." *See* Patient Protection and Affordable Care Act (2010)

obstacles to health care reform. *See* national health care in the US

Ochsner Foundation Hospital, 116–17

Office of Management and Budget [OMB], 45, 206, 273, 276, 342, 390

Offices of the Actuary, 390–91

Omnibus Reconciliation Act of 1989, 227

open enrollment period, 40, 73, 391

Organisation for Economic Co-operation and Development [OECD], 239, 240–41

Orszag, Peter, 273, 342

outliers, 219–20, 391

Owen, Jack, 218

Packwood, Bob, 55

Palin, Sarah, 281, 282, 324

Panetta, Leon, 36, 41

parliamentarian, 317–18, 391

patient-centered medical home [PCMH], 340

Patient-Centered Outcome Research Institute [PCORI], 283, 391

Patient Protection and Affordable Care
Act (2010), 7, 8
abortion issue, impact of, 269–70,
287–91
changing health care delivery and
finance, 338–42
early stages of developing, 254–73
framework for, 247–53
work of Baucus, Grassley, and the
Gang of Six, 274–77
financing of, 286–87, 302–308, 313,
326–27
estimated costs of over ten years,
344
need to not add to deficit, 19, 21,
246, 251, 253, 277, 286, 302,
308
learning strategy for passage from
history, 330–37
passage of, 291, 313
final reconciliation of bills and
passage into law, 316–26
and Harry Reid, 295–302, 308–312
impact of Scott Brown's election,
315
and Nancy Pelosi, 285–91, 320,
322, 325, 326–27
Senate's Christmas Eve vote on, 8,
292–313
signed into law, 326
summary of final legislation,
326–29
poll on public views on, 324
proposed Independent Payment
Advisory Board, 266–67, 271,
273
public reaction to (summer of the
death panels), 278–84
See also public option
Pauley, Jane, 223

Paulson, Henry, 46
Payne, L. F., 78
Pell, Claiborne, 260
Pelosi, Nancy, 76, 262, 276, 306, 315,
332
and Obama health care plan, 285–91,
316, 320, 322, 325, 326–27
pension plans, protecting, 169–70
Pepper, Claude, 155
per diem cost basis, 147, 205–206,
207–209, 385
Perkins, Henry, 99
Perot, Ross, 32
Pfizer Inc., 259
pharmaceutical companies
fears of comparative effectiveness
research, 284
government prohibited from negotiating prices, 20, 187–88, 246, 258
and Medicare Part D
benefits for supporting, 192
protection of in the legislation,
187–88
and Obama's health plan, 257–60
opposition to universal health coverage, 20
Pharmaceutical Research and Manufacturers of America [PhRMA], 254,
257, 258–60, 266, 267, 391
Physician Payment Review Commission [PPRC], 226
physicians
and the American Medical
Association
fears of regulation and price-
controls on doctors, 20, 29, 98,
127, 128, 224, 226, 227, 228
opposing any cuts to Medicare
reimbursement for physicians,
228, 271–72

cost of specialist care, 339
and end-of-life counseling, 281–82
growth of numbers between 1970
   and 1990, 229
Medicare Physician Payment bill,
   227–28
Physician Payment Reform, 224–26
primary care physicians [PCPs], 38,
   339–41
Resource-Based Relative Value Scale,
   226
splitting hospital and physician care
   in Medicare, 139–40, 144–45
Planned Parenthood, 310
play-or-pay systems, 69–70
point of service plan [POS], 38, 391
Poling, Harold "Red," 230–31
*Politico* (newspaper), 256
politics
   and Barack Obama, 29, 77–78,
      330–37
   and Bill Clinton, 74–75, 77, 78,
      82–85, 90–96
   presidential politics, 31–32, 41
   "Southern strategy," 33, 41
   and Richard Nixon, 28–35
Pollack, Ron, 254–55
poor, subsidizing health care for, 51–52,
   57
   and Medicare Part D, 188
   in Obama's health plan, 262–63, 276
   *See also* Hill–Burton Program; Med-
      icaid; State Children's Health
      Insurance Program
preexisting condition, 19, 54, 86, 92,
   163–64, 168, 245–46, 248, 253, 260,
   280, 336, 391
preferred provider organizations
   [PPOs], 38, 234–35, 391
premiums, insurance plans spending as

a percentage on health care, 263,
   341
premium support, 178, 184, 190, 197
prepaid group practices, 29, 35, 36, 39,
   73, 391
   *See also* capitation; Health Mainte-
      nance Organizations; prospective
      payment system
prescription drugs
   originally left out of Medicare, 142
   stand-alone drug plans and the Medi-
      care Advantage program, 186–87
   *See also* Medicare, Medicare Part D;
      pharmaceutical companies
preventive health care, 51, 338–39
Pricewaterhouse Coopers study, 264
pricing according to age, 263
pricing according to health status, 248,
   260
primary care and prevention as a way
   to cut costs, 338–39
primary care physicians [PCPs], 38,
   339–41
private employee pension plans, protecting, 169–70
private insurance
   and American Association for Labor
      Legislations failed health plan,
      98
   American Medical Association pre-
      ferring to work with, 144
   and a catastrophic health plan, 44
   developing HMO-type managed care
      plans, 231–32
   employer mandates sustaining the
      industry, 48–49
   growth of Americans having, 107
   how insurance industry works, 85–88
   insurance reform in Obama's health
      plan, 248

large insurance companies liking
Clinton's health plan, 82
Medicare Advantage plans, 193
providing 15% more than regular
Medicare, 304
providing 15% more than regular
Medicare to, 280
and Medicare Part D
benefits for supporting, 192–93
and Obama's health plan
limiting pricing differences for age,
263
reasons for opposing, 86
required to spend certain percentage of premiums on
direct medical care, 263, 341
receiving antitrust exemption to pool
risks for elderly, 135
role of in health care, 13–14
starting to use experience rating, 125
*See also* subsidies for insurance
private Medicare programs. *See*
Medicare, Medicare Advantage
Professional Standards Review Organizations [PSROs], 54
Prospective Payment Assessment Commission [ProPAC], 159, 221, 391
Prospective Payment Review Commission [PPRC], 221, 226, 391
prospective payment system [PPS],
217, 219, 220–21, 222–25, 226, 229,
391–92
*See also* prepaid group practices
Protestant Hospital Association, 103
Public Health Service Act of 1975, 118,
119
public option, 21, 268, 392
and Obama's health plan, 75, 130,
245, 251, 253, 286, 290, 291,
296–302, 299, 313

giving up on, 246, 271, 273, 276,
300–301, 310
opposition to, 261, 267, 269, 272,
275, 286, 296, 299
use of trigger to begin if costs rose,
275, 300
public relations as a political strategy
tool, 335–36

quality-adjusted life year [QALY], 238,
392

rating bands, 263, 392
rationing health care, 87, 237, 239,
283–84
Rayburn, Sam, 127, 133
Reagan, Ronald, 41, 90, 149, 214
efforts to control health care costs,
215–21, 228–29
Medicare Prospective Payment
System, 219–24
Physician Payment Reform,
224–26
and Medicare Catastrophic Health
Bill, 149–61, 178, 180, 330
reconciliation, 9, 76, 77–78, 227, 302,
316–20, 321, 322, 323, 324, 326, 392
how reconciliation changed Obama's
health care bill, 326–29
Reid, Harry, 274, 276, 285, 294, 332
final negotiations and Reid's manager's amendment, 295–302,
308–312
Reischauer, Robert "Bob," 79–80, 90,
178, 213, 318
Republicans, 106
and the Golden Rule Insurance
Company, 167
and Medicare, 129–30, 140, 155,
303–304

trying to substantially reduce, 233–34

and Medicare Part D, 191, 193–94

opposition to Clinton health plan, 21, 90–94

opposition to Medicare Catastrophic Health Bill, 160

opposition to Obama health plan, 21, 246, 277, 291, 293–95, 310–12, 319–20, 323–24

Republican In Name Only [RINO], 275

on social insurance, 153

support of tort reform, 272

unwilling to negotiate, 92

rescissions of coverage, Obama plan eliminating, 248, 253, 260

Resource-Based Relative Value Scale [RBRVS], 226, 392

retrospective payment, 224, 392

Reuther, Walter, 28, 260

Ribicoff, Abraham, 57

Rice, Dorothy, 205

Richardson, Bill, 256–57

Richardson, Elliott, 42, 45, 111, 112, 117, 120–21, 204, 206

RINO, 275

risk, need to spread, 49, 248

risk adjustment, 73, 392

Rivlin, Alice, 79

Rockefeller, Jay, 62, 74, 227

Rockefeller, Nelson, 41, 91, 127

Rodham, Hillary, 74. See also Clinton, Hillary

Roemer, Milt, 211

Roe v. Wade, 288, 392

Rohack, James, 272

Romney, Mitt, 253

Rooney, J. Patrick, 166–67

Roosevelt, Franklin D., 14, 18, 76, 330

and a national health proposal, 99–102, 105–106

Roosevelt, James, 159–60

Roosevelt, Theodore "Teddy," 7, 97, 333

Rose, Marilyn, 115–17, 118, 119, 120

Rostenkowski, Dan, 18, 84, 95, 156, 158–59, 219

Rother, John, 78, 157, 177, 197

Rubin, Bob, 62

Rumsfeld, Donald, 204

rural areas, health care in

Burton–Hill hospital construction, 113, 114

and Medicare Advantage plans, 186–87, 193, 304

and Medicare Part D, 184, 192, 193, 251

and Medicare + Choice plans, 181, 184

Medicare reimbursements, 69, 222–23, 226, 235

only one or two companies dominating markets in, 251

and the Patient Protection and Affordable Care Act (2010), 266, 268, 270, 286

physician shortages in, 226

sole community hospitals, 223

Sanders, Bernie, 294, 310, 318

scandals, effects of on passing health care reform, 17–18, 45, 60, 61

See also Watergate scandal

Schultz, George, 206

Schumer, Chuck, 262, 308–309, 310

Schwarz, Tony, 137

Schweiker, Richard, 216, 219

Scully, Tom, 186, 195, 198

Seattle Times (newspaper), 317

Sebelius, Kathleen, 257
self-insured plans, 169–70
Shactman, David, 15, 19
Shriver, Sargent, 116
shutdowns, federal government, 233
"Single-Payer System in Jackson Hole
    Clothing, A" (Enthoven), 90
single-payer systems, 60, 68–69, 71, 86,
    87, 102, 144, 241, 294, 301, 392
    and Barack Obama, 246, 247, 321,
        333, 344
    and Bill Clinton, 68, 71, 89–90, 102
    "Medicare for all," 154, 171, 246,
        298–99, 300
    in other countries, 86
    and Richard Nixon, 29–30, 56, 344
    support of
        by Bernie Sanders, 294, 318
        by Ted Kennedy, 29–30, 44, 55–56
Sloan, Frank, 210–11
Smathers, George, 136, 137
Smith, Nick, 193–94
Snowe, Olympia, 262, 263, 275, 276,
    277, 300
social insurance, 102, 103, 124, 126, 129,
    142, 150, 152–54, 183, 191, 392
    non-social social insurance, 156–58,
        183, 189. See also Medicare Cata-
        strophic Health Bill (1989)
    See also Medicare; Social Security Act
        (1935)
socialized medicine, claims of, 280
Social Security Act (1935), 7, 99–100,
    113, 150
Social Security Act Amendments
    (Medicare and Medicaid) (1965),
    7, 140
    attaching King–Anderson bill to
        Social Security Act, 134–35
    See also Medicaid; Medicare

Social Security Administration, 56, 205,
    208
Social Security Trust Fund, 132, 138,
    141, 393
Social Security withholding tax, 247,
    393
sole community hospitals, 223, 393
southern Democrats. See Democrats
"Southern Manifesto," 132
"Southern strategy," 33, 41
special interests. See businesses and
    health care; interest groups; phar-
    maceutical companies; private
    insurance
Specter, Arlen, 64–65, 278
Stark, Pete, 155
Starr, Paul, 81
State Children's Health Insurance Pro-
    gram [SCHIP], 23, 163, 171–76,
    250, 317, 343
states
    regulating health care costs in the
        '70s, 210–12
    and SCHIP program, 174–75
    and self-insure plans, 169–70
    and state-based insurance exchanges
        in Obama's health plan, 250–51,
        253, 280, 301
Stein, Herb, 204
Stephanopoulos, George, 62
Stockman, David, 220
Studds, Gerry, 91
Stupak, Bart, 289, 290, 313, 322–23, 325
subsidies for insurance, 51–52, 92, 99,
    103, 105, 124, 129, 139, 153, 212,
    237
    under Assisted Health Insurance
        Plan, 54
    and Medicare Advantage plans, 187,
        197, 305, 328

and Medicare Part B, 148, 154
and Medicare Part D, 70, 187, 188,
190, 192–93
Nixon calling for, 8, 42–43, 105
under Obama health plan, 20, 245,
246, 248, 250–51, 255, 261, 276,
280, 287, 291, 326, 329
problem if it involves covering abortions, 21, 288–89
and State Children's Health Insurance Program, 173
supplemental insurance, 56
Supreme Court, 169
sustainable growth rate [SGR], 228,
271–72, 273, 393

Taft, Robert, 103, 104
Taft, William Howard, 113, 114, 115
Tauzin, Billy "Swamp Fox," 257–60,
261, 266
tax advantage of employer-provided
health care, 101, 106–107
tax credits, 130, 247, 328
tax deductible health benefits, 52–53,
236–37, 307–308
tax-deferred savings accounts for health
care, 165–66
Tax Equity and Fiscal Responsibility
Act of 1982 [TEFRA], 216–17, 393
tax incentive plans, 70
teaching adjustments for hospitals,
220–21
Tea Party, 279, 282, 323, 324
third party administrator, 393
third party reimbursement, 393
Thomas, Bill, 178, 184, 191, 195, 198
Thompson, Frank, 123
Thompson, John, 207–208, 217
Thompson, Tommy, 194
Thorburgh, Dick, 64

Thorpe, Ken, 62, 63, 74
"three-layer cake strategy," 59, 139–40
*See also* Byrnes bill; Eldercare bill;
King–Anderson bill; Medicare
Thurmond, Strom, 41
Tiberi, Patrick, 281
*Time* (magazine), 74
tobacco industry
AMA siding with in fight against
Medicare, 123, 133, 134, 333
impact on Clinton health plan, 78
increase in cigarette tax funding
SCHIP, 174
*Today Show* (TV program), 223
Trial Lawyers Association, 272
trillion dollars, dramatizing the magni-
tude of, 203
Truman, Harry, 140, 330
and national health insurance,
102–105, 106, 113, 163
Tyson, D'Andrea, 179

Umbdenstock, Richard, 265, 269
uncompensated care, 112, 114, 115, 116,
118, 119, 235, 252, 254, 265, 280, 393
*See also* Hill–Burton Program
underwriting practices and Obama's
health plan, 248, 249–50, 253
uninsured, 11–12, 18, 53, 171–76
unions, 58
concerns about run-away health
costs, 28
not interested in universal coverage,
56
opposition to taxing "Cadillac"
health plans, 21, 286–87,
307–308
United Auto Workers [UAW], 28
United Kingdom use of cost effectiveness analysis, 238

unit of care, definition of, 205
universal access, 393
  and universal coverage, 49
universal coverage, 8–9, 13, 28–29, 70,
    96, 141, 213–14, 293, 335, 393
  and Bill Clinton, 71, 81, 89
  Carter pursuing cost control instead,
    163
  and Clinton's health plan, 75
  and Obama's health plan, 75, 246,
    247, 249, 252, 253, 255, 261,
    264–65, 268, 290, 334. *See also*
    public option
  opposition to, 20, 22, 44, 66, 271
  and Richard Nixon, 48, 52, 53, 64,
    163, 247
  and universal access, 49
upcoding. *See* Diagnosis Related Group
  creep
urban areas, health care in
  Medicare reimbursements, 69,
    222–23
    higher for teaching hospitals,
      220–21
  and the Patient Protection and
    Affordable Care Act (2010), 266,
    268, 286
US Conference of Catholic Bishops,
  269–70, 288–89, 310, 321
US government shutdown and Newt
  Gingrich, 93
utilization review, 87, 237, 393

Vanderbilt University Hospital, 118,
  119
Vatican on Obama health plan, 270
Veneman, John, 36, 41
Veterans Administration, 14, 188
"Volume Performance Standard," 227
vote-o-rama, 319

Voting Rights Act, 41
vouchers, 178

Wagner, Robert, 101, 102, 113
Wagner–Murray–Dingell bill, 102–105,
  113
waiver, 175, 210, 393
Wallace, Henry, 104
Wallack, Stanley, 213
*Wall Street Journal* (newspaper), 56
War Labor Board, 101
*Washington Post* (newspaper), 80, 312
Watergate scandal, 8, 31, 32, 41, 45, 46,
  58, 61
Watson, Tony, 261
Watts, John C., 122, 123, 131–32, 133–34
Waxman, Henry, 156, 160, 316
Weicker, Lowell, 91
Weinberger, Casper "Cap the Knife,"
  34, 35, 44–46, 47, 52, 206
Weinstein, Michael, 72
Whelan, John, 167
Whitehouse, Sheldon, 312
White House Office of Health Reform,
  256, 257
Whitewater affair, 17
Wilensky, Gail, 234
Wilhelm (Kaiser), 98
Wilson, Woodrow, 97
withholding tax. *See* Medicare,
    Medicare withholding tax; Social
    Security withholding tax
Wofford, Harris, 64–65, 68, 72, 88, 314
Workhorse Group, 254–55, 257, 271,
  334
Wright, Jim, 156
Wyden, Ron, 296

Zelman, Walter, 81
zero-premium plan, 186, 305, 393